Hyperacusis and Disorders of Sound Intolerance

Clinical and Research Perspectives

Hyperacusis and Disorders of Sound Intolerance

Clinical and Research Perspectives

Marc Fagelson, PhD
David M. Baguley, BSc, MSc, MBA, PhD

Plural Publishing Inc.

PLURAL PUBLISHING INC.

5521 Ruffin Road
San Diego, CA 92123

e-mail: info@pluralpublishing.com
website: http://www.pluralpublishing.com

FSC
www.fsc.org
MIX
Paper from responsible sources
FSC® C011935

Typeset in 11/13 Adobe Garamond by Achorn International
Printed in the United States of America by McNaughton & Gunn

Library of Congress Cataloging-in-Publication Data

Names: Fagelson, Marc, editor. | Baguley, David (David M.), editor.
Title: Hyperacusis and disorders of sound intolerance : clinical and research perspectives / [edited by] Marc Fagelson, David M. Baguley.
Description: San Diego, CA : Plural Publishing, [2018] | Includes bibliographical references and index.
Identifiers: LCCN 2017058142| ISBN 9781944883287 (alk. paper) | ISBN 1944883282 (alk. paper)
Subjects: | MESH: Hyperacusis—diagnosis | Hyperacusis—therapy | Tinnitus—diagnosis | Tinnitus—therapy
Classification: LCC RF293.7 | NLM WV 270 | DDC 617.8/9—dc23
LC record available at https://lccn.loc.gov/2017058142

Contents

SECTION IV. MANAGEMENT

Preface

For most of us, life is full of sound. While there are some individuals who lead a solitary, silent, or contemplative life, the more common path is replete with auditory stimulation. On an early morning walk in a North American city before conference presentations, the two editors of this book were intentionally attentive to the sounds around them, including sirens, engine sounds, phones ringing, and shouting. Many of the sound alerts in common use have been designed so as to be as compelling, and in a sense, as annoying as possible, cutting through distractions and other sounds to demand immediate and sustained attention (Patterson, 1990; Vastfjall et al., 2014).

For many years substantial scientific and clinical effort has been expended in understanding and ameliorating the impact of reduced hearing, resulting in sophisticated technologies such as hearing aids and auditory implants, advanced surgical techniques, and intensive rehabilitation strategies. Far, far less attention and scrutiny have been given to the experiences of individuals for whom the world of sound is more intense, more vivid, and perhaps perceived as more toxic than is usual. Most audiologists and otologists know of patients for whom everyday sound evokes discomfort, distress, aversion, and in some, pain.

This book seeks to explore and help the reader begin to understand those experiences. Some challenges will be encountered. The vocabulary used to describe such experiences is varied and imprecise, including decreased, reduced, or collapsed sound tolerance, and hyperacusis. Definitions of each of these terms varies; given such fundamental differences, it is not surprising that data regarding the epidemiology and natural history of hyperacusis is sparse, and inconsistent where it does exist. Some aspects of the physiological mechanisms of loudness or sound intensity perception in the auditory brain remain obscure, and there is a disconnect between the auditory neuroscience and the clinical communities that remains difficult to bridge. The experiences of individuals with reduced sound tolerance is heterogeneous, and can vary on a day to day, or hour to hour basis, and in some this is modulated by emotional and psychological state as well as the auditory environment. Tools to assess the extent and severity of loudness tolerance symptoms are crude, and in some cases may be deeply uncomfortable for the patient, as may be the case in some methods of ascertaining the threshold of loudness discomfort using sound stimulation. There is little in the way of hard evidence regarding therapy, and which interventions might be optimal for which type of patient.

All this may seem daunting, and lead one to consider that the topic of decreased sound tolerance cannot sensibly be addressed at all. However, looking at other fields would lead us to disagree. The field of pain studies was, until recently, in a similar state to that which is observed regarding hyperacusis (Chen, 2011), but systematic and focused endeavor has led to deeper understanding of mechanisms and the development of therapies that can be rigorously assessed in well-designed clinical trials. The present volume represents an attempt to take a first step on a similar journey, and it is our hope that it will inspire and provoke colleagues in both the auditory neuroscience and the clinical (especially audiology, otology, and neurology) communities to discuss, explore, and research hyperacusis and related phenomena. Given the present state of knowledge, different authors have used different terminology, and have varied opinions, in their chapters: while we have edited with a goal of improving clarity and consistency, we have preserved some of these variations so that distinctive opinions, interpretations, and hypotheses might be heard.

Thanks are due to each of the authors for their fine contributions, and the time and effort expended on them, to Plural Publishing for agreeing to support this work, and to our families and colleagues for their support and forbearance. We would like to express our appreciation also to the many patients who have shared their experiences of hyperacusis and other phenomena of disordered loudness perception, from whom we have gleaned knowledge, experience, and inspiration.

—Marc Fagelson
David M. Baguley

References

Chen, J. (2011). History of pain theories. *Neurosci. Bull., Oct, 27*(5), 343–350. doi: 10.1007/s12264-011-0139-0.

Patterson, R. (1990). Auditory warning sounds in the work environment. *Philos. Trans. R Soc. Lond. B Biol. Sci., 327*(1241), 485–492.

Vastfjall, D., Bergman, P., Sköld, A., Tajadura, A., & Larsson, P. (2012). Emotional responses to information and warning sounds. *J. Ergonomics, 1*, 106. doi:10.4172/2165-7556.1000106.

Note. DB is funded through the NIHR Biomedical Research Centre program, however, the views expressed are those of the authors and not necessarily those of the NIHR, the NHS, or the Department of Health.

Contributors

Gerhard Andersson, PhD, Dr. Med. Sci.
Professor in Clinical Psychology
Department of Behavioural Sciences and Learning
Linköping University
Linköping, Sweden
Department of Clinical Neuroscience
Karolinska Institute
Stockholm, Sweden
Chapter 10

David M. Baguley, BSc, MSc, MBA, PhD, FAAA
Professor of Hearing Services
President, British Tinnitus Association
Nottingham Biomedical Research Centre
University of Nottingham
Otology and Hearing Group
Division of Clinical Neuroscience
University of Nottingham
Honorary Consultant Clinical Scientist (Audiology)
Nottingham University Hospitals NHS Foundation Trust
Nottingham, United Kingdom
Chapters 1, 3, 11, and 16

Claire Benton, MSc
Consultant Clinical Scientist (Audiology)
Nottingham Audiology Services,
Nottingham University Hospitals NHS Foundation Trust
Nottingham, UK
Chapter 13

Ian C. Bruce, PhD, PEng, FASA
Professor and Associate Chair for Graduate Studies
Department of Electrical and Computer Engineering
McMaster University
Hamilton, Ontario, Canada
Chapter 6

Jos J. Eggermont, PhD
Emeritus Professor
Physiology and Pharmacology, and Psychology
University of Calgary
Calgary, Alberta, Canada
Chapter 8

Kathryn Fackrell, PhD
Research Fellow
University of Nottingham
Nottingham, United Kingdom
Chapter 4

Marc Fagelson, PhD
Professor
Department of Audiology and Speech Language Pathology
East Tennessee State University
Johnson City, Tennessee
Chapters 1, 2, 12, and 16

Frederick J. Gallun, PhD
Research Investigator, VA RR&D
National Center for Rehabilitative Auditory Research
Assistant Professor
Department of Otolaryngology—Head and Neck Surgery
Oregon Health and Science University
Portland, Oregon
Chapter 9

Derek J. Hoare, PhD
Senior Research Fellow
University of Nottingham
Nottingham, United Kingdom
Chapter 4

Veronica Kennedy, FRCS(Oto), FRCP, FRCPCH
Consultant Audiovestibular Physician
Bolton NHS Foundation Trust
Bolton, United Kingdom
Chapter 13

Rosie Kentish, MA
Consultant Clinical Psychologist
Royal National Throat Nose and Ear Hospital
London, United Kingdom
Chapter 13

Rob Littwin, MA
Musician
Producer
Arranger
Atlanta, Georgia
Chapter 15

Don McFerran, MA, FRCS
Consultant ENT Surgeon
Colchester Hospital
University NHS Foundation Trust
Colchester, United Kingdom
Chapter 7

Melissa A. Papesh, PhD, AuD
Research Investigator, VA RR&D
National Center for Rehabilitative Auditory Research
Portland, Oregon
Chapter 9

Larry E. Roberts, PhD
Professor Emeritus
Department of Psychology Neuroscience and Behaviour
McMaster University
Hamilton, Ontario, Canada
Chapter 6

Prof. Dr. Tanit Ganz Sanchez, MD, PhD
Associate Professor of Otolaryngology
University São Paulo School of Medicine
Founder of Instituto Ganz Sanchez
São Paulo, Brazil
Chapter 6

Roland Schaette, PhD
Lecturer
University College London, Ear Institute
London, United Kingdom
Chapter 5

Grant D. Searchfield, BSc, MAud(Hons), PhD
Associate Professor, Audiology
Director, Hearing and Tinnitus Clinic
The University of Auckland
Member, The University of Auckland Centre for Brain Research and Brain Research New Zealand
Scientific Director, TinnitusTunes
Auckland, New Zealand
Chapter 14

Caroline Selvaratnam, BSc, MAud, MNZAS
Audiologist
University of Auckland Clinics
Hearing and Tinnitus Clinic
University of Auckland
Auckland, New Zealand
Chapter 14

Sarah M. Theodoroff, PhD
Research Investigator, VA RR&D
National Center for Rehabilitative Auditory Research
Assistant Professor
Department of Otolaryngology—Head and Neck Surgery

Oregon Health and Science University
Portland, Oregon
Chapter 9

Glynnis A. Tidball, MSc, RAUD
Clinical Instructor
School of Audiology and Speech Sciences
University of British Columbia
Audiologist
Department of Audiology
St. Paul's Hospital
Vancouver, Canada
Chapter 2

Marc and David, as well as many other professionals and the contributors to this text, continue to learn what it means for people and their families to live with hyperacusis and other forms of sound intolerance; this book is dedicated to the many individuals, patients, and providers, who sparked and continue to nurture that interest.

SECTION I

Definitions, Measurement, and Epidemiology

1

Disorders of Sound Tolerance: History and Terminology

Marc Fagelson and David M. Baguley

Introduction

Traditionally the discipline of audiology has been concerned with the challenges faced by people with reduced hearing abilities in order to alleviate the effects associated with hearing loss. While there is a multitude of such people, and the burdens they face are certainly substantial, in recent years there has been increasing awareness of a population of people who have the experience of sound being too intense for them, rather than being too quiet. In this chapter we introduce this topic, and critically examine the various definitions and models that have been proposed, and identify where present knowledge is inadequate.

The impact of hearing loss, particularly of sensory and/or neural origin on the auditory system's loudness processing, is difficult to predict, and prone to the influence of many non-auditory factors. Although hearing aid use often improves an individual's communication ability and quality of life, the lack of a straightforward relation between a patient's sensitivity and their behavior on specific audiologic tests or routine activities precludes development of interventions for individuals with hearing impairment that are consistently as effective as, for example, glasses for myopia. A similar, complex and multifactorial relation appears to exist between disorders of loudness perception, their impact, and the handicap that is associated. This chapter will focus specifically on basic elements related to disorders of sound tolerance—items such as terminology and models, both auditory-based and psychology-based, that support the terminology—that continue to vex providers, patients, and students who seek clarity when managing patients in distress.

History

The concept that human hearing varies with the sound environment and context in which the person is listening has long been accepted, the English phrase, 'I could hear a pin drop' articulating the experience of intense and active listening. The experience of hearing becoming acute at times of emotional intensity is also known, and used extensively in horror films: for example, the trope of increasing the loudness of an enemy's footsteps as they approach along a gravel drive is widespread. The fact that an increase in the perceived intensity of the sound environment can be involuntary is less well known, however. This forms a major plot device in the novel *The Woman in White* by Wilkie Collins (1860), although the symptom is un-named. The heroine of the novel is Miss Laura Fairlie, who as the novel opens has recently been orphaned, and has inherited some money, which renders her attractive to predatory suitors, and she seeks the protection of her uncle, Mr Frederick Fairlie. Unfortunately, he is unable to support her, as he is living as a reclusive invalid, due to a number of symptoms, one of which is a decreased ability to tolerate sound. In the first conversation between niece and uncle, held at some distance across a semi-darkened room, Frederick Fairlie articulates his situation thus:

> *Pray excuse me. But could you contrive to speak in a lower key? In the wretched state of my nerves, loud sound of any kind is indescribable torture to me. You will pardon an invalid?*

Mr. Fairlie thus describes intense sound-evoked pain, leading to invalidity. While Laura eventually transcends the multiple adverse events that befall her, her uncle's situation, which is normally seen by literary critics as an abrogation of his male responsibilities, is a major setback.

Sound intolerance, such as that described by the unfortunate Mr. Fairlie, often accompanies hearing loss across patient groups of all ages, backgrounds, and auditory history, although it may also be present in individuals with hearing thresholds within the range of normal. In practice, this situation is described in terms of dynamic range, or the signal intensities that comprise the range of values spanning the patient's threshold of sensitivity to their threshold of pain or discomfort. In hearing impaired listeners, the dynamic range is reduced in one of two ways. First, in the presence of loudness recruitment thresholds of sensitivity may be elevated while thresholds of discomfort remain essentially unchanged. Alternatively, in cases of hyperacusis, the threshold of discomfort may change over time, and become abnormally low; regardless of absolute sensitivity, the patient's dynamic range would be reduced. In extreme cases, perhaps such as that described by Mr. Fairlie, the patient's dynamic range may collapse and become limited to such a narrow range of intensities that the patient develops aversions to most routine sounds and curtails life activities accordingly.

No mention is made of Mr. Fairlie having a hearing loss, and he is probably an illustration of decreased sound tolerance with normal or age-appropriate hearing thresholds. In the case of a person with hearing loss, it is valuable to consider the paradox at work, as the presence of that hearing loss should, at least on the surface, allow a person to tolerate moderate sound levels without feeling discomfort. However, many patients with hearing loss experience inordinate loudness in the presence of what should be acceptable sound levels, powerful negative emotions in the presence of sounds that most other people do not find objectionable, or sounds that cause pain in and around the ears. Patients affected by such sounds may practice avoidance strategies to minimize their discomfort; we must also consider that strategy's shortcomings.

We hope to expand upon the idea, expressed in the book's preface, that patients would benefit from greater consensus among professionals regarding terms and definitions related to unusual sound experiences. If a patient avoids situations and environments because of aversions to specific sounds or sound levels, then that patient's discomfort and emotional response could be exacerbated by seemingly inconsistent advice and counseling from health care providers. Accurate and effective counseling relies upon many factors; certainly, the list would include an agreed-upon lexicon. In this regard, audiologists have much to learn from the psychological and trauma literatures in which a variety of clinical approaches that target patients' beliefs and understanding take a primary role in the intervention. When basic terminology cannot be agreed upon, the potential for patient learning and adapting to a challenging condition likely decreases. In this chapter, we will review definitions and terms currently in use; our intent is to move the conversation forward in a way that prioritizes lexical items supporting the needs of patients and practitioners.

Hearing Loss and Loudness Growth

Loudness Recruitment

The development of the audiometer improved the precision with which auditory thresholds were estimated. Audiometers generated signals covering a broad range of frequency and intensity, and in addition to threshold measures facilitated identifying the relation between sound intensity and the perception of loudness. Early investigators (Fowler, 1936; Steinberg & Gardner, 1937) reported that patients with hearing loss experienced, in addition to elevated thresholds, an unusual relation between the intensity of a stimulus and the loudness it evoked. For some patients with hearing loss, a signal 10 dB SL regarding the puretone threshold (that is, signal level 10 dB higher than the patient's threshold of hearing) was rated as a loudness (i.e., on a 1 to 100 scale) higher than the value provided by a normal-hearing person. Further, the rating provided by the listener with hearing loss increased by a greater amount than that of the normal hearing listener given identical increases in stimulus level. When loudness rating was graphed as a function of stimulus level, the hearing-impaired listener functions were steeper than those for normal hearing listeners. Investigators also found that, in general, at stimulus levels higher than 90 to 95 dB SPL, regardless of the hearing loss magnitude, the loudness functions as rated by hearing-impaired listeners approached and often could be superimposed upon those functions from normal hearing listeners. This loudness growth pattern was termed "loudness recruitment" by Fowler.

The loudness recruitment label captured a few interesting aspects of auditory system function. First, Fowler and other investigators employed the term to describe the way that an array of auditory nerve fibers would be influenced by damage to the cochlear hair cells. Given that not all fibers in the auditory nerve displayed identical thresholds, the loss of hair cells should have the most substantial effect on fibers with low thresholds, or those that would under normal conditions respond to audible signals of low intensity. The change in nerve innervation would commonly follow damage to some of the cochlea's most vulnerable components, the outer hair cells. While the sensory fiber population serving the outer hair cells would not be expected to influence audibility, the weakened contribution of the outer hair cells to basilar membrane mechanics would result in reduced stimulation of inner hair cells, thereby producing mild-moderate hearing loss.

At stimulus levels exceeding 50 to 60 dB, however, the relative contribution of the outer hair cell system to cochlear mechanics decreases under normal conditions, and the displacement along the basilar membrane is sufficient to activate inner hair cells and generate an audible response regardless of the outer hair cell component. The higher stimulus levels would increase the likelihood that fibers with higher thresholds would be stimulated. Therefore, the ensuing neural activity would be dominated by fibers that respond exclusively to moderate or high-level signals. Because these fibers code high-intensity stimuli, the ensuing perception would feature the sensation of high or perhaps excessive loudness even though the sound did not exceed the listener's threshold by a substantial amount.

At the upper limit of loudness tolerance, the hearing-impaired listener's experience of loudness mimicked that of normal hearing listeners even though the stimulus did not exceed their thresholds by a similar amount, or sensation level. Such patient reports were consistent with the idea that the high-threshold fibers were "recruited" into action even though the lower-threshold, more sensitive fibers were no longer capable of encoding low intensity sounds. Hence, the observation that, for high level signals, while the relation between loudness and stimulus is similar across populations with different amounts of hearing loss, the relation is substantially different at low-to-moderate levels.

As discussed in Chapter 4, the measures of loudness tolerance may be of more value for decisions regarding intervention than those of absolute threshold despite the lack of a method for loudness measures as reliable and replicable as that used for puretone thresholds. The loudness growth pattern described above would correspond to cochlear hearing loss; indeed, many audiology students were taught that loudness recruitment was the "hallmark" of a cochlear hearing loss. However, hearing loss may produce an unusual perception that was described as a loss of ability to hear sounds as soft (Buus & Florentine, 2002), as patients reported sounds in the hearing loss region, usually the high frequency region, produced substantial loudness even at intensity levels that barely exceeded threshold. A sound was louder for such patients at threshold than it would be for an unaffected listener; patients either did not hear a sound in the hearing loss region, or, when they did, even at low sensation levels, the sound was never soft. Rather, the ability to hear a sound as soft appeared beyond the patient's processing ability, and Buus and Florentine (2002) suggested that the unusual experience of pronounced loudness at threshold was likely a better way to describe the effect of recruitment than that provided by the traditional definition of abnormal growth of loudness accompanying suprathreshold signals. Additionally, patients with trauma histories, or combat exposure, often reported the exaggerated startle response that they experienced when sounds would appear to "come out of nowhere" and grow to painful loudness instantaneously. The potential value of hearing aids may be limited for such patients, and the reader is urged to consider a listening program such as that provided by Rob Littwin in Chapter 15.

Unfortunately, many patients who experience routine events that produce unusual loudness experiences often respond to the discomfort by avoiding what they perceive as unsafe areas, or by wearing hearing protection even when sound levels pose no threat. As the patients often have hearing loss, the use of hearing protection seems intuitive, and may be urged by an audiologist or other professional. After all, if the loss of ability to hear soft sounds is related to hearing loss, then protecting the remaining hearing must be a priority. It therefore surprises many patients, and even some professionals, to learn that hearing protection may be overused, or even abused by patients whose intention is merely to protect what hearing they have left.

Hyperacusis

Although recruitment is a typical consequence of cochlear hearing loss, the term is sometimes used interchangeably with hyperacusis. This situation is unfortunate because the two disorders are profoundly different with respect to their prevalence and effect on a patient's quality of life. Although recruitment is consistent with reduced dynamic range of hearing, hyperacusis suggests a more substantial reduction, perhaps a collapse, of loudness tolerance, and by extension, dynamic range. Patients may experience pain when they hear sounds that were once pleasant, such as conversations or amplified music. The change in auditory processing associated with hyperacusis can arise from many potential sources. Patient narratives and passages in literature illuminate the confounding and existential thoughts accompanying offending sounds (Baguley, 2016).

One recent example is provided by the poet Ruby Robinson who incorporated her challenges with sound tolerance in a poem entitled *Internal Gain* (2016), from which this is an excerpt:

> *My room was vibrating with electricity sockets*
> *and light beams*
> *and I could hear every little sound my*
> *mouth made.*
>
> *Outside my window*
> *a butterfly, miniscule on a roof tile*
> *rubbed its wings together*
> *excruciatingly.*

Such literary depictions of decreased sound tolerance chime with written descriptions of the experience. Dan Malcore is the founder of the Internet community at www.hyperacusis.net, which is an invaluable resource for people with what is described as "collapsed sound tolerance." His difficulties with sound began at a long-anticipated sports event, attended with his children. His family was seated close to a blaring loudspeaker, and Dan soon realized he was being injured as an immediate reduction in his ability to tolerate sound became increasingly apparent, exacerbated by further accidental exposure to loud sound. His description of his troubles is moving and lucid:

> *My symptoms were severe and my life was collapsing around me. In a matter of only a few days I could no longer tolerate the normal sounds of life (conversation, telephone, television). Even my young children whispering to me or the sound of turning my head on my pillow at night was distressing.* Malcore (2013)

Adults who experience hyperacusis are often able to articulate their situation verbally, but this may not be the case for children. In such a situation, it is possible to ask them to draw a picture of themselves with their symptoms, and an example is given in Figure 1–1. This young man experiencing severe sound tolerance issues, picturing himself as buffeted by sound, assailed by it as it strikes him. Such pictures enable the patient to be heard, and so can be empowering: they also allow parents, teachers, and clinicians to see inside the lived experience of hyperacusis.

One can imagine the lure that hearing protection devices would afford a person going through what the people above describe. If sounds were painful, logic would dictate that they were also potentially damaging. As the patient may experience hearing loss concurrent with their difficulties tolerating reasonable sound levels, they may be encouraged by a professional to protect their ears in order to preserve residual hearing. The patient may be convinced that hearing protection is needed in an increasing number of situations,

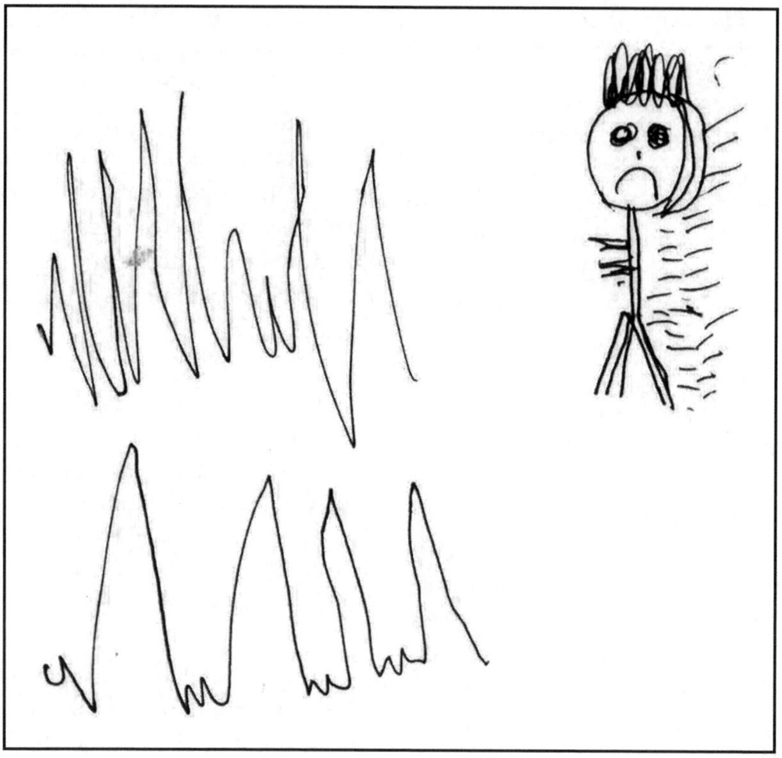

Figure 1–1. A young patient's depiction of the hyperacusis experience.

again to minimize the probability that they will incur additional damage. Unfortunately, for patients in both clinics and experimental protocols, hearing protection often was not the panacea it initially appeared to be.

Use of earplugs was linked to changes in loudness tolerance in innovative experiments by Formby and colleagues (Formby et al., 2003). Participants wore an earplug in one ear and a low-level in-ear masking device in the other ear throughout the day. At the end of two weeks, loudness discomfort levels (LDLs) were compared to the pre-experiment values. In two weeks' time, the plugged ears displayed a lowering (less tolerance) than pre-experiment levels while the masker ears displayed an increased LDL relative to baseline. The changes occurred relatively quickly, and reversed themselves within a few days after the experiment's termination. Clearly, the auditory pathway's loudness processing evolved rapidly to changing conditions in the environment, or with respect to the peripheral system's integrity; this finding illustrated that hearing protection could be overused, thereby exacerbating the problem for which it was intended.

Indeed, for some individuals, habitual hearing protection use reduces loudness tolerance to the point that routine activities cannot be managed or endured. Again, it is as if the ability to tolerate most sound collapses. To date, medical terminology and definitions of decreased sound tolerance have not quite been able to articulate the depth of patient experiences, and the anguish that may be associated. The term *hyperacusis* derives from the Greek words for "over" or "above" and "hearing." This translation may be misleading for our purposes as it implies better than average sensitivity, but at the threshold level; our interest is at the other end of the dynamic range. Interestingly, Google translation of hyperacusis into Greek, and then back to English, yields the term "infrared," another example of the inadequacies of unsophisticated translation. Hyperacusis refers to a general perception of the sound environment as intense and adverse. An early mention of the hyperacusic response to sound was reported by Paul of Aegina (625 to 690 AD) (Adams, 1844, cited in Stephens, 2000). When writing about individuals who experienced persistent tinnitus, the physician indicated that some of those patients also suffered from what he termed "increased sensibility," or an experience of inordinate loudness to sounds that others could tolerate easily. It must be noted that Paul wrote during a time when there were few intense sounds produced by humans; perhaps a blacksmith, or a child shouting/screaming would fit the bill.

Laurence Turnbull (1881) identified several aspects of hearing loss whose remediation would continue to frustrate clinicians to this day. In addition to a prescient review of electrical stimulation to ameliorate the effects of tinnitus, Turnbull described patients who reacted powerfully to sound levels that should not produce excessive loudness. He did not specifically link such behavior to the term hyperacusis. Later, a description of reduced sound tolerance was offered in the otolaryngology medical literature in 1938 by Perlman, who used the hyperacusis term. The addition of a suffix led to the term *hyperacusis dolorosa* by Mathieson in 1969, referring to the profound sadness experienced by some individuals with reduced sound tolerance, but this phrase did not achieve widespread acceptance.

Several definitions of hyperacusis exist in the literature, perhaps due in part to the varied and sometimes intense nature of patients' reports. Note in those cited below components of both auditory and psychological state. First, Jack Vernon was a pioneer of the clinical understanding of tinnitus who noticed that some of his tinnitus patients experienced decreased sound tolerance, though his estimates of this fall considerably short of that which is presently believed (see Chapter 11). Vernon defined hyperacusis as "unusual tolerance to ordinary environmental sounds" (Vernon, 1987). Vernon's neutral definition contrasts with a contemporary account from the otology literature, which has a pejorative tone:

> *consistently exaggerated or inappropriate responses or complaints to sounds that are neither intrinsically threatening or uncomfortably loud to a typical person.* (Klein et al., 1990)

In a further attention to strike a neutral or cautiously positive tone, a partnership between an audiologist and a psychologist resulted in:

> *experience of inordinate loudness of sound that most people tolerate well, associated with a component of distress.* (Baguley & Andersson, 2007)

In a scoping review, Fackrell et al. (2017) considered definitions of hyperacusis in 43 published papers, finding that 14 (33%) did not provide a working definition of hyperacusis. Of those that did, the definitions used variously focused on *reductions* in sound tolerance, on *increased sensitivity* to sound, on *intolerance* to sound, and on *reaction* to sound. Underpinning all these themes was a concept of the tolerance to sound being different from 'normal.'

The potential for sound to produce such responses should remind us that one person's hyperacusis may be another person's enjoyable night out on the town, in that some people will seek out hyperintense and discordant sound experiences for pleasure. This is analogous to the dissonance between the distressing experience of a patient with vertigo, and the exhilarating experience of riding a rollercoaster.

Auditory status alone cannot predict the sounds that will prove aversive to a listener, rather experience and mental health status influence in powerful ways any perceptual event. The one source of security to which many patients may turn, namely hearing protection, seemingly tricks the auditory pathway into an acceleration of the processing that contributed to the excessive loudness in the first place. If avoidance and hearing protection fail to address loudness intolerance, then an effective method for desensitizing listeners must be considered. Rob Littwin's chapter expands upon many elements indicated on Dan Malcore's network for managing negative responses to sound. We are fortunate to share his work in Chapter 15.

Beyond Audibility: Phonophobia and Misophonia

Patients may experience a variety of other aversive reactions to sound, in addition to hyperacusis and loudness recruitment. Phonophobia, from the Greek words *phone* meaning voice, or sound, and *phobia* referring to fear, is a vague term applied to sounds that provoke responses of fear. While some sounds evoke fear in the majority of hearers, for example, screams or approaching large vehicles producing a warning sound, other sounds are innocuous to most people, yet provoke fear in others. The response to a sound can change over time, and it is common in clinical settings for patients to express that certain sounds, once pleasing, no longer provide relief, they produce distress. Such patients may indicate that a bedside sound generator, for use to facilitate sleep, may exert the opposite effect when it is turned on. The chapter's first author has abundant experience with patients who are military Veterans, startling and immediately moving to leave the room when the sound of a small creek, or stream, is played out on the sound generator. When asked about the response, the patient may reveal that the sound is reminiscent of a stream that flowed by the location of a war-time facility at which the patient was a prisoner. Juxtaposed against the typical patient response, the jarring and immediate discomfort demonstrated by the affected Veteran affirms that one sound may be processed in profoundly different ways by two observers with identical hearing sensitivity, but different lifetime experiences. The sound is not excessively loud; however, it produces substantial arousal.

Phonophobia has been specifically associated with migraine, and this situation is explored in Chapter 7, by Don McFerran, wherein the issues of a terminology based on fear, or phobia, when the migraineurs experience may be of irritation or annoyance, is described.

Another form of negative patient response to sound is termed misophonia (Jastreboff & Jastreboff, 2004); while this term has not yet gained wide acceptance among professionals (although consensus is growing), its presence on a number of self-help Internet boards ensures that its use will continue. The term's Greek roots are somewhat vague; *misos* connoting hatred, and *phone*, as above, referring to voice or sound. Following its initial use by Jastreboff and Jastreboff (2004) as a blanket term for any annoying sound (fingers on a chalkboard, the sound of someone coughing uncontrollably, an annoying dog barking hour after hour), the term has been applied primarily to individuals whose lives have been altered by a powerful aversion to the sound of people chewing, sipping drinks, or clattering silverware on a plate (see McFerran, 2016, for review). In a sense, most humans have specific sounds that trigger sensations of anger or discomfort; however, the patient with misophonia will report an inventory of additional sounds that trigger similar, or more powerful, emotional responses.

The possibility that patients complaining of misophonia were demonstrably different from those who do not was long supported by patient narratives and comments on online discussion boards. However, evidence supporting specific neural mechanisms underlying the powerful psychological responses was lacking. Kumar et al. (2016) compared 20 patients with specific complaints of misophonia to 22 age-matched control subjects. The participants were presented with three types of sound: neutral sounds that were presumed to evoke a minimal response (such as rain falling), unpleasant sounds that would be disliked by most listeners (such as a baby crying), and sounds that misophonic patients routinely cite as triggers (such as people eating or loud breathing). The investigators measured levels of distress by patient report. Additionally, they measured a variety of physiologic responses to the sound, including heart rate and skin conductivity, as well as activity in brain regions associated with arousal, monitoring of emotions, and interoception, here referring to a signal's salience and identity that may contribute to the modification of a person's monitoring of body functions such as the heart rate and respiration rate.

The investigators reported substantial group differences between the patient ratings of sound, as well as the neural centers activated by the sounds. For example, the patients in the misophonia group rated the trigger sounds as substantially more distressing than the unpleasant sounds whereas the nonmisophonic participants not only expressed a minimal difference between the two, on average, they rated the unpleasant sounds as more annoying than the sounds serving as triggers for the misophonics. Both groups rated neutral sounds as neither distressing nor annoying.

Physiologic data also delineated the two groups effectively. In particular, the investigators noted a consistent functional connectivity between areas associated with the aforementioned interoception, or the anterior insular cortex, and the brain areas regulating arousal and emotional state. The finding reiterated Garfinkel et al.'s (2016) report that misophonics, as well as individuals on the autism spectrum, displayed an unusual awareness and attention to internal sensations. Kumar et al. (2016) asserted that the group differences could explain the unusual patient reports that stymied rehabilitation efforts of clinicians from a variety of professions. In conclusion, the investigators reported their data "suggest that abnormal salience attributed to otherwise innocuous sounds, coupled with atypical perception of internal body states, underlies misophonia" (p. 532).

Patients with either phonophobia or misophonia illustrate that sounds do not have to be loud to be distressing, or to provoke avoidance. Routinely experienced, everyday sounds can induce in certain listeners powerful emotions, such as anger, fear, or disgust; at the same time, other sounds may evoke annoyance, and in others, pain. The provider is essentially at the patient's mercy when trying to categorize or understand the patient's reports as the clinician has little or no confirmatory evidence with which to work. Patients' hearing thresholds add little to the rehabilitative effort, although accurate and replicable measurement of LDLs could provide valuable information.

A model that attempted to describe the space occupied by a patient with hyperacusis was proposed by Baguley and Andersson (2007), with a particular aim to delineate the influences on life imposed by decreased sound tolerance (Figure 1–2). The factors described were noise sensitivity, fear of sound and injury, and irritation/annoyance. In an alternative proposal, the spectrum of patients' complaints and resulting challenges for clinicians was addressed to some degree by a loudness labeling scheme proposed by Tyler et al. (2014).

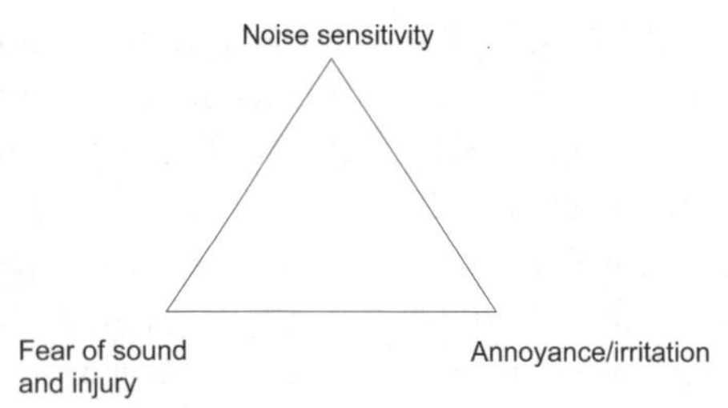

Figure 1–2. Model describing the space occupied by a patient with hyperacusis including the patient's noise sensitivity, fear of sound and injury, and irritation/annoyance.

Types of Hyperacusis

Tyler et al. (2014) proposed four distinct types of hyperacusis in an attempt to simplify terminology, and by doing so, firm the field's definitions of these challenging conditions to terms that could enjoy broader acceptance, online discussion boards notwithstanding. Tyler et al. suggested four distinct types of hyperacusis, all of which capture one or more of the sound-related challenges to patients summarized above.

Tyler et al.'s four hyperacusis labels included loudness, annoyance, fear, and pain. Loudness hyperacusis was the broadest of the terms, indicating that some patients experience uncomfortable loudness idiosyncratically. Although a patient might display a recruitment-like (i.e., typical) experience with loudness, it would be possible for some sounds to appear louder than others due to their spectral content and the uniqueness of the patient's hearing loss. In such cases, a patient would complain about certain sounds being uncomfortably loud without necessarily mentioning powerful emotions being triggered by such sounds.

Fear hyperacusis was described by Tyler et al. (2014) as a response to sound that was not only aversive, it also provoked stress of anticipation. As such, patients experiencing fear hyperacusis would display avoidance behaviors and would limit their activities when they were concerned the offending sounds would be present. Fear hyperacusis could be considered an analog of phonophobia, as described above, with the same negative consequences for the patient who gives in to temptation to avoid sound or overprotect hearing.

The definition of annoyance hyperacusis focused on emotions and reactions to certain sounds. As with some cases of fear hyperacusis, the offending sounds might not be excessively powerful or damaging. Yet despite the knowledge that the sounds would not hurt hearing, the patient avoided such sounds as though they were toxic and emotionally scarring. Sounds that evoke annoyance hyperacusis would contribute to a patient's state of mind by inducing anxiety, irritation, and stress in a manner outlined convincingly by Kumar et al. (2016). Similarly, annoyance hyperacusis may be considered an analog of misophonia.

Pain hyperacusis was the fourth label provided by Tyler et al. (2014) and referred to observers experiencing pain in the presence of certain sounds. Although the mechanism by which ear pain would be generated in response to sound remained unclear in Tyler et al.'s scheme, Eggermont (in Chapter 8) provides a review of current experimentation linking inner ear damage in mice to avoidance behaviors via a special class of pain receptors (nociceptors) located in the cochlear nuclei and activated by cochlear hair cells. Although the inner ear does not employ pain receptors per se, damage to inner ear sensory cells may activate pain receptors in the brainstem, thereby resulting in a sensation of pain deep in the ear in response to loud sounds.

While Tyler and colleagues undertook a robust attempt to survey the available literature, the four-category model of hyperacusis has not yet been empirically verified, and the clinical experience of the present authors indicates that patients may easily inhabit two or more of the categories, and that these are not distinct nor mutually exclusive. Perhaps the experience of hyperacusis, like that of pain, defies simple categorization or description, in which case, the final reflections of this chapter should go to a patient.

A Patient Summarizes

The magnitude of distress experienced by patients is probably best described by the patients themselves. What follows is a brief report from a patient whose experiences encapsulate many aspects of the information above. The lived experience of reduced sound tolerance, when chronic, as indicated in this excerpt from a female hyperacusis patient, in her 4th decade, make it possible for the reader to view the patient as a "prisoner" of her symptoms: the purpose of this book is to try to understand how this can happen, and how the situation can be improved.

> *My partner and I were still unaware what this hypersensitivity to noise was and began to be very anxious, wondering what was wrong with me, and wondering if it might be a brain tumour. By now, I couldn't bear to be in the kitchen (couldn't tolerate the noise of the kettle, boiler, microwave, fridge, etc.), or use the vacuum cleaner, listen to music, TV, play piano. At its worst I couldn't bear the noise of the hair dryer, or the sound of cutlery on the crockery. Equally, I couldn't bear to be outside and tolerate noises such as birds chirping, traffic (either close to or in the distance), planes flying overhead, lawn mowers, [with] the last of these triggering panic attacks. When we finally saw the Ear Nose and Throat Specialist, he allayed our fears by giving it a name (Hyperacusis) and telling us that it was non-life threatening. However, it took away many aspects of life because it is SO limiting. I was unable to continue in my job, as well as in my voluntary work and all my social activities. I was unable to travel either by car, bus, train or plane, unable to go anywhere, other than for quiet walks 'round the village; unable to visit family or friends (near or far), unable to work, difficult to talk to anyone on the phone, couldn't cook meals in the kitchen, etc. It was like being a prisoner in my own home. Thankfully, my husband was able to arrange to work from home where he had to do the cooking, as well as go with me wherever I went in case I had a panic attack.* (Quoted from Baguley, 2008)

References

Baguley, D. M. (2008). Hyperacusis. In R. S. Tyler (Ed.), *The consumer handbook on tinnitus.* Auricle Ink: Sedona, AZ.

Baguley, D. M. (2016). Tinnitus in literature. In D. M. Baguley and M. Fagelson (Eds.), *Tinnitus: Clinical and research perspectives* (pp. 1–12). San Diego, CA: Plural.

Baguley, D. M. & Andersson, G. (2007). *Hyperacusis mechanisms, diagnosis, and therapies.* San Diego, CA: Plural.

Buus, S. & Florentine, M. (2002). Growth of loudness in listeners with cochlear hearing losses: recruitment reconsidered. *J. Assoc. Res. Otolaryngol, 3,* 120–139. doi: 10.1007/s1016 20010084

Collins, W. (1860). *The woman in white.* London, UK: Penguin Classics.

Fackrell K., Potgeiter I., Shekhawat G. S., Baguley D. M., Sereda M., & Hoare D. J. (2017). Clinical interventions for Hyperacusis in Adults: a scoping review to assess the current position and determine priorites for research. *BioMed Research International,* doi.org/10.1155/2017/2723715

Formby, C., Sherlock, L. P., & Gold, S. L. (2003). Adaptive plasticity of loudness induced by chronic attenuation and enhancement of the acoustic background. *Journal of the Acoustical Society of America, 114*, 55–58.

Fowler, E. P. A method for the early detection of otosclerosis. *Arch Otolaryng, 24*, 731–734.

Garfinkel, S. N., Tiley, C., O'Keeffe, S., Harrison, N. A., Seth, A. K., & Critchley, H. D. (2016). Discrepancies between dimensions of interception in autism: implications for emotion and anxiety. *Biol. Psychol., 114*, 117–126.

Jastreboff, P. J., & Jastreboff, M. M. (2004). Decreased sound tolerance. In: J. B. Snow (Ed.), *Tinnitus: Theory and management* (pp. 8–15). London, UK: BC Decker.

Klein, A. A. J., Armstrong, B. L., Greer, M. K., & Brown, III, F. R. (1990). Hyperacusis and otitis media in individuals with Williams syndrome. *Journal of Speech and Hearing Disorders, 55*, 339–344.

Kumar, S., Tansley-Hancock, O., Sedley, W., . . . Griffiths, T. D. (2016). The brain basis for misophonia. *Current Biology, 27*, 527–533.

Mathiesen, H. (1969). Phonophobia after stapedectomy. *Acta Oto-Laryngologica (Stocklhom), 68*, 73–77.

Malcore, D. (2013). The hyperacusis network. *ENT and Audiology News, 21*(6), 72–73. Available at http://www.entandaudiologynews.com/assets/Uploads/Pdfs/Hyperacusis-JF13.pdf

McFerran, D. (2016). Misophonia and phonophobia. In D. M. Baguley & M. Fagelson (Eds.), *Tinnitus: Clinical and research perspectives* (pp. 245–260). San Diego, CA: Plural.

Perlman, H. B. (1938). Hyperacusis. *Annals of Otology, Rhinology, Laryngology, 47*, 947–953.

Robinson, R. (2016). *Every little sound.* Liverpool, UK: Liverpool University Press.

Steinberg, J. C. & Gardener, M. B. (1937). The dependency of hearing impairment on sound intensity. *J. Acou. Soc. Am., 9*, 11–23.

Stephens, D. (2000). A history of tinnitus. In R. Tyler (Ed.), *Tinnitus handbook* (pp. 437–448). Clifton Park, NJ: Thompson Learning.

Turnbull, L. (1881). *Imperfect hearing and the hygiene of the ear*. Philadelphia, PA: JB Lippincott & Co.

Tyler, R. S., Pienkowski, M., Roncancio, E. R., . . . , Moore, B. C. J. (2014). A review of hyperacusis and future directions: Part I. Definitions and manifestations. *Am. J. Aud.*, (23), 402–419.

Vernon, J. A. (1987). Pathophysiology of tinnitus: A special case—hyperacusis and a proposed treatment. *Am. J. Otol., 8*, 201–202.

2

Audiological Assessment of Decreased Sound Tolerance

Glynnis A. Tidball and Marc Fagelson

Introduction

Decreased sound tolerance (DST), here defined as an abnormal physical and emotional response to routinely experienced everyday sounds, is an auditory complaint arising from damaging sound exposure, physical disease or dysfunction, mental health conditions or injury, or as a side effect of some medications. DST has also been reported in individuals with certain genetic syndromes such as William's syndrome (Katzenell & Segal, 2001).

Sounds can be deemed intolerable by patients because they are perceived as overly loud, annoying, fear-inducing, or painful (Tyler et al., 2014). General usage of the term in medical, psychological, and audiological texts suggests that DST is a subjective complaint without an objective or easily measured correlate. Behaviors reported or observed in those with DST include sound avoidance, over-use of hearing protection, exaggerated startle response to sound, and increased awareness of ambient sounds. The means by which DST can be identified, measured, and managed in an audiological setting, as well as the merits and limitations of current assessment techniques and tools, provide the focus of this chapter. The discussion of assessment here is meant to apply to both adult and pediatric populations; issues specific to pediatric assessment will be considered later in the chapter.

Rationale for Assessment of Decreased Sound Tolerance

Given the multidimensional challenges faced by patients with DST, a successful intervention approach likely must consider input from an inter-professional team of providers. Patients with DST are likely to access care for their condition through an audiologist and/or otolaryngologist. The lack of specific measures precludes definitive statements regarding the prevalence of DST; however, the reported overlap of tinnitus, hearing loss and DST (see Chapter 3, Epidemiology) suggests that audiologists should be equipped to diagnose, manage, and direct patients to appropriate care in order to establish and act upon the causes and effects of DST and thus optimize opportunities for intervention.

Any patient being assessed for hearing function has the potential to present with DST. Routine audiological tests may involve high-level sound stimulation that individuals with DST find uncomfortable or painful (e.g., vestibular-evoked myogenic potential, auditory brainstem responses, acoustic reflex thresholds). Patients with DST may report that these and other routine audiological tests exacerbate tinnitus or contribute to and heighten sound-provoked anxiety. Indeed, Aazh and Moore (2017b) found that 21% of patients at a clinic specializing in management of tinnitus and hyperacusis experienced stimulus levels exceeding loudness discomfort levels (LDLs) when completing the basic audiologic test battery performed according to the British Society of Audiology recommended procedures. Screening or interviewing the patient for DST prior to testing is advisable in the interest of preserving patient comfort and clinical rapport, and to avoid possible iatrogenic effects of testing such as provoking reactive tinnitus. If DST is suspected, the test battery should be modified accordingly. If a test using high-intensity stimuli is attempted, the rationale for performing the test should be explained to the patient beforehand, giving the patient the choice of opting out of or terminating the test. Indeed, test battery adjustments, as suggested by Aazh and Moore (2017b), should be considered for these patients following a rationale similar to that provided when performing pediatric audiological assessment under normal conditions; the audiologist's goal is to complete the test battery, but not at the expense of the patient's well-being, psychological state, and with care not to render the patient fearful of the audiometric test suite.

Identification of DST is informative from a diagnostic perspective as its presence may be symptomatic of significant medical pathology, including both otological and non-otological causes (see Chapters 7 and 9). Otological conditions that include DST as a possible accompanying symptom include acoustic shock disorder and superior canal dehiscence (SCD). SCD frequently alters sound tolerance due to the enhanced transmission of sounds via bone conduction, labelled "conductive DST" (Banerjee, 2005) or "bone hyperacusis" (Ward et al., 2017). Patients with SCD may experience their own voice, heel strikes as they walk or run, and even eye movements as unusually loud, and may report that loud sounds or pressure changes evoke a spinning sensation or nausea (the so-called Tullio phenomenon) as well as the perception that still objects are moving. An example of SCD appears as the second case in this chapter.

The diagnostic significance of DST underscores the need to ask patients not only if they are intolerant of certain sounds, but also to describe the quality or nature of sounds that are not well tolerated, the effect that the sounds elicit, and the circumstances under which DST developed. Patients may not volunteer this information during the case history unless specifically asked about sound tolerance as they may believe the symptoms are unusual or incidental. Therefore, it is essential for audiologists to interpret case history information thoroughly and to consider the possibility that DST influences the patient's auditory behaviors by provoking, for example, avoidance strategies, modifications of lifestyle, or over-use of hearing protection.

From the perspective of hearing loss management, identification and measurement of DST is essential for patient satisfaction, acceptance of new devices, and optimal speech performance when hearing aids are fit. Indeed, several studies have indicated that loudness in tolerance contributes to dissatisfaction with amplification for many users. Kochkin (2000) found that 25.3% of survey respondents cited loudness of amplified sound as a reason they did not use their hearing aids. Specifically, respondents reported that amplification made noise painful, annoying, distracting, or unacceptable. In a subsequent survey of hearing aid users, Kochkin (2002) found that 58% of survey respondents indicated that they would like to see new hearing aid technology make "loud sounds less painful." A scoping review by McCormack and Fortnum published in 2013 suggests that noise and comfort is still an issue with regard to patients' rejection of hearing aids. Humes et al. (2003) found that successful hearing aid users judged low-level sounds as less loud and had higher loudness discomfort levels (LDLs) overall when compared to patients who used their hearing aids less frequently.

While none of these surveys identified individuals with DST, they suggested that dissatisfaction with loudness of amplified sound contributed to hearing aid returns. The rate of returns for hearing aids in the United States in 2014 was 19.4%. Approximately 60% of all hearing aids returned to the manufacturer were returned with "first-fit" settings (Kochkin, 2000), which suggested that in most cases the output of the returned hearing aids was set according to predicted loudness tolerance, or that the patient was not consulted regarding sounds that caused pain or discomfort.

Individuals with DST who find that output of amplification uncomfortably or painfully exceeds loudness tolerance may be reluctant to wear their instruments, or insist that the gain be reduced to accommodate DST. When tinnitus and DST are present, patients may also report that amplification exacerbates tinnitus. It is reasonable to expect that DST will be an impediment to acceptance of amplification, or that tolerance problems may compel users to set their hearing instruments below target gain and therefore at levels inadequate to support optimal speech intelligibility. Because hearing aid output can be easily measured, there is no excuse for professionals fitting hearing aids to abrogate their responsibility to consider patient reports and tolerance limits. Further, hearing aid returns are costly to the dispenser and manufacturer and worse, there is a cost to the patient who has a poor first experience with hearing aids and concludes that, "I tried hearing aids and they didn't work." Such patients may then be reluctant to pursue instruments in the future.

A fitting protocol that includes management of DST could improve user satisfaction and ultimately allow patients to use amplification at settings optimal for speech intelligibility rather than wearing hearing aids set with lower outputs, as are often preferred by patients at initial fittings. A treatment approach described by Formby et al. (2015) employed wideband sound therapy, delivered via ear-level sound generators, and counseling that prioritized increasing loudness tolerance and expanding dynamic range in hearing-impaired individuals. As the use of wideband sound fostered desensitization to offending sounds in patients, the authors postulated that the added sound decreased central auditory gain, considered a putative mechanism by which the auditory pathway would compensate for loss of sensitivity. The authors reported that subjects preferred a higher presentation level of speech (most comfortable level, or MCL) after using the devices for several weeks. Subjects tolerated target gain values and related audibility of speech sounds more consistently and with fewer complaints of uncomfortable loudness at the end of the study period.

Investigations of DST prevalence indicate that DST frequently co-occurs with tinnitus, and affects an estimated 40% of tinnitus patients (Baguley & Andersson, 2008). Individuals presenting with both DST and tinnitus frequently report that tinnitus reacts (i.e., worsens) following intense sound exposures. Schecklmann et al. (2014) indicate that 86% of individuals with intrusive tinnitus and DST (defined in the study as "sounds cause pain or physical discomfort") report increased tinnitus loudness following exposure to noise. Given that amplification and sound therapy are routinely used in tinnitus management (e.g., Henry et al., 2008; Jastreboff & Jastreboff, 2000; Searchfield, 2015), tinnitus intervention should include assessment of DST to ensure that neither amplification nor sound used for sound therapy exacerbate tinnitus. Jastreboff and Jastreboff (2000) assert that DST should be managed prior to tinnitus intervention. Patients will be more likely to accept masking noise, amplification, and other sound therapies used in specific tinnitus interventions when loudness tolerance or specific aversions to sounds have been addressed.

The rationale for sound therapy in tinnitus management is that sound, if acceptable to the patient, will ultimately reduce tinnitus distress. When patients experience reduced sound tolerance, however, their willingness to use sound therapy may be limited due to an aversive response to the very sounds whose intent is therapeutic. In cases of tinnitus accompanying hearing loss, the potential value of hearing aids or combination instruments may be reduced when patients discover the devices produce uncomfortable sound levels that provoke avoidance rather than participation. Sound therapy can utilize sounds that mix with or mask tinnitus, or it can prioritize the use of environmental sounds, or other information-bearing signals, to interfere with tinnitus perception. However, those patients affected by DST will have, by definition, a limited palate of sounds from which to choose, and within the limited set of acceptable sounds, tolerable sound levels may restrict further the options available to patient and clinician. A careful process of desensitization, perhaps similar to that offered by Rob Littwin in Chapter 15 can support the patient's efforts to obtain relief from tinnitus through acceptance of masking sounds.

Perhaps the most compelling reason to identify DST in an audiology setting is the significant and detrimental impact on quality of life for patients and those around them (see Chapter 10). Individuals with DST are likely to avoid situations in which intolerable sounds are anticipated; their worlds can become functionally and metaphorically very small. Patients' ability to function at work and at home may be compromised, and they may feel isolated, misunderstood, and unsupported. Identifying and acknowledging the presence of DST and its impact is an important first step toward patient management and helping the audiologist gain the patient's trust.

Assessment Components

Case History

Individuals may present to their care provider with DST as their primary complaint and concern. Others may not volunteer that they have difficulty tolerating sound, especially when the focus of assessment is hearing loss or tinnitus. Patients may feel that DST is not relevant to their assessment, or believe that their complaints are unusual or untreatable. Given the prevalence of DST in the general population and especially in clinical populations in which tinnitus is present (see Chapter 3), including a general question in the standard case history is recommended.

Asking the patient, "Are you bothered by sound in any way?" is a simple question that allows the patient to acknowledge whether sound tolerance and/or routinely experienced sounds or environments present consistent problems. It is useful to remember that sound tolerance will vary depending on sound characteristics (intensity, frequency, rise time, and context), the patient's psychological health status, including levels of stress and arousal, and the patient's beliefs about sound. Some questions for clinicians to consider may be drawn from examples below.

Description of Problem

How and when did this start?

DST may develop secondary to an acoustic event such as exposure to music, occupational noise, unanticipated sound proximal to the ear; health event (such as an otologic or neurologic condition or event, physical injury, prescribed and/or illicit drug use); or psychological event, perhaps after trauma or a period of high stress or anxiety (Anari et al., 1999). The conditions under which DST began provide insights into possible mechanisms or contributing factors to DST. When tinnitus is present, DST may arise coincidental to tinnitus, or before or after tinnitus onset. Sudden-onset DST, similar to sudden-onset tinnitus, likely produces a more severe disruption to daily life and greater levels of psychological stress for the patient than those same conditions emerging in a gradual manner (Fagelson, 2007; Kreuzer et al., 2014).

Describe sounds that bother you.

Patients may easily recall specific sounds or sound qualities that they find bothersome, or they may struggle to identify any examples of problematic sounds. Providing patients with examples of sounds that are commonly identified as problematic can help them to describe their experience. Anari et al. (1999) surveyed 100 patients with DST to determine sounds most commonly identified as problematic from a closed list of 13 sounds. The list below summarizes the authors' findings.

Hypersensitivity to:	*Yes answers (%)*
Low frequency sounds	
• Drilling machine	83
• Traffic noise	72
• Dog barking	62
High frequency sounds	
• Rattling of dishes	88
• Child crying	84
• Paper rustling	71
• Applause	47
• Dentist's drill	44
• Birdsong	24
Broad band noise	
• TV	49
• Speech	44
Sudden sounds	
• Hammering	87
• Door slamming	72

Some individuals will have lowered tolerance of sound because sounds provoke a negative emotional response such as annoyance, rage, or fear. Often it is the context or association of the sound rather than its acoustic characteristics that drives the response. The term "misophonia" as defined by Jastreboff and Jastreboff (2002) is intended to describe an intense dislike of sounds, and approximates the definition of annoyance hyperacusis (Tyler et al., 2014). "Selective sound sensitivity syndrome" is used to describe an aversive reaction to a specific subset of "trigger" sounds (Bernstein et al., 2013). Misophonia also appears in the psychiatric literature to describe this subset of DST reports (Schröder et al., 2013). Examples of bothersome or trigger sounds include oral or eating sounds (chewing, swallowing, lip smacking, etc.), breathing sounds, and repetitive sounds (e.g., clicking of keyboard keys or a pen, leg jostling) (Schröder et al., 2013). The same sounds may not be reported as problematic when made by the patients themselves (Edelstein et al., 2013). Identification of misophonia during assessment is critical in order to establish appropriate counselling and treatment options.

What happens when you hear these sounds?

Tyler et al. (2014) proposed using hyperacusis as an umbrella term for DST, and using additional subcategories of annoyance (described above), loudness, fear, and pain DST to categorize the impact of sound on the listener. These subcategories could provide structure to the case history interview, although we must acknowledge that the subcategories overlap with other terms and definitions as outlined in Chapter 3. Patients may experience overwhelming feelings of aversion or may experience a variety of strong emotions related to sound exposures. Their ability to put such feelings into words, or being provided a lexicon that supports understanding of such feelings, can be beneficial. In a manner similar to that employed during psychological counseling, the patient can be educated regarding their responses to sound, and most effectively when the patient uses prior knowledge or logic to shape their approach to managing challenging problems (Bandura, 1986). For example, a patient who avoids going to a coffeehouse because the music is experienced as annoyingly loud can be counseled to observe the reactions of others in the same environment. If other patrons did not appear to be disturbed, or if nobody else made their way, hands to their ears, to the door, then it would be likely that the sound level was not damaging, and although uncomfortable, could contribute to a process of desensitization that should be the patient's long-term goal.

"Pain hyperacusis" has been described as pain occurring in the ear or head in response to sound levels well below 120 dB SPL, the pain threshold for individuals with normal loudness tolerance (Hood & Poole, 1966). Both peripheral and central mechanisms for a pain response to sound have been proposed. Liu et al. (2015) demonstrated that Type II afferent neural fibers terminating on the outer hair cells were selectively activated when hair cell damage occurred in the cochlea. These Type II fibers activated neurons in the cochlear nucleus when damaging sounds were subsequently presented to the cochlea, and Flores et al. (2015) proposed activation of these Type II nerve fibers might serve as a mechanism for pain hyperacusis (see Chapters 5 and 8).

Patients with pain hyperacusis frequently describe a sharp or "jabbing" pain, as well as a variety of other symptoms associated with offending sounds. Additional symptoms include dull ear ache, burning or numbness in or around the ear or face, pain that radiates down the neck, tinnitus, transient aural fullness, "muffled" or distorted hearing, slight nausea or dizziness/vertigo, headache, popping, clicking, or a fluttering sensation in the ear (Westcott et al., 2013). Klockoff (1978) first described this cluster of symptoms as "tonic tensor tympani syndrome" (TTTS). He suggested an anxiety-based condition developed involuntarily from a lowered threshold of activation of the tensor tympani muscle in the middle ear, resulting in spasm or rhythmic contraction of the muscle. These symptoms could arise from and worsen with sound exposure, particularly sound pressures that caused acoustic trauma or acoustic shock. A similar cluster of symptoms—otalgia, tinnitus, vertigo, and subjective hearing loss—was described in individuals with temporomandibular dysfunction (TMD), which may be present when there is history of head and/or neck injury or dysfunction (Kisnisci et al., 1999). These symptoms are challenging for both patient and clinician; it is also possible that any or all occur in the absence of any identifiable underlying otologic pathology.

When a patient experiences these somatic symptoms and associates them with sound exposure, the symptoms are likely to contribute to the patient's fear and avoidance of sound as well as the belief that routine and moderate levels of sound are damaging. Inquiring about somatic complaints associated with DST can provide direction for referrals, counseling, and reassurance. When head/neck injury or dysfunction is reported, the presence of somatic complaints may suggest that referral to dental, physiotherapy, or other relevant health care provider is indicated; unfortunately, clinical guidelines on the treatment pathway for pain DST do not yet exist.

Patients reporting sound- and pressure-induced spinning sensations upon hearing loud sounds should be queried for other commonly reported symptoms of SCD such as increased loudness of internally generated sounds including their own voice (autophony) and pulsatile tinnitus.

How does this problem influence your daily life at home? At work?

The impact of DST will depend on patients' circumstances at home and at work. Individuals may find that activities of daily living regularly expose them to sounds that they find uncomfortably loud, painful, fear-inducing, and that worsen DST and tinnitus, when present. In some cases, patients may feel the need to remove themselves temporarily or permanently from their work environment and to modify their home and social environments to limit exposure. The audiologist or other health care professional needs to assess the appropriateness of patients' adaptations to sound exposure—for example, are patients' avoidance behaviors reasonable or overly protective? Littwin (Chapter 15) provides several examples of such behaviors, as well as strategies for managing patients' perceived need to avoid certain environments. When patients are involved in a medicolegal or workplace dispute in which DST is a factor, clinicians may be asked to provide an opinion on what level and type of sound exposure is appropriate for the patient in the short and long term.

How important is it to you to do something about your difficulty with sound?

Assessing patient motivation and readiness to address DST, as any disorder, informs the clinician about how to proceed with recommendations and provides an opportunity to open discussion. Patients may feel that their adaptations to DST are reasonable, perhaps due to fear of exposure or satisfaction with their choices. As discussed by Veronica Kennedy (Chapter 14), a child affected by DST influences the activity level and options of the family. The presence of DST in adults can also influence family life when childcare, family activities and household chores are experienced as difficult to tolerate. Counseling and identification of strategies, therefore, may need to address the concerns of a family, not just the individual. On a positive note, the involvement of family members will illustrate for all stakeholders the challenges experienced by the patient. The load carried by the patient may then be shared in a more reasonable manner by the people supporting the patient rather than by the patient alone, particularly as the condition could make the patient feel isolated from potential sources of assistance.

When and how do you use hearing protection?

Audiologists often find indications that an individual with DST misuses hearing protection; indeed, Formby et al. (2003) demonstrated that overuse of hearing protection may induce DST. Beyond DST effects, overuse or unwarranted doubling up of hearing protection in an occupational or military setting can put the individual and those around them in jeopardy by attenuating warning signals including verbal alerts from co-workers. Asking patients about their use of hearing protection provides an opportunity to discuss safe levels of sound and appropriate hearing protection, as well as alternatives to conventional hearing protection such as electronic hearing protection devices that permit warning sounds and speech to reach the ears while attenuating hazardous noise. The key to managing the use of hearing protection may rely upon the clinician confirming that most environments specified by the patient as troublesome likely do not contain damaging levels of noise unless, as indicated previously, others in the vicinity are required to shout to people standing within one meter to be understood, or are holding their ears and fleeing the environment. Patients may feel reassured with this knowledge but may still prefer to keep hearing protection at hand or have an exit strategy in case noise levels become intolerable.

Do you have a history of anxiety, depression, or other mental health concerns? Do you feel that you may be anxious or depressed now?

Several investigators have demonstrated a positive correlation between mental health disorders and sound tolerance. Jüris et al. (2013) found that 56% of individuals with DST also had at least one psychiatric disorder, most frequently an anxiety disorder. DST was also associated with higher risk of co-morbid depressive symptoms.

With DST, as with tinnitus, mental health has the potential to contribute to the magnitude of the symptoms. Patients commonly report that DST worsens with stress and anxiety levels. Sahley and Nodar (2001) propose that emotional and/or physical stress can exacerbate DST through the excitatory effects of stress on the auditory system. Mood can also alter attentional processes, and such changes are observed in conditions such as anxiety or high stress, obsessive compulsive disorders, and post-traumatic stress disorder. The patient's mental health status, particularly in cases associated with hyperarousal such as PTSD, may enhance awareness and increase startle responses to external sounds in a manner that contributes to DST (Fagelson, 2007). The relation between DST and psychological state is bidirectional; not only can the psychological state amplify sound tolerance problems, DST can also negatively influence mental health by contributing to stress arousal, hypervigilance, feelings of persecution, and isolation through sound avoidance. DST, like tinnitus, thus differs from other auditory disorders such as loss of sensitivity, which can reasonably be managed and rehabilitated using hearing aids or other assistive devices with appropriate orientation. The amount and depth of counseling differs greatly in cases of tinnitus and DST. While hearing loss may contribute to feelings of isolation and depression (Arlinger, 2003), pure tone sensitivity does not worsen with mental health disorders. This mutually reinforcing dynamic between DST and mental health conditions underscores the value of discussion of mental health in DST assessment, and management of DST should benefit from identification and treatment of co-morbid mental health disorders such as anxiety.

Unfortunately, hearing health care professionals may feel unqualified or uncomfortable broaching the topic of mental health with patients. Our experience is that an open and neutral approach to discussing mental health in the context of DST is often welcomed by patients and can motivate them to consider options such as behavioral therapies or sound therapy in their treatment plan. Screening tools for psychological disorders, such as the Hospital Anxiety and Depression Scale (HADS; Zigmond & Snaith, 1983), Patient Health Questionnaire-9 (PHQ-P; Martin et al., 2006), and the Generalized Anxiety Disorder-7 (GAD-7; Spitzer et al., 2006), can indicate when referral to the family physician or mental health care provider is warranted.

Pure Tone Audiometry

Pure tone audiometry is essential in determining the severity, nature, and possible etiology of disordered hearing in patients with DST. The relation between hearing loss and DST as indicated by pure tone audiometry is, however, unclear (Tyler et al., 2014). Research indicates that pure tone threshold loss at conventional test frequencies is not required for development of DST. Sheldrake et al. (2015) report that a third of patients with a primary complaint of DST present with clinically normal hearing thresholds (<25 dB HL for test frequencies up to 8 kHz), while the remainder of patients demonstrate pure tone thresholds in the range of mild to severe hearing loss. Brandy and Lynn's (1995) comparison of pure tone thresholds of 25 individuals with DST to those of 13 controls without DST demonstrate no significant difference in hearing thresholds between groups. Andersson et al.'s (2002) survey of individuals about their DST and hearing impairment via an Internet and postal questionnaire asserts that the majority of individuals reporting DST do not identify having a hearing impairment; however, those reporting DST are more likely to also report hearing impairment than respondents without DST complaints.

Conventional pure tone audiometry does not accurately predict auditory function in everyday situations nor does it reflect the integrity of the auditory system as a whole. Conventional diagnostic audiometry measures threshold of audibility at 250 to 8000 Hz (ASHA, 2005) but does not capture pure tone threshold loss at the upper frequency range of human audibility. Furthermore, pure tone thresholds may fall into the range of normal hearing despite changes in auditory function for suprathreshold stimuli. Cochlear synaptopathy, the loss of the synapses between inner hair cells and cochlear neurons due to noise exposure or ageing, is believed to contribute to "hidden hearing loss" cases in which sensitivity to low intensity sounds is preserved but coding of high-intensity signals in continuous noise is impaired (Liberman et al., 2016). Cochlear synaptopathy has been proposed as a generator for DST as changes in central auditory gain may occur secondary to the peripheral damage (Knipper et al., 2013). Future developments in the assessment of cochlear synaptopathy may provide valuable insights into mechansims of DST and assist DST assessment and treatment.

Pure tone audiometry for patients reporting DST merits a few modifications to conventional diagnostic testing. Extending the frequency range of pure tone testing to include thresholds at 10 to 16 kHz may help to identify "hidden hearing loss" (Liberman et al., 2016). When patient DST symptoms are consistent with SCD, inclusion of 250 Hz air and bone conduction threshold measures with testing of bone conduction below 0 dB HL is necessary to identify possible changes in transmission of sound via bone conduction secondary to third window pathology (Ward et al., 2017). Finally, pure tone thresholds can be measured by using an ascending technique rather than a descending method, thereby minimizing patient discomfort.

Behavioral Measures of Loudness

A patient's loudness tolerance is derived by assessing the upper limit of the auditory system's dynamic range. Measurement of behavioral threshold of sensitivity is a well-agreed upon metric and one that has remained unquestioned and unchanged for decades. Threshold of sensitivity defines the lower limit of the patient's dynamic range, but as has been pointed out in a variety of investigations, audiometric thresholds do not necessarily correlate with the integrity of an individual's hearing pathway (Kujawa & Liberman, 2009; Myers et al., 2009). Paradoxically, the measure of loudness tolerance is not standardized, and its interpretation may be complicated by non-auditory factors such as patient psychological health. This said, loudness measurements may provide results that illuminate in more useful ways a patient's auditory status. For example, during the fitting of hearing aids in which loudness tolerance must be considered, a patient's reduced dynamic range is more substantially limited by DST than by elevated absolute thresholds alone.

The measure of loudness tolerance appears on the surface a straightforward proposition. A patient can be provided a list of descriptors, such as "soft," "loud but OK," or "uncomfortably loud" to describe a signal controlled by a clinician, researcher, or the patient. Alternatively, patients can employ a numerical scale, or some other form of categorization scheme that allows them to map their perceptual experiences to stimuli of various magnitudes and spectral composition. In either case, it is clear from dozens of studies that the ratings upon which a patient settles will be affected by, among other things, instructions (Hawkins, 1980), number of times the test was conducted, and/or training that was provided (Silverman, 1947; Sherlock & Formby, 2005), as well as concurrent drug use (Globus et al., 1978), presence of tinnitus, and history of traumatic brain injury (Fagelson, 2007; Myers et al., 2009). Despite thorough reviews of techniques and findings since Silverman's work was published, the labile nature of loudness measures continues to stymie the audiologist who seeks patient responses that are as easy to obtain, and as consistent over time, as the measures of threshold of sensitivity. Despite their imperfections, loudness tolerance measures remain important because loudness perception contributes to success of hearing aid fittings (Formby et al., 2017) and is an important consideration when managing tinnitus (Jastreboff & Jastreboff, 2000).

One of the more widely recognized techniques for establishing LDLs remains Cox et al.'s (1997) contour test of loudness perception. The contour test utilizes patient ratings of loudness similar to those employed previously by Hawkins (1980). The test employs sound presentations across a wide range of stimulus intensities and spectra and establishes loudness growth characteristics covering a patient's dynamic range. Formby et al. (2017) recently proposed streamlining this test as they determined signal levels corresponding to patients' ratings of "soft," "comfortable," and "loud, but OK" were most relevant to rehabilitation efforts. The authors stress that such patient ratings could substantially improve hearing aid fittings as uncomfortable loudness is a frequent patient complaint, particularly for first-time users. Such conclusions reinforce the notion that understanding a patient's loudness tolerance is at least as relevant to clinical practice as the measure of absolute threshold.

In addition to loudness measures and ratings, the reaction time of humans and animals to sounds of various levels illustrates the relation between signal strength and the response it evokes. Recently, Radziwon et al. (2017) reported that salicylate-induced hyperacusis decreased relative to controls in the response times in rats. Their work presented various doses of salicylate and assessed reaction times to tones of a wide range of frequencies. The authors reported that the influence of high doses of salicylate, 150 mg/kg or higher, shortened reaction times of the animals across all stimulus frequencies tested. The authors concluded that the drug-induced hyperacusis related to central mechanisms whose excitability was influenced by the drug across a wide range of stimuli.

Behavioral or psychoacoustic measures of loudness tolerance for pure tones and speech are commonly used by audiologists when fitting hearing aids. The threshold of pain for most people is typically reached when sound intensity reaches 120 dB SPL (Hood & Poole, 1966), whereas permanent hearing loss can arise following a single exposure to 140 dB SPL (Chandler, 2006). In a clinical setting, typical loudness tolerance is often found between 90 and 105 dB HL for pure tones presented via earphones.

LDLs are used in some tinnitus and hyperacusis centers (Aazh et al., 2016) as a method of identifying and quantifying DST. Unfortunately, the evidence for use of LDL in assessment of DST is lacking. Zaugg et al. (2016) found only weak correlations between patients' subjective report of DST and LDL for pure tones and speech in a Veteran population with co-morbid tinnitus. Meeus et al. (2010) found no correlation between audiological measurements and DST complaints in a cohort of ENT clinic patients using questionnaire scores. Jüris et al. (2013) did not find a consistent correlation between LDL and other DST measures although there was a correlation between the Hospital Anxiety and Depression Scale anxiety scale scores and LDLs. The utility of LDL measurements is further limited by test-retest variability across and within individuals (Stephens et al., 1977). It may be that speech or pure tones of varying frequencies presented in a test booth do not capture the complexity of sounds in the real world. At the same time, "real world" sound may be poorly tolerated because of characteristics other than intensity and frequency such as sound duration, rise time, or because of acoustical and situational contexts or memories associated with such sounds.

It is important to consider the patient perspective when performing LDL measurements. Individuals with DST are likely to find that entering a sound booth and submitting to listening to sounds that reach or approximate the point of discomfort is an extremely unpleasant or fearful experience. This experience can undermine clinical rapport and ensure that the patient considers the test suite an unsafe environment, thereby complicating future contact. Alternatively, patients may feel that measurement of LDLs validates their complaints. Given the potential for patient distress, the decision to perform loudness measures in assessment of DST should be a joint decision between the clinician and the patient.

Immittance

Acoustic reflex threshold testing can provide valuable diagnostic information during audiological assessment (see Musiek & Rintelmann, 1999 for full discussion of ART in diagnostic audiology). In cases when loss of the stapedial reflex is suspected such as with Bell's palsy, or when there is normal tympanometry in an ear with a conductive hearing loss such as with superior canal dehiscence, ARTs may provide insight into an underlying audiological mechanism of DST. For identifying or measuring DST, however, the rationale for inclusion of ART in assessment is limited. Changes in ART secondary to DST due to mechanisms other than dysfunction of the stapedial reflex have not been demonstrated as significantly altered in patients with DST (Anari et al., 1999). Inclusion of the ART test specifically for assessment of DST is not warranted and should be carefully considered and discussed with patients during routine audiological testing.

Otoacoustic Emissions

The utility of otoacoustic emissions in DST assessment has been previously proposed (Jastreboff & Jastreboff, 2000). Bartnik et al. (2008) compared input-output function of distortion product otoacoustic emissions (DPOAEs) of normal-hearing controls to those of subjects with tinnitus only, hyperacusis only, and both tinnitus and hyperacusis. Input-output functions only partially distinguished hearing disordered subjects from controls, and did not distinguish between the three hearing disordered groups.

A measure that more effectively distinguished subject groups was reported by Attias et al. (2005) following assessment of transient evoked otoacoustic emissions (TEOAE) in the presence of contralateral masking noise. The use of contralateral masking during OAE measurement targets auditory efferent activity that is known to have a suppressive effect on cochlear and associated neural activity (Berlin et al., 1993). The absence of such an effect could contribute to auditory complaints associated with loudness intolerance. Attias et al. compared patients with traumatic brain injury (TBI) histories and loudness tolerance issues to those with TBI but without loudness complaints, as well as to a group of normal controls. They reported 87% of the patients in the group with loudness intolerance lacked the typical suppression effect that was present in the patients who did not report the auditory problem. Amplitudes of TEOAEs across groups differed as well, which complicated interpretation of the findings; however, the authors concluded that dysfunction of the efferent, and putatively suppressive effect was at least partially responsible for the observed loudness tolerance issues expressed by the participants.

Questionnaires

Questionnaires can aid in identification of DST, measurement of DST severity, and provide a baseline measure for treatment efficacy, and are discussed in detail in Chapter 5. Of note, Khalfa et al. (2002) developed the Hyperacusis Questionnaire to identify individuals with DST. However, several studies have found lack of correlation between DST as identified through the Hyperacusis Questionnaire and LDL measurements (Aazh & Moore, 2017; Meeus et al., 2010; Aazh & Moore, in press). Sherlock and Formby (2017) developed the Sound Tolerance Interview and Questionnaire Instrument (STIQI) to qualify and quantify sound tolerance in individuals considering hearing aids. Although the STIQI had not yet been validated at the time of this writing, this assessment tool has the potential to measure the effects of treatment of DST and changes in sound tolerance that occur with hearing aid use and provides additional guidance for case history of DST. The reader is referred to Chapter 5, Scales and Questionnaires for DST, for further discussion of available instruments.

DST in Children

Coelho et al. (2007) reported that 43.5% (222/506) of children aged 5 to 12 years answered "yes" to the question, "Are you bothered by loud sounds?," although only a subset of children that answered "yes" (40 of 222) had LDLs below 90 dB HL in at least one test frequency in one ear. In a smaller sample of pediatric patients aged 7 to 18 years, Aazh and McFerran (personal communication) found the average LDL, measured at 0.25, 0.5, 1, 2, 4, and 8 kHz, was below 80 dB HL in at least one ear for 90.5% (19/21) of patients tested. Seventy-one percent of patients (17/24) had LDLs of 60 dB HL or less for at least one of the measured frequencies for at least one ear. LDLs of less than 60 dB HL were most frequently found at 8000 Hz. There was no correlation between LDLs and results from the Hyperacusis Questionnaire (HQ; Khalfa et al., 2002); however, the authors reported a significant correlation between the HADS questionnaire and the HQ. This latter finding demonstrated the potential that co-morbid mental health issues existed in children, as with adults, and that psychological evaluation should be considered when hyperacusis has been identified.

In practice, clinicians may opt out of LDL testing to preserve patient comfort and clinical rapport, and because LDLs may be of limited value in terms of management (see Chapter 14). As with adults, it is therefore important to engage the pediatric patient and his or her family in order to identify the sounds they find bothersome, when and under what circumstances DST began, what they experience when they hear offending sounds, and how DST may be limiting activities and influencing family dynamics. Indeed, in a problem-based approach to assessment, children are encouraged to recount their story and thoughts regarding DST, such as is described by Veronica Kennedy in Chapter 14. Younger children may have an easier time describing their experience by drawing a picture to illustrate how sounds affect them.

Finally, it is essential for the clinician to get a sense of whether there is any exaggeration of DST complaints that may result in secondary gain, such as absence from school, and whether the family understands the validity of DST complaints and can constructively support their child.

Future Developments in Audiological Assessment of DST

There is no unique clinical presentation of DST and no test or test battery that can adequately identify and quantify DST at present. Audiological assessment of DST will continue to develop as the components and mechanisms of DST are better understood and as a consensus on the ideal set of DST test instruments and definitions emerges. Currently identification of DST relies heavily on patient report and behavioral measures, with little in the way of audiological testing to confirm the presence of DST or its severity through objective measures. Measurement of DST using electrophysiological tests such as auditory brainstem response (ABR), middle latency response (MLR; Formby et al., 2017), as well as auditory steady-state response (ASSR; Ménard et al., 2008) has been proposed and may ultimately augment current clinical tools used to assess DST. Aron et al. (2015) reported changes in intra-subject tympanometric measurements that reflected voluntary engagement of the tensor tympani muscle and which could prove useful in identification of tonic tensor tympani syndrome. Establishing normative data in objective testing for subjects with DST should lead to more options for clinical assessment of DST in audiology.

Case Examples

Case Example 1

KL was a 62-year-old male who presented to a tinnitus and hyperacusis clinic with suicidal ideations, distressing tinnitus, and hearing loss. He summarized his experience of hearing loss and tinnitus as feeling "stuck in a bubble with air hissing into it through a hole and no way to escape." KL reported extreme irritability that was affecting relationships at work and at home, and said he was suffering financial distress as he was unable to work full-time due to excessive fatigue and difficulty with concentration. KL indicated that he tried hearing aids several years earlier but found that they aggravated his tinnitus; he returned the instruments to his dispenser at that time. Upon further questioning, he said he was aware that loud and especially high-frequency sounds contributed to his irritability but did not identify that he had lowered tolerance of sound per se. When asked about his mental health, KL revealed a significant history of anxiety and depression that had worsened with antidepressant medication in the past.

Pure tone audiometry revealed a moderate to severe high-frequency sensorineural hearing loss that was apparently long-standing and secondary to occupational noise exposure. LDLs were obtained bilaterally at 70 to 90 dB HL. Acoustic reflex testing was not attempted as the audiologist felt that the information would not add to the assessment and could exacerbate the patient's stated concerns.

KL's worsening of tinnitus with amplification suggested the presence of DST, confirmed by further questioning of the patient and LDL measurements. KL was fit with hearing instruments with amplification and built-in sound generator for tinnitus masking. Amplification was set initially below target gain to accommodate LDLs and eventually increased to optimal settings for speech understanding. KL also received informational counseling regarding DST, tinnitus, and hearing loss. KL chose to try mindfulness-based stress reduction to address emotional health but found quiet reading provided greater sense of relaxation once the tinnitus was manageable.

Seven months after his initial fitting, KL reported that sounds were now "crisp and wonderful" and that his "brain was finally able to relax" when using his hearing instruments. He was eventually able to resume full-time work and reported little tinnitus distress or reaction to the sounds that had bothered him previously. While tinnitus and hearing loss were KL's primary complaints, his case illustrates the value of inclusion of DST assessment with respect to the rehabilitative aims regarding flexibility in hearing aid fitting and related patient expectations.

Case Example 2

Patient DM was referred to a hospital-based tinnitus clinic for a group session for patients with tinnitus and DST. Her accompanying referral documents included an otolaryngology consult note, audiometry results, and a report from a community hearing instrument clinic. The otolaryngologist noted tinnitus and dizziness secondary to a head injury. Audiological assessment indicated essentially normal pure tone air- and bone-conduction thresholds for all measured frequencies. Acoustic immittance results (tympanometry, acoustic reflex thresholds) were reported as normal.

DM's primary complaints in the group session were DST, "ringing" tinnitus centered in her head, and dizziness since her head injury. She denied any difficulty hearing sound or pulsatile quality to her tinnitus, although she noted hearing her heart beat in the left ear. When asked about the effect sound had on her, she said loud sounds made her feel "off." Further probing revealed that she perceived her own voice (autophony) and footsteps as louder in the left ear.

DM was brought in for a full diagnostic audiogram, including bone conduction thresholds at 250 Hz and vestibular-evoked myogenic potential (VEMP) testing. Pure tone thresholds indicated a 15-dB air-bone gap for the left ear at 250 Hz with normal tympanometry and reflexes bilaterally. Vestibular testing indicated a subthreshold cervical VEMP response (65 dB nHL) on the left and an asymmetrical ocular VEMP (50% asymmetry ratio), with a higher amplitude response on the left. Video head-impulse test results revealed corrective saccades when the left anterior canal was assessed. A 512-Hz tuning fork placed on the left ankle bone (lateral malleolus) was reported by the patient as audible in the left ear. DM was referred back to ENT and a high-resolution temporal bone CT scan was ordered (Figures 2–1 and 2–2).

The radiology report confirmed a dehiscence of the right superior canal. DM's report illustrates the value of a comprehensive case history following complaints of DST, as such information gathering can support identification

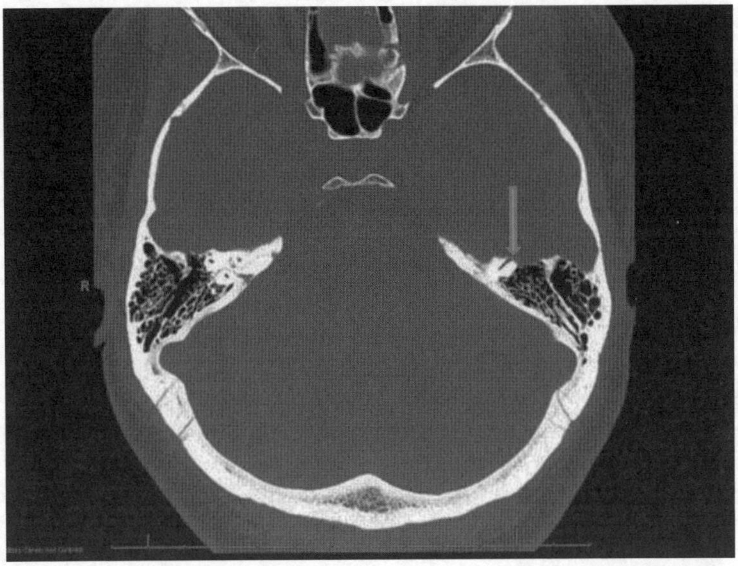

Figure 2–1. High resolution axial CT image showing left superior canal dehiscence of the anterior limb (arrow).

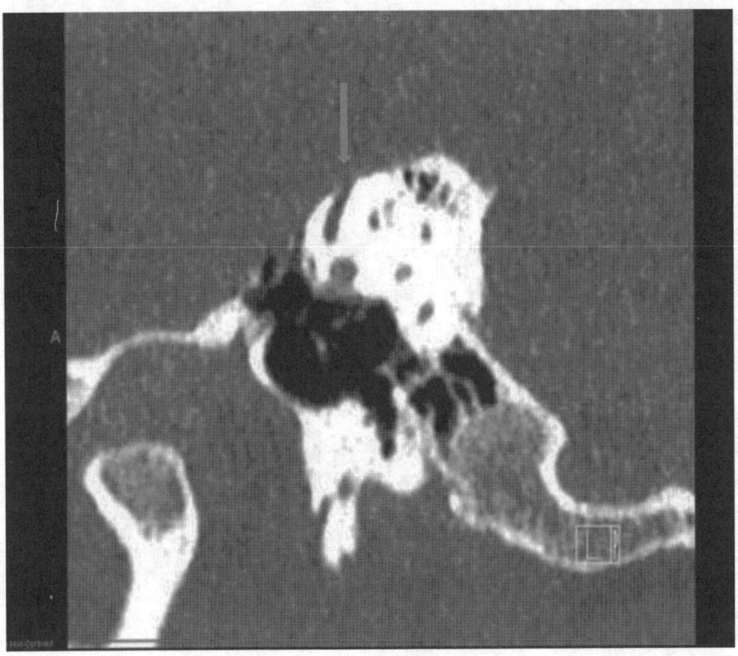

Figure 2–2. Oblique CT scan showing dehiscence of the left superior canal of the anterior limb/apex.

of superior canal dehiscence, with corresponding intervention considerations.

References

Aazh, H., & McFerran, D. (2017). Factors related to tinnitus and hyperacusis handicap in children and adolescents (personal communication).

Aazh, H., & Moore, B. C. J. (2017a). Thoughts about suicide and self-harm in patients with tinnitus and hyperacusis. *Journal of American Academy of Audiology, in press.*

Aazh, H., & Moore, B. C. J. (2017b). Incidence of discomfort during pure-tone audiometry and measurement of uncomfortable loudness levels among people seeking help for tinnitus and/or hyperacusis. *American Journal of Audiology, in press.*

Aazh, H., & Moore, B. C. J. (2017c). Usefulness of self-report questionnaires for psychological assessment of patients with tinnitus and hyperacusis and patients' views of the questionnaires. *International Journal of Audiology*, Mar 09, 1–10.

Aazh, H., Moore, B. C. J., Lammaing, K., & Cropley, M. (2016). Tinnitus and hyperacusis therapy in a UK National Health Service audiology department: Patients' evaluations of the effectiveness of treatments. *International Journal of Audiology, 55*(9), 514–522.

Aazh, H., & Allott. R. (2016). Cognitive behavioral therapy in management of DST: a narrative review and clinical implementation. *Auditory and Vestibular Research, 25*(2), 63–74.

Anari, M., Axelsson, A., Eliasson, A., & Magnusson, L. (1999). Hypersensitivity to sound: questionnaire data, audiometry and classification. *Scandinavian Audiology, 28*(4), 219–230.

Arlinger, S. (2003). Negative consequences of uncorrected hearing loss—a review. *International Journal of Audiology, 42*, 2 S17–2 S20.

Axelsson, A., & Hamernik, R. P. (1987). Acute acoustic trauma. *Acta Oto-laryngologica, 104*(3–4), 225–233.

Baguley, D. M., & Andersson, G. (2007). DST: Mechanisms. In *Diagnosis and therapies*, San Diego, CA: Plural.

Baguley, D., Andersson, G., McFerran, D., & McKenna, L. (2007). Hyperacusis. In *Tinnitus: A multidisciplinary approach* (2nd ed.) (pp. 133–147). London, UK: Whirr.

Bandura, A. (1986). *Social foundations of thought and action: A social cognitive theory*. Englewood Cliffs, NJ: Prentice-Hall, Inc.

Bartnik, G., Hawley, M., Rogowski, M., Raj-Koziak, D., Fabijanska, A., & Formby, C. (2008). Distortion product otoacoustic emission levels and input/output-growth functions in normal-hearing individuals with tinnitus and/or hyperacusis. *Otolaryngologia Polska (The Polish Otolaryngology), 63*(2), 171–181.

Berlin, C. I., Hood, L. J., Wen, H., Szabo, P., Cecola, R. P., Rigby, P., & Jackson, D. F. (1993). Contralteral suppression of nonlinear click-evoked otoacoustic emissions. *Hearing Research, 71*, 1–11.

Bernstein, R. E., Angell, K. L., & Dehle, C. M. (2013). A brief course of cognitive behavioural therapy for the treatment of misophonia: A case example. *The Cognitive Behaviour Therapist, 6*, e10.

British Tinnitus Association. Annual Tinnitus Research Review 2016. Available from www.tinnitus.org.uk/ATRR2016. (Accessed October 16, 2016.)

Canlon, B., Theorell, T., & Hasson, D. (2013). Associations between stress and hearing problems in humans. *Hearing Research, 295*, 9–15.

Ceranic, B. J., Prasher, D. K., Raglan, E., & Luxon, L. M. (1998). Tinnitus after head injury: Evidence from otoacoustic emissions. *Journal of Neurology, Neurosurgery & Psychiatry, 65*(4), 523–529.

Chandler, D. (2006). Blast-related ear injury in current U.S. military operations. *ASHA Leader, 11*, 9–29.

Coelho, C. B., Sanchez, T. G., Tyler, R. S. (2007). Hyperacusis, sound annoyance, and loudness hypersensitivity in children. *Progress in Brain Research*, 166, 169–178.

Edelstein, M., Brang, D., Rouw, R., & Ramachandran, V. S. (2013). Misophonia: Physiological investigations and case descriptions. *Childhood, 3*, 27.

Fackrell, K., Fearnley, C., Hoare, D. J., & Sereda, M. (2015). Hyperacusis questionnaire as a tool for measuring hypersensitivity to sound in a tinnitus research population. *BioMed Research International.*

Fagelson, M. A. (2007). The association between tinnitus and posttraumatic stress disorder. *American Journal of Audiology, (16),*107–117.

Flores, E. N., Duggan, A., Madathany, T., Hogan, A. K., Márquez, F. G., Kumar, G., . . . & García-Añoveros, J. (2015). A non-canonical pathway from cochlea to brain signals tissue-damaging noise. *Current Biology, 25*(5), 606–612.

Formby, C., Korczak, P., Sherlock, L. P., Hawley, M. L., & Gold, S. (2017). Auditory brainstem and middle latency responses measured pre-and posttreatment for hyperacusic hearing-impaired persons successfully treated to improve sound tolerance and to expand the dynamic range for loudness: Case evidence. *Semin. Hear., 38,* 71–93.

Formby, C., Payne, M. S., Yang, X., Wu, D., & Parton, J. M. (2017). Repeated measurement of absolute and relative judgments of loudness: Clinical relevance for prescriptive fitting of aided target gains for soft, comfortable, and loud, but OK sound levels. *Semin. Hear., 38,* 26–52.

Globus, G. G., Cohen, H. B., Kramer, J. C., Elliott, H. W., & Sharp, R. (1978). Effect of marijuana induced 'altered state of consciousness' on auditory perception. *Journal of Psychedelic Drugs, 10(1),* 71–76.

Hawkins, D. B. (1980). Loudness discomfort levels: A clinical procedure for hearing aid evaluations. *J. Speech Hear. Disord., 45(1),* 3–15.

Henry, J. A., Zaugg, T. L., Myers, P. J., & Schechter, M. A. (2008). Using therapeutic sound with progressive audiologic tinnitus management. *Trends in Amplification, 12(3),* 188–209.

Hood, J. D., & Poole, J. D. (1966). Tolerable limit of loudness: Its clinical and physiological significance. *J. Acoust. Soc. Am., 40,* 47–53.

http://www.hearingreview.com/2015/01/hearing-aid-sales-increase-4-8-2014-rics-continue-market-domination/.

http://www.hearingreview.com/2015/10/best-practices-best-results/

Jastreboff, P. J., & Jastreboff, M M. (2000). Tinnitus retraining therapy (TRT) as a method for treatment of tinnitus and hyperacusis patients. *J. Am. Acad. Audiology, 11(3),* 156–161.

Jastreboff, M. M., & Jastreboff, P. J. (2002). Decreased sound tolerance and tinnitus retraining therapy (TRT). *Australian and New Zealand Journal of Audiology, 24*(2), 74.

Jüris, L., Ekselius, L., Andersson, G., & Larsen, H. C. (2013). The Hyperacusis Questionnaire, loudness discomfort levels, and the Hospital Anxiety and Depression Scale: A cross-sectional study. *Hearing, Balance and Communication, 11(2),* 72–79.

Katzenell, U., & Segal, S. (2001). Hyperacusis: Review and clinical guidelines. *Otology & Neurotology, 22(3),* 321–327.

Khalfa, S., Dubal, S., Veuillet, E., Perez-Diaz, F., Jouvent, R., & Collet, L. (2002). Psychometric normalization of a hyperacusis questionnaire. *ORL; Journal for Oto-Rhino-Laryngology and Its Related Specialties, Nov–Dec, 64(6),* 436–442.

Kisnisci, R., Onder, E., & Tuz, H. (1999). Prevalence of otologic complaints in temporomandibular disorder patients. *International Journal of Oral and Maxillofacial Surgery, 28*:101–102.

Klochoff, I. (1978). The tensor tympani syndrome—a source of vertigo. *Abstracts, Barany Society Ordinary Meeting; Uppsala, Sweden,* 31–32.

Kochkin, S. & MarkeTrak, V. (2000). "Why my hearing aids are in the drawer": The consumers' perspective. *The Hearing Journal, 53(2),* 34–36.

Kochkin, S. (2002). Consumers rate improvements sought in hearing instruments. *Hearing Review, 9(11),* 18–22.

Kreuzer, P. M., Landgrebe, M., Schecklmann, M., Staudinger, S., & Langguth, B. (2012). Trauma-associated tinnitus: Audiological, demographic and clinical characteristics; The TRI Database Study Group. *PLoS One, 7*(9), e45599. Retrieved from www.plosone.org.

Liu, C., Glowatzki, E., & Fuchs, P. (2015). Unmyelinated type II afferent neurons report cochlear damage. *Proceedings of the National Academy of Sciences USA, 112(47),* 14723–14727. doi: 10.1073/pnas.1515228112.

Martin, A., Rief, W., Klaiberg, A., & Braehler, E. (2006). Validity of the brief patient health questionnaire mood scale (PHQ-9) in the general population. *General Hospital Psychiatry, 28*(1), 71–77.

McCormack, A., & Fortnum, H. (2013). Why do people fitted with hearing aids not wear them? *International Journal of Audiology, 52(5),* 360–368.

McFerran, D. J., & Baguley, D. M. (2007). Acoustic shock. *The Journal of Laryngology & Otology, 121*(04), 301–305.

Meeus, O. M., Spaepen, M., Ridder, D. D., & Heyning, P. H. V. D. (2010). Correlation between hyperacusis measurements in daily ENT practice. *International Journal of Audiology, 49(1)*, 7–13.

Ménard, M., GallÈgo, S., Berger-Vachon, C., Collet, L., & Thai-Van, H. (2008). Relationship between loudness growth function and auditory steady-state response in normal-hearing subjects. *Hearing Research, 235*(1), 105–113.

Mueller, G. H., & Bentler, R. A. (2005). Fitting hearing aids using clinical measures of loudness discomfort levels: An evidence-based review of effectiveness. *Journal of the American Academy of Audiology, 16(7)*, 461–472.

Musiek, F. E., & Rintelmann, W. F. (1999). *Contemporary perspectives in hearing assessment.* Needham Heights, MA: Allyn & Bacon.

Radziwon K., Holfoth, D., Lindner, J., Kaier-Green, Z., Bowler, R., Urban, M., Salvi, R. (2017). Salicylate-induced hyperacusis in rats: Dose- and frequency-dependent effects. *Hearing Research, 350*(1), 133–138. doi: 10.1016/j.heares.2017.04.004. Epub 2017 Apr 27.

Sahley, T. L., & Nodar, R. H. (2001). A biochemical model of peripheral tinnitus. *Hearing Research, 152*(1), 43–54.

Schecklmann, M., Landgrebe, M., Langguth, B., & TRI Database Study Group. (2014). Phenotypic characteristics of DST in tinnitus. *PLoS One, 9(1)*, e86944.

Searchfield, G. D. (2015). Hearing aids for tinnitus. In *Tinnitus: Clinical and research perspectives.* San Diego, CA: Plural.

Sheldrake, J., Diehl, P. U., & Schaette, R. (2015). Audiometric characteristics of hyperacusis patients. *Frontiers in Neurology, 6*, 105.

Sherlock, L. P., & Formby, C. (2005). Estimates of loudness, loudness discomfort, and auditory dynamic range: Normative estimates, comparison of procedures, and test-retest reliability. *J. Am. Acad. Audiol., 16(2)*, 85–100.

Sherlock, L. P., & Formby, C. (2017). Considerations in the development of a sound tolerance interview and questionnaire instrument. *Seminars in Hearing, 38(01)*, 53–70.

Silverman, S. R. (1947). Tolerance for pure tones and speech in normal and defective hearing. *Ann. Otol. Rhinol. Laryngol., 56(3)*, 658–677.

Spitzer, R. L., Kroenke, K., Williams, J. B., & Löwe, B. (2006). A brief measure for assessing generalized anxiety disorder: The GAD-7. *Archives of Internal Medicine, 166(10)*, 1092–1097.

Stephens, S. D. G. (1970). Personality and the slope of loudness function. *The Quarterly Journal of Experimental Psychology, 22(1)*, 9–13.

Stephens, S. D. G., Blegvad, B., & Krogh, H. J. (1977). The value of some suprathreshold auditory measures. *Scandinavian Audiology, 6(4)*, 213–221.

Tyler, R. S., Pienkowski, M., Roncancio, E. R., Jun, H. J., Brozoski, T., Dauman, N., & Martin, N. (2014). A review of DST and future directions: Part I. Definitions and manifestations. *American Journal of Audiology, 23(4)*, 402–419.

Ward, B. K., Carey, J. P., & Minor, L. B. (2017). Superior canal dehiscence syndrome: Lessons from the first 20 years. *Frontiers in Neurology, 8*, 177.

Westcott, M., Sanchez, T. G., Diges, I., Saba, C., Dineen, R., McNeill, C., Chiam, A., O'Keefe, M., & Sharples, T. (2013). Tonic tensor tympani syndrome in tinnitus and DST patients: A multi-clinic prevalence study. *Noise and Health, 15(63)*, 117.

Zaugg, T. L., Thielman, E. J., Griest, S., & Henry, J. A. (2016). Subjective reports of trouble tolerating sound in daily life versus loudness discomfort levels. *American Journal of Audiology*, 1–5.

Zigmond, A. S. & Snaith, R. P. (1983). The hospital anxiety and depression scale. *Acta Psychiatr. Scand., 67(6)*, 361–370.

3

The Epidemiology and Natural History of Disorders of Loudness Perception

David M. Baguley

Introduction

For any clinical condition, reliable data about the prevalence, incidence, and natural history of the disorder is invaluable, both for caring for the individual patient, for a wide and deep understanding of the condition, and for public health planning and commissioning of clinical services. Unfortunately, our knowledge in this regard is incomplete for each of the subtypes of the disorders of loudness perception defined in Chapter 1 (Tyler et al., 2014), and this is a major shortcoming as scientists and clinicians try to understand the lived and shared experience of people with sound tolerance challenges. In this chapter we will delineate the present state of knowledge, and indicate where there are opportunities for focused and highly relevant research in this regard. The specific issue of how hyperacusis and tinnitus are associated is discussed in detail in Chapter 11.

Recruitment

As described in Chapter 2, loudness recruitment is a cochlear phenomenon, associated with outer hair cell (OHC) dysfunction (Smeds & Leijon, 2011). The prevalence of recruitment has not been formally determined, but it is reasonable to expect that it will be in tandem with that of cochlear hearing loss, although it is apparent that not all individuals with this condition also experience loudness similarly. The reasons why some individuals have abnormal loudness growth, whereas others with similar audiograms do not, are obscure. The natural history of recruitment has also not been formally determined, although it is reasonable to expect that as cochlear hearing loss progresses with age, the loudness perception dysfunction, particularly the patient's observation regarding the inability to hear sounds in the hearing loss region as "soft" (Buus & Florentine, 2002) would progress also. While recruitment does vary with the sound environment (e.g., the intensity of sound being heard), it does not vary with emotion or mood: in some cases this can be useful to disambiguate the contribution of recruitment from that of hyperacusis (which can be modulated by mood state) in an individual patient.

Hyperacusis in Adults

There have been a small number of epidemiological studies of hyperacusis in the adult population, generally using a random postal questionnaire methodology. One issue with such research is that response rates are generally rather low, and as a result the findings may overestimate the prevalence of hyperacusis, as human nature dictates that a person is more likely to complete a questionnaire on a symptom or condition of which they have some experience.

Two conference reports were the first to raise the issue. The first was from Sweden, where Rubinstein and colleagues (1996) undertook a postal study which sought to identify the prevalence and associations between hyperacusis, headaches, temporomandibular disorders, and amalgam fillings. Data from 1023 female respondents was reported, indicating a point prevalence of 23%, but unfortunately information in the conference proceedings about the definition of hyperacusis, and the response rate of the study, are both so scant that this study is only of note as the first in the area.

In Poland, Fabijanska and colleagues (1996) undertook a postal questionnaire on hyperacusis, again with an unspecified index question. There were 10,349 respondents, of whom 15.2% reported hyperacusis, with a slightly higher prevalence in females. Interestingly, some regional differences were reported, though no supporting information shed light on the cultural or socioeconomic variations that may have led to that.

The first study on the epidemiology of hyperacusis published in the peer-review literature originated in Sweden, and for many years the work of Andersson et al. (2002) was definitive in this area. They used the following definition of hyperacusis (translation in Baguley and Andersson, 2007):

> *In our society we are surrounded by sounds of many kinds. Some of these sounds can be annoying or even unpleasant in character. We all differ in how vulnerable we are to these sounds. In this survey we study sensitivity to everyday sounds in the sense that they evoke adverse reactions. By this we mean, for example, reactions to a conversation, chirping of birds, paper noises (rustle), the ringing sound at a pedestrian crossing, or the sounds of a running water tap. In other words, we ask about sounds of moderate loudness that most people experience daily without being annoyed. Our interest in this is not restricted to loud sounds such as drilling machines or low flying aircraft.*

The methodology was twofold. The first strategy was to recruit respondents through the website of a major and reputable Swedish newspaper, where readers were invited to click through to the survey via a banner on the front page. The Swedish population were early adopters of the Internet, even in 2002, and uptake was equitable across class and gender (Andersson, personal communication). While 1167 people clicked on the web banner, only 595 responded; thus, the response rate was 52%, although many more people may have seen the banner and been uninterested. The second arm was a postal survey in Uppsala, Sweden, where 987 people were mailed the questionnaire pack, and 589 responded (60%). With the aim of sampling hyperacusis rather than recruitment, the authors excluded anyone self-identifying as hearing impaired from the analysis. A point prevalence rate of 7.7% was determined for the Internet group, and 5.9% in the postal survey. Of the individuals with hyperacusis, in the Internet group 51% were female, and in the postal group, 55% were female, indicating a slight preponderance.

Of interest was the fact that Gerhard Andersson and colleagues reported both the types of sound the respondents found aversive, and the reactions that were reported, both of these being chosen from provided lists. These are detailed in Tables 3–1 and 3–2, respectively.

While ostensibly a study about hyperacusis, a number of reflections can be made. The list of annoying sounds did not include eating or breathing sounds, but potentially the category of "other everyday sounds" included these, and thus could represent misophonia. Also, most reactions were irritation, distraction, and annoyance, which also map more onto a modern conception of misophonia than hyperacusis.

Table 3–1. Ranking of sounds considered aversive in Andersson et al. (2002). The question was "What kind of sounds do you consider aversive?" and the number of respondents 1151.

	n	%
Noise	660	57
Mechanical, monotonous sounds	326	28
Music	309	27
Other everyday sounds	274	24
Clatter	171	15
Paper noises	55	5
Talk	39	3

Source: Adapted from Baguley and Andersson (2007).

Table 3–2. Reactions to sounds from Andersson et al. (2002). The question was "How do you feel when you are being exposed to disturbing sounds?", again with 1157 respondents.

	n	%
Irritated	862	75
Poor concentration	479	41
Angry	141	12
Tense	199	10
Pain	57	5
Afraid	16	1

Source: Adapted from Baguley and Andersson (2007).

The fact that a number of respondents, albeit small, reported sound-induced pain was also of interest. This was higher in those self-reporting reduced sound tolerance than those who did not (12.5% vs. 4.5%, respectively), and the sound-induced pain and/or fear reports may represent what would now be classified as hyperacusis. As suggested in Chapter 1, such patients likely endured symptoms associated with more than one of the Tyler et al. (2014) categories, as sounds could induce pain in the short term, and a durable sensation of fear over time.

Another postal questionnaire study from Scandinavia, this time from Finland, included a question about hyperacusis in a wider consideration of self-reported hearing problems in older adults (Hannula et al., 2011). A cohort of adults were sampled (n = 1428, aged 54 to 66 years, respondents n = 850, response rate 59.5%). Participant selection was said to be random, but the report indicated that the individuals were also participating in a large multicenter trial of hearing impairment, and had undergone otoscopy and audiometry as part of that. Four questions were asked in the survey, and that pertaining to sound tolerance was presented as follows:

> *Are you particularly sensitive to loud sounds?*

A total of 146 individuals responded *yes* (17.1%), but this data was of limited value as the question was rather nonspecific, and would capture individuals with recruitment as well as hyperacusis. Of these individuals, 102 (70%) were female.

In a study with the main focus on hyperacusis, Paulin et al. (2016) reported data from a cohort of adult individuals who were ongoing participants in the Vasterbotten Environmental Health Study in Sweden. Of the 8520 people (aged 18 to 79 years) contacted by post, 3406 agreed to participate (40.0%), and were asked the following questions:

> *Have you been diagnosed with sound intolerance by a physician?*
>
> *Do you have a hard time tolerating everyday sounds that you believe most other people can tolerate?*

As with other studies reviewed above, it is difficult to rule out the possibility that the sound tolerance question might also capture persons with recruitment. Of the cohort, 66 (1.9%) identified as having been diagnosed by a physician, and 313 (9.2%) self-identified with reduced sound tolerance: this latter group also included all the people that responded "yes" to the physician question. The physician-diagnosed group was found to be older, to have more frequent problems and for longer duration, and a slightly longer history than the self-identified group although no statistical analysis was undertaken. There was a statistically significant preponderance of women over men in both the physician-diagnosed and self-identified groups (66% and 70% female, respectively).

Given the generally low response rate, and the motivational issue regarding nonresponse by people with no experience of reduced sound tolerance, a skeptical view would be to recalculate prevalence rates with the assumption that nonresponse equates to no sound tolerance problems, and this is undertaken in Table 3–3.

Once undertaken, this reanalysis brings the estimates closer in line with previous clinician-based estimates of 2 to 3% of the adult population having troublesome hyperacusis (Jastreboff, 2000; Baguley & Andersson, 2007).

One further reflection on the population studies described above is the possible implication that patients experience reduced sound tolerance along a continuum. Many adults appear to experience aversion or intolerance to some sounds, at least at some times, and troublesome hyperacusis may then be an extreme and persistent form of that.

Until recently, little attention has been paid to hearing thresholds in patients with hyperacusis. Anari et al. (1999) noted that pure tone audiograms "show normal hearing or a slightly high tone loss," and Hannula and colleagues (2011) found that while patients with hyperacusis had statistically significantly worse hearing than controls, the hyperacusis was not associated with increased hearing handicap, unlike tinnitus, or self-reported problems with hearing in noise. A study with the audiometric characteristics of patients with hyperacusis as its main focus was a welcome addition to the literature (Sheldrake et al., 2015). Audiometric findings, both pure tone audiometry (PTA) and loudness discomfort level (LDL) in a series of 381 patients (170 female – 45%, and 211 male – 55%) with a primary complaint of hyperacusis were retrospectively analyzed. The mean age was 43.9 years (s.d. 15.0). The clinic at which they were seen was in the U.K. independent sector; therefore, they were self-pay, or had private insurance; in the United Kingdom,

Table 3–3. Prevalence rates recalculated on the assumption that non-response equates to no sound tolerance problems.

Authors (year)	Method	Response Rate	Reported Prevalence Rate	Recalculated Prevalence Rate
Andersson et al. (2002)	Internet cohort	52%	7.7%	4.0%
	Postal cohort	60%	5.9%	3.5%
Hannula et al. (2011)	Postal cohort	60%	17.1%	10.3%
Paulin et al. (2016)	Postal cohort	40%		
	Physician diagnosed		1.9%	0.76%
	Self-identified		9.2%	3.68%

this might bias the results as the patients might have been more severely affected than a more general hyperacusis population. Pure tone audiometry was undertaken up to 8 kHz, using standard techniques, and LDLs performed using pure tones of 0.5 sec duration, increasing intensity in increments of 5 dB, and the patient indicating verbally when they wished not to be presented with the next sound. The authors found that patients presented normal hearing thresholds (i.e., =<20dB HL) at low frequencies with mild hearing loss (specified as 20 to 40 dB HL) at 4 to 8 kHz; no comparison was made with age-matched normative audiometric data. The LDL data was compared with a normative data set from Sherlock and Formby (2005), and group data indicated that the hyperacusis patients had lower LDLs (e.g., reduced dynamic range) on the order of 15 dB: this effect was noted across the frequency range. Some anomalies in individual LDL patterns were noted: an unspecified but small number of patients had LDL measurements at 30 dB HL, whereas others did not reach an LDL at the upper limit of the audiometer. This may call the diagnostic reliability of LDL into question, a situation covered in more detail in Chapter 2. The conclusions that can be drawn from this study, which was by far and away the largest series of hyperacusis patients reported upon, included the finding that cochlear hearing loss was not required to develop hyperacusis, distinguishing it from recruitment, and that reduced dynamic range in hyperacusis occurred across the frequency range.

In the introduction to this chapter it was proposed that knowledge about the natural history of a symptom or condition is important for the effective counseling and treatment of the patient. Unfortunately, this information was not available for hyperacusis, and no longitudinal studies have been published. While one of the population surveys described above did collect information about length of history (Paulin et al., 2016), that information only pertained to those individuals in whom sound tolerance issues persisted, and participants were not asked, "Did you have reduced sensitivity to sound that has now resolved?" Andersson et al. (2002) did reflect on a longitudinal study of a cohort of tinnitus patients in whom the incidence of "sensitivity to noise" increased from 38% to 85% over a 5-year period. There are opportunities for robust longitudinal studies of the natural history of hyperacusis.

Hyperacusis in Childhood

As is the case with adults, data regarding the epidemiology of hyperacusis in childhood is sparse, and characterized by major differences in definitions, populations studied, and hence in the magnitude of prevalence estimates. An attempt at systematic review was made by Nemholt Rosing et al. (2016), and while the team identified three relevant articles (Coeho et al., 2007; Landalv et al., 2013; Widen & Erlandsson, 2004), they reluctantly concluded that the heterogeneity of the literature was so high that it was not feasible to pool the studies.

In a study of self-reported tinnitus and "noise sensitivity" among adolescents (13 to 19 years) in Sweden, Widen and Erlandsson (2004) included the question, "Do you consider yourself to be oversensitive to noise?" in their questionnaire. Of the 1547 young people to whom it was issued, data from 1238 individuals (77.8%) was complete and was analyzed. Of this cohort, it was reported that 17.1% answered the noise sensitivity question positively, and of these, 4.0% indicated they had both noise sensitivity and tinnitus; this group was also more likely to worry about their hearing, and to use hearing protection. The young people were stratified into two groups (13 to 15 and 16 to 19 years) on the basis of schooling, and the older group was reported to be more likely to experience noise sensitivity.

The same noise sensitivity question was used by another Swedish research group (Landalv et al., 2013) who reported data from 281 youths aged 15 to 19 years. A modification was that the participants were asked to rank the frequency of this experience, as never (0% of the time), seldom (<25% of the time), relatively often (about 50% of the time), often (>50% of the time), or always (100% of the time). Of the participants, 39.2% reported noise sensitivity 50% of the time or more. The authors considered 50% or more as the point of clinical significance, although they acknowledged that they sampled the frequency of the experience rather than severity.

The Avon Longitudinal Study of Parents and Children (ALSPAC) (Golding et al., 2001) is a large prospective study based in the Bristol district of the United Kingdom. More than 14,000 pregnant women were recruited in 1991/1992, and the health and socioeconomic status of the children and mothers has been sampled regularly since that time. Audiological aspects of the children were studied at age 11, and this included questions on hyperacusis and tinnitus (reported in Hall et al., 2016 and Humphriss et al., 2016, respectively). The relevant questions used were: "Do you ever experience over-sensitivity or distress to particular sounds?" and "Do you ever get noises in your ears? (not associated with noise exposure)" (Humphriss et al., 2016). Of the 7097 children that were sampled, 7092 answered the question about sound tolerance, and 261 reported that they were oversensitive to sound. Of these, 157 were male, and 104 were female. This group was also asked about behavioral avoidance of activities or places due to over-sensitivity to sound, and 112 young people (42.9%) responded affirmatively; 21 (8.0%) used hearing protection for some sounds. The possibility of sensitivity to other sensory stimuli was also investigated, the most common being to light/colors (n = 22, 8.4% of those with hyperacusis), touch (n = 17, 6.5%), and smell (n = 14, 5.4%). Information was available on the presence or absence of tinnitus in 260 of the 261 young people with hyperacusis, and a strong association was reported with 109 (41.9%) of the individuals with hyperacusis also experiencing tinnitus.

No association was found between hyperacusis and birth weight, housing status (rented or owned), or social class, but there were associations identified with being male, an admission to hospital within the first four weeks of life (but not admission to a Special Care Baby Unit in the neonatal period), and, surprisingly, a higher level of maternal education. Regarding otologic/audiologic status, the children with hyperacusis were not more likely to have had a history of otitis media with effusion, or elevated stapedial reflex thresholds, and no significant associations were found with hearing thresholds on PTA. An interesting association was found with larger otoacoustic emission amplitudes to low-intensity stimuli, but not to higher-intensity stimuli. Unfortunately, data was not available on diagnoses of autistic spectrum disorder (see Chapter 7). The authors noted that the associations with hyperacusis that were identified raised as many questions as answers, but also that the lack of a link with otitis media with effusion ran counter to some previous reports (Sun et al., 2011).

With the aim of researching both childhood tinnitus and hyperacusis, Coelho et al. (2007) reported data from a cohort of 506 children (240 female – 47.4%, 266 male – 52.6%) with a mean age of 9.46 years (SD 2.1). The presence of hyperacusis was sought using the question "Are you bothered by any kind of sound or noise?", and that of phonophobia by "Are you afraid of sounds?" Hyperacusis was identified in 16 of the children (3.2%), and phonophobia in 47 (9.3%); phonophobia was reported to be present in 5 (1.2%) of the children with hyperacusis. Of the 16 children with hyperacusis, 8 (50%) experienced tinnitus, but no mention was made of severity; of the 490 children without hyperacusis, 96 (19.6%) experienced tinnitus. Having a mild hearing loss in the left ear was associated with an elevated risk of hyperacusis.

Hyperacusis was mentioned tangentially in a study by Basjo et al. (2016), which focused on the listening habits in 9-year-old children, and the association with hearing thresholds and tinnitus. While 21 of the 411 children (5.3%) reported tinnitus, hyperacusis (not defined) was said to be present in only one child (0.2%), although it was not clear if issues with sound tolerance were formally sought.

Regarding the incidence of hyperacusis in childhood, two studies are of note. In a survey of clinical practice regarding childhood tinnitus, Baguley et al. (2012) reported data from 4 expert centers in Europe. Of the 88 children that had been referred to these centers in a calendar year, data on the presence of hyperacusis was available in 87, and in these cases hyperacusis was present in 34 (39%), but no other information was collected. In a study from Southern Denmark, Nemholt-Rosing (2016) reported data from 15 ENT clinics over a 5-year period regarding children and adolescents referred for care for tinnitus and/or hyperacusis. In that period 69 children were referred, and of those 9 (12.8%) had a primary complaint of hyperacusis, and a total of 11 cases (15.7%) experienced both tinnitus and hyperacusis, leaving 58 (84.3%) cases with tinnitus alone.

To the author's knowledge there are no studies that have described the natural history of hyperacusis in childhood. Whether the onset is abrupt or insidious, the nature of the relation with tinnitus (see Chapter 11), and the progression over time, all remain obscure. As with the situation regarding adult hyperacusis, the opportunities for research abound.

Misophonia

Given the relatively recent consideration of misophonia as a discrete clinical entity, it is not a surprise that there is a paucity of published data on the epidemiology and natural history. The experience of misophonia is usually associated with a specific sound (eating or sniffing, for example) (McFerran, 2016), and it has been suggested that there are three characteristic elements (Jastreboff & Jastreboff, 2014; Rouw et al., 2017):

- Disproportional aversive responses to the trigger
- Awareness that this response is disproportionate
- No clear physical feature (such as loudness of the sound) to explain the response

Minimal prevalence data is available. Wu et al. (2014) studied misophonic experiences in a group on university undergraduates. The report was that nearly 20% had experiences of misophonia, which is several orders of magnitude higher than that which is seen in psychiatry or audiology clinics. The popular press in the United Kingdom have raised concerns that some reports or apparent experiences of misophonia may be examples of misanthropic behavior (Figure 3–1). This does not honor the extreme distress and aversion some clinical patients with misophonia experience. As with hyperacusis, if there exists a continuum of such experiences, with clinical misophonia at the extreme end, then patient complaints must be analyzed carefully and given the benefit of the doubt; the possibility must be considered that a dismissive view from society or professionals could exacerbate unnecessarily the patient's suffering.

Some data is becoming available about the natural history of clinical misophonia. Rouw and Erfanian (2017) report data from a group of 300 self-identified people with misophonia, who responded online to their enquiries. While by definition, such persons may be at the extreme end of such experiences, and their natural history has not been one of a reversion to non-misophonia, the fact that the experience of the majority of this group (n = 232, 77%) was one of a worsening over time of their symptoms is of note. It was also noted that the most common age of onset was in childhood or early adolescence, as has been noted elsewhere (McFerran, 2016), and that participants spanned the age range, with broadly equal impact of symptoms across ages.

Following the identification of a family with 15 members who were misophonic, Sanchez et al. (2017) raised the possibility that there might be an inherited component. However, in the study by Rouw et al. (2017), only a minority of participants had another family member with similar symptoms (n = 67, 22%) so familial inheritance may not be responsible for the usual pattern.

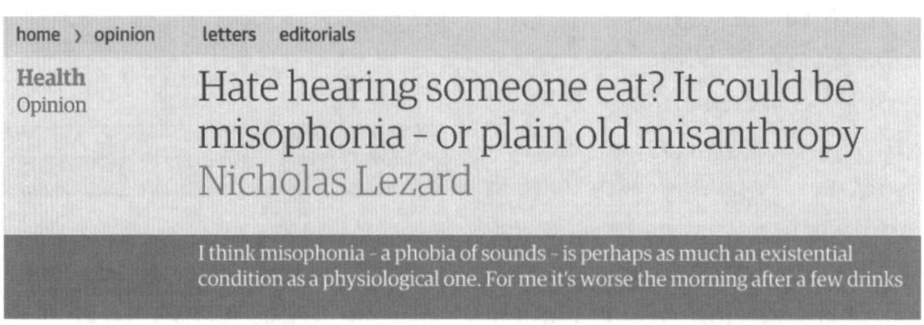
home › opinion letters editorials

Health
Opinion

Hate hearing someone eat? It could be misophonia - or plain old misanthropy
Nicholas Lezard

I think misophonia - a phobia of sounds - is perhaps as much an existential condition as a physiological one. For me it's worse the morning after a few drinks

Figure 3–1. From the U.K. Guardian newspaper, August 18, 2017. https://www.theguardian.com/commentisfree/2017/aug/18/hate-hearing-person-eat-sound-misophonia-misanthropy.

While information about misophonia is emerging, there is also evidence that opinions on some aspects are polarized. Examples are whether this is a primary psychiatric disorder, or an auditory dysfunction (see Cavanna & Seri, 2015, for discussion), and also whether the characteristic emotional state is annoyance/irritation (Rouw & Erfanian, 2017; Kumar & Griffiths, 2017), or anger/rage (Schröder et al., 2017). This is a literature to be watched with interest.

Summary

Data regarding the epidemiology and natural history of disorders of sound tolerance is sparse, and opportunities for research are plentiful. As will be discussed elsewhere (Chapter 16), one major constraint is the lack of available research funding in this area, which is certainly worthy of urgent clinical and scientific research.

References

Anari, M., Axelsson, A., Eliasson, A., & Magnusson, L. (1999). Hypersensitivity to sound–questionnaire data, audiometry and classification. *Scand. Audiol.*, *28(4)*, 219–230.

Andersson, G., Lindvall, N., Hursti, T., & Carlbring, P. (2002). Hypersensitivity to sound (hyperacusis): A prevalence study conducted via the Internet and post. *Intl. J. Audiol.*, *41(8)*, 545–554.

Baguley, D. M., & Andersson, G. (2007). *Hyperacusis: Mechanisms, diagnosis, and therapies*. San Diego, CA: Plural.

Baguley, D. M., Bartnik, G., Kleinjung, T., Savastano, M., & Hough, E. A. (2013). Troublesome tinnitus in childhood and adolescence: Data from expert centres. *Intl. J. Pediatr. Otorhinolaryngol.*, *Feb*, *77(2)*, 248–251. doi: 10.1016/j.ijporl.2012.11.009.

Båsjö, S., Möller, C., Widén, S., Jutengren, G., & Kähäri, K. (2016). Hearing thresholds, tinnitus, and headphone listening habits in nine-year-old children. *Intl. J. Audiol.*, *Oct*, *55(10)*, 587–596. doi: 10.1080/14992027.2016.1190871.

Buus, S., & Florentine, M. (2002). Growth of loudness in listeners with cochlear hearing losses: recruitment reconsidered. *J. Assoc. Res. Otolaryngol.*, *3*, 120–139. DOI: 10.1007/s1016200 10084.

Cavanna, A. E., & Seri, S. (2015). Misophonia: Current perspectives. *Neuropsychiatr. Dis. Treat.*, *18(11)*, 2117–2123. doi: 10.2147/NDT.S81438.

Coelho, C., Sanchez, T. G., & Tyler, R. S. (2007). Hyperacusis, sound annoyance, and loudness hypersensitivity in children. *Progress in Brain Research*, *166*, 168–178.

Degeest, S., Corthals, P., Dhooge, I., & Keppler, H. (2016). The impact of tinnitus characteristics and associated variables on tinnitus-related handicap. *J. Laryngol. Otol.*, *130(1)*, 25–31.

Fabijanska, A., Rogowski, M., Bartnik, G., & Skarzynski, H. (1999). Epidemiology of tinnitus and hyperacusis in Poland. In *Proceedings of the sixth international seminar* (pp. 569–571). J. W. P. Hazell (Ed.). London, U.K.: Tinnitus and Hyperacusis Centre.

Golding, J., Pembrey, M., & Jones, R. (2001). ALSPAC Study Team (ALSPAC): The Avon longitudinal study of parents and children. I. Study methodology. *Paediatr. Perinat. Epidemiol.*, *15*, 74–87.

Hall, A. J., Humphriss, R., Baguley, D. M., Parker, M., & Steer, C. D. (2016). Prevalence and risk factors for reduced sound tolerance (hyperacusis) in children. *Int. J. Audiology*, *55(3)*, 135–141.

Hannula, S., Bloigu, R., Majamaa, K., Sorri, M., & Maki-Torkko, E. (2011). Self-reported hearing problems among older adults: Prevalence and comparison to measured hearing impairment. *J. Am. Acad. Audiol.*, *22 (8)*, 550–559.

Humphriss, R., Hall, A. J., & Baguley, D. M. (2016). Prevalence and characteristics of spontaneous tinnitus in 11-year-old children. *Int. J. Audiol.*, *55(3)*, 142–148. doi: 10.3109/14992027.2015.1120890.

Jastreboff, P. J. (2000). Tinnitus habituation therapy (THT) and tinnitus retraining therapy (TRT).

In Tyler, R. S. (Ed.). *Tinnitus handbook* (pp. 357–376). San Diego, CA: Singular.

Jastreboff, P., & Jastreboff, M. (2014). Treatments for decreased sound tolerance (hyperacusis and misophonia). *Sem. in Hear., 35(02),* 105–120.

Kumar, S., & Griffiths, T. D. (2017). Response: Commentary: The brain basis for misophonia. *Front. Behav. Neurosci., 29(11),* 127. doi: 10.3389/fnbeh.2017.00127.

Landälv, D. L., Malmström, L., & Widén, S. E. (2013). Adolescents' reported hearing symptoms and attitudes toward loud music. *Noise Health, 15(66),* 347–354. doi: 10.4103/1463-1741.116584.

McFerran, D. J. (2016). In Baguley, D. M., & Fagelson, M. (Eds.). *Tinnitus: clinical and research perspectives.* San Diego, CA: Plural.

Nemholt-Rosing, S., Hvass Schmidt, J., Wedderkopp, N., & Baguley, D. M. (2016). Prevalence of tinnitus and hyperacusis in children and adolescents: A systematic review. *BMJ Open, 6,* 1–20.

Paulin, J., Andersson, L., & Nordin, S. (2016). Characteristics of hyperacusis in the general population. *Noise & Health, 18(3),* 178–184.

Rosing, S. N., Kapandais, A., Schmidt, J. H., & Baguley, D. M. (2016). Demographic data, referral patterns and interventions used for children and adolescents with tinnitus and hyperacusis in Denmark. *Int. J. Pediatr. Otorhinolaryngol., Oct, 89,* 112–120. doi: 10.1016/j.ijporl.2016.07.036.

Rouw, R., & Erfanian, M. (2017). A large-scale study of misophonia. *J. Clin. Psychol.,* epub ahead of print.

Rubinstein, B., Ahlqwist, M., & Bengtsson, C. (1996). Hyperacusis, headache, temporomandibular disorder and amalgam fillings—an epidemiological study. In Reich, G. E., & Vernon, J. A. (Eds.). *Proceedings of the fifth international tinnitus seminar* (pp. 657–658). Portland: American Tinnitus Association.

Sanchez, T. G., & Silva, F. E. D. (2017). Familial misophonia or selective sound sensitivity syndrome: Evidence for autosomal dominant inheritance? *Braz. J. Otorhinolaryngol., pii: S1808–8694(17),* 30114–30113. doi: 10.1016/j.bjorl.2017.06.014. [Epub ahead of print]

Schröder, A., van Wingen, G., Vulink, N. C., & Denys, D. (2017). Commentary: the brain basis for misophonia. *Front. Behav. Neurosci., Jun 2, 11,* 111. doi:10.3389/fnbeh.2017.00111.

Sheldrake, J., Diehl, P. U., & Schaette, R. (2015). Audiometric characteristics of hyperacusis patients. *Front. Neurol., May 15, 6,* 105. doi: 10.3389/fneur.2015.00105.

Sherlock, L. P., & Formby, C. (2005). Estimates of loudness, loudness discomfort, and the auditory dynamic range: Normative estimates, comparison of procedures, and test-retest reliability. *J. Am. Acad. Audiol., 16(2),* 85–100.

Smeds, K., & Leijon, A. (2014). Loudness and hearing loss. In Florentine, M., Popper, A. N., & Fay, R. R. (Eds.). *Loudness* (pp. 223–259). New York, NY: Springer.

Sun, W., Manohar, S., Jayaram, A., Kumaraguru, A., Fu, Q., Li, J., & Allman, B. (2011). Early age conductive hearing loss causes audiogenic seizure and hyperacusis behavior. *Hear Res., Dec, 282(1–2),* 178–183. doi: 10.1016/j.heares.2011.08.004.

Tyler, R. S., Pienkowski, M., Roncancio, E. R., Jun, H. J., Brozoski, T., Dauman, N., Dauman, N., Andersson, G., Keiner, A. J., Cacace, A. T., Martin, N., & Moore, B. C. (2014). A review of hyperacusis and future directions: part I. Definitions and manifestations. *Am. J. Aud., 23(4),* 402–419.

Widén, S. E., & Erlandsson, S. I. (2004). Self-reported tinnitus and noise sensitivity among adolescents in Sweden. *Noise Health; Oct–Dec, 7(25),* 29–40.

Wu, M. S., Lewin, A. B., Murphy, T. K., & Storch, E. A. (2104). Misophonia: Incidence, phenomenology, and clinical correlates in an undergraduate student sample. *J. Clin. Psychol., 70(10),* 994–1007.

4

Scales and Questionnaires for Decreased Sound Tolerance

Kathryn Fackrell and Derek J. Hoare

Introduction

Reliable measurement of decreased sound tolerance (DST) problems, including hyperacusis and misophonia, is important to both determining the nature and severity of the problem, and to the evaluation of any treatment-related change. For assessment of these conditions, clinicians and researchers rely on audiometric measures of DST (e.g., uncomfortable loudness levels [ULLs], most comfortable listening levels [MCLs], loudness scaling), and/or patient self-reported measurement tools (i.e., questionnaires).

Audiometric Measures of Decreased Sound Tolerance

Measurements of ULLs have long been used by hearing health professionals (Liu & Chen, 2000) and an evidence-based recommended procedure for the measurement of ULLs is provided by the British Society of Audiology (2011). This document describes the objective of ULL measurement as being to "identify the minimum level of sound that is judged to be uncomfortably loud by the subject." It refers also to the term loudness discomfort level (LDL) as being used synonymously with ULL but expressly recommends ULL as the preferred term.

The ULL is effectively an absolute judgment often used by clinicians, for example, as a threshold for sound tolerance when deriving information for limiting hearing aid output (Morgan, Dirks, Bower, & Kamm, 1979). In a standard clinical set-up, ULLs are estimated using an audiometer and measured in both ears at 500, 1000, 2000, and 4000 Hz. Sound stimuli are presented with a duration of about 1000 msec, and an inter-stimulus interval of about 400 msec. Patients are instructed to either press a handheld response button or to inform the investigator by other means (i.e., hand raise or verbal acknowledgment) when the signal level becomes uncomfortable.

In determining their clinical value, Stephens, Blegvad, and Krogh (1977) examined the reliability of various audiometric measures including ULLs in a sample of 10 adults with normal hearing. They found a high level of variance in ULLs both within and between subjects, although within subject variance was smaller, and similar to that observed for an objective measure (the acoustic reflex threshold) in the same participants. For 5 of their 10 participants, ULLs for low frequency sound (250 Hz) exceeded the output limit of the audiometer.

Sherlock and Formby (2005) conducted a series of experiments to estimate normative values for absolute and relative judgments of ULLs, and to evaluate the reliability of within- and between-subject variability in a test-retest situation in a group of 59 younger adults (21 males, 38 females) with normal hearing and without sound tolerance problems. The resulting estimated normative value of the ULL was about 100 dB HL and was deemed sufficiently reproducible for the authors to conclude that a simple ULL estimate of loudness discomfort would be a valid clinical measure of the "threshold of discomfort" for sound. More recently, however, Sheldrake, Diehl, and Schaette (2015) measured hearing thresholds and ULLs in 381 patients with hyperacusis and mild high-frequency hearing loss or normal hearing thresholds. They found ULLs to be significantly decreased compared to a normal-hearing reference group, at an average of 85 dB HL across frequencies. Using receiver operating characteristic (ROC) analysis they showed that ULL measurements were not sufficiently sensitive or specific for them to be considered a conclusive test for hyperacusis. Interestingly, ULLs tended to be higher at hearing loss frequencies suggesting that hyperacusis was unlikely to be triggered by increased hearing threshold. Rather, they concluded that hyperacusis might be due to a general increase in auditory gain.

Goldstein and Shulman (1996) examined correlations between tinnitus, hyperacusis complaint, and ULLs in 42 consecutive patients with a primary complaint of severely disabling tinnitus, providing a methodology for hyperacusis assessment and severity classification. They recommended performing (1) pure tone audiometry, Feldmann masking curves and the Metz test for recruitment, and (2) ULL measurement at frequencies from 250 to 8000 Hz, and at a frequency matched to tinnitus confirmed over three trials. For diagnosis, they recommended that ULLs of 90 dB HL or less at two or more frequencies, or a dynamic range (the difference between thresholds of audibility and ULLs) of 55 dB or less at any frequency should be taken as indicative of hyperacusis. Conversely, hyperacusis was not evinced if ULLs were 95 dB HL or greater at all frequencies and if the dynamic range was 60 dB or greater at all frequencies. How measurements might be interpreted using the classification system proposed by Goldstein and Shulman (1996) is summarized in Table 4–1.

It is important to say here that unless ULLs are performed with care, exposing an individual who suffers from hyperacusis or tinnitus to sounds at or close to an intensity that evokes pain or discomfort can be unpleasant. When this is the case, there is a risk that the therapeutic relationship between patient and clinician is undermined by using the procedure. In general, clinicians are advised to proceed with great caution when performing ULLs.

ULLs are affected by various factors including the choice of stimulus (Beattie & Boyd, 1986; Walker, Dillon, Byrne, & Christen, 1984), the instruction given to the patient (Beattie, Svihovec, Carmen, & Kunkel, 1980; Borstein & Musiek, 1993; Hawkins, Walden, Montgomery, & Prosek, 1987), and the psychophysical method used (Hawkins, 1980; Morgan, Wilson, & Dirks, 1972).

Anari, Axelsson, Eliasson, and Magnusson (1999) compared ULLs for pure tone and real-life sounds in 100 consecutive patients complaining of severe oversensitivity to envi-

Table 4–1. Interpretation severity of sound tolerance problems.

Problem Level	Loudness Discomfort Level	Dynamic Range
Severe hyperacusis	≤60 dB (at least 2 frequencies)	≤35 dB (at least one frequency)
Moderate hyperacusis	Up to 75 dB (at least 2 frequencies)	Up to 45 dB (at least one frequency)
Mild hyperacusis	Up to 90 dB (at least 2 frequencies)	Up to 55 dB (at least one frequency)
No problem	≥95 dB (at all frequencies)	≥60 dB (at all frequencies)

Source: Adapted from Goldstein & Shulman, 1996.

ronmental sounds. ULLs for pure tones were tested at 500, 1000, 2000, 3000, and 4000 Hz. Tone pulses were started at 50 dB or 30 dB above hearing threshold, and raised in 5 dB steps until the patient reported discomfort. The authors then measured ULLs for everyday sounds such as a baby crying, a dog barking, a bird singing, and speech-weighted noise. Meaningful comparison of the different stimuli was achieved by measuring long-term sound spectra and short-term levels in narrow bands with center frequencies from 250 to 8000 Hz. They found that, far from being a consistent measure, ULLs of pure tones varied between patients from extreme hypersensitivity (ULLs between 35 and 45 dB HL) to apparently normal ULLs sometimes exceeding 110 dB HL at all frequencies. ULLs for the everyday sounds were generally lower and not directly relatable to the ULLs for pure tones. Interestingly, there was a clear relation between the ULLs for everyday sounds and those sounds to which patients self-reported as being most (baby crying) and least (dog barking) sensitive.

In an earlier study, Filion and Margolis (1992) tried to determine whether clinical-derived ULLs were valid predictors of subjective impressions of uncomfortable loudness in real-life environments. Groups of individuals who socialized or worked in noisy environments were recruited directly from being in those environments, underwent ULL testing, and completed a multi-item questionnaire. The questionnaire involved participants rating the percentage of time in the environment they recalled the noise level being of a particular comfort level, using a 9-point scale from "very soft" to "painfully loud." Their results indicated large discrepancies in measures from which they concluded that ULLs may not accurately predict a patient's impression of uncomfortable loudness. They concluded the procedure may not provide a reliable basis for setting the sound level of hearing aids, for example.

Bornstein and Musiek (1993) measured ULLs for a 12-speaker babble in 20 participants with normal hearing sensitivity using two different sets of participant instructions and a simple up/down adaptive procedure. In one set of instructions, participants were asked to identify a loudness level at which they would choose "not to listen for any period of time." In the second set of instructions, participants were asked to identify a loudness level at which they "would choose not to listen for 15 minutes or longer." Data were collected on four occasions over 13 weeks. The difference in results was striking; ULLs generated using the "not to listen for any period of time" were 9 dB higher than those using the "not to listen for 15 minutes or longer" instruction. There was also a clear difference in the reliability of ULLs; for the "not to listen for any period of time" repeated measure correlations ranged from 0.90 to 0.97, but for the criterion "not to listen for 15 minutes or longer" correlations ranged from 0.62 to 0.89. This study clearly demonstrated that ULLs could be reproducible, particularly at levels approximating the upper limit of the dynamic range, and it highlighted the importance of knowing the impact of instruction on both the estimate and reliability. Johnson (1999) also reiterated the importance of consistent testing and instructions. In addition to consistent use of the wording described by Bornstein and Musiek (1993), Johnson recommended a slow ascending approach to measuring ULLs to avoid exceeding tolerance levels, and to use 1-dB or 2-dB steps when there was an indication of severe hyperacusis, for example, if the patient often wore earplugs or went to great lengths to avoid noise exposure.

Another audiometric measure of sound tolerance is the "most comfortable listening level (MCL)." This was defined as "the level at which the listener would set the stimulus were he obliged to listen to it for a long time" (Stephens et al., 1977, p. 213). As with ULLs, various instruction sets have been used in estimating MCLs. Variants of MCL tests have included the use of semantic or nonsemantic (unintelligible) speech signals or pure tone stimuli. For example, Brännström et al. (2014) described testing for MCLs using nonsemantic signals in a group of 32 normal hearing adults. In their procedure, participants were instructed to first listen to a speech signal presented diotically through headphones at 48 dB SPL. The participants then adjusted the sound level to their MCL using an up-and-down procedure. Participants were required to adjust the loudness of the signal by first increasing it until they judged the signal to be too loud, and then decreasing the signal level until they judged it to be too soft, ultimately increasing and decreasing the loudness until an MCL level was selected. Brännström et al. (2014) found a highly significant order effect, in that the first MCL estimate was significantly different from the estimates derived from repeated measures, an outcome attributed to procedural learning effects. Other studies found MCL estimates to be reproducible over time regardless of the specific methodology used (Kopra & Blosser, 1967), or to have a trend toward increasing over time (Sammeth, Birman, & Hecox, 1989). Others have observed MCL estimates to be affected by variables such as age (Coren, 1994), hearing loss (Kamm, Dirks, & Mickey, 1978), and phonological working memory (Brännström et al., 2014).

A third audiometric method sometimes used to estimate DST is loudness scaling. Loudness scaling methods involve either magnitude estimation or category rating (Hellman & Meiselman, 1990; Elberling & Nielsen, 1993). In magnitude estimation, participants listen to sound stimuli of different intensity levels and provide loudness ratings using a scale typically ranging from 0 to 100 in response, from which a ratio scale can be derived. This method is associated with logarithmic response bias; for example, it is typically found that a patient rating of loudness doubling corresponds to a 10 dB increase in level, which is a value that does not correspond to a doubling (or 3 dB increase) in signal intensity. In contrast, category rating involves participants producing responses to stimuli that are based on what is presumed to be units that more closely represent linear intervals, thus avoiding logarithmic response bias. The relative validity of these two methods is long-debated with published loudness scaling data obtained with various procedures, and from participants with normal hearing or hearing loss, producing both substantially different or remarkably similar estimates (Elberling, 1999).

Questionnaires

Health-related questionnaires that are clinically useful should ideally (1) provide thorough assessment of the relevant presenting symptoms of the construct (i.e., decreased sound tolerance), (2) provide reliable characterization and quantification of individual differences in terms of the perceived severity, and/or (3) have the capacity to responsively estimate changes in health status pre- and post-intervention to provide evidence for clinical efficacy of interventions. To have confidence that a given questionnaire is performing as anticipated, it is essential to critically evaluate its ability to fulfill these requirements, and to ask whether there is sufficient evidence that the questionnaire is fit for its intended purpose (i.e., diagnosing decreased sound tolerance in clinic or measuring changes in a clinical trial) as well as to determine its appropriateness for use in the intended population (Terwee et al., 2007). Just because a questionnaire has been found to be a reliable measure in one population does not necessarily mean that the same questionnaire will be reliable for use with a different population. Outlined in Table 4–2 are four validation topics with 10 quality criteria proposed by Terwee et al. (2007) as essential in questionnaire validation. These quality criteria should be assessed to ensure the integrity of study findings and clinical interpretations for a given population.

Given that decreased sound tolerance is associated with physiological, behavioral, cognitive, and emotional complaints (Baguley & Andersson, 2008; Tyler et al., 2014; Pienkowski et al., 2014), clinical questionnaires should provide a means of measuring these complaints. When effective, questionnaires may yield a single severity value that identifies varying levels of problems with avoidance of social situations, fear, anxiety, and annoyance across patients. Questions addressing similar symptoms can also form subscales, with separate and statistically independent scores that help clinicians and researchers identify specific areas of concern and target interventions accordingly. That said, only a few questionnaires have been developed that specifically quantify decreased sound tolerance, and for those in use, the evidence of appropriately established psychometric properties that would ensure instrument validity and generalizability is limited. Here we review some commonly used questionnaires and others that are less cited or in development.

Hyperacusis Questionnaire (HQ)

The Hyperacusis Questionnaire (HQ) was developed in France by Khalfa et al. (2002). Its primary function is to quantify and characterize hypersensitivity to sound, but it has also been used as an outcome measure of changes in sound tolerance (e.g., Jüris, Andersson, Larsen, & Ekselius, 2014; Mertens, Bodt, & Van de Heyning, 2016). The HQ was developed as a two-part questionnaire. The first part consists of binary questions collecting general information on noise exposure history and auditory disorders. These questions are not scored. The second part of the HQ consists of 14 negatively worded items. For each item, individuals indicate their level of agreement by rating one of four response options on a 4-point Likert scale: "no" (0 points), "yes, a little" (1 point), "yes, quite a lot" (2 points), and "yes, a lot" (3 points). The mean global score reflects the sum of all responses with a maximum possible score of 42, and a global score of >28 indicative of significant hyperacusis.

The development procedure of the HQ is not fully documented. Khalfa et al. (2002) based the questionnaire's construct on dimensions of behavioral and adaptive consequences of offending noise, as well as cognitive and emotional aspects of aversive listening experiences as reported in the literature. No information was provided on how the items were derived from this information and the authors did not conduct item reduction. From initial conception, the HQ appears to have consisted exclusively of 14 items and three binary questions.

Examination of questionnaire structure is recommended during development to establish the degree of variance explained by the interrelationships between the set of observed variables. Exploratory factor analysis is used to determine the structure without postulating a theoretical structure. In their exploratory factor analysis, Khalfa et al. (2002) identified three factors (subscales) for the HQ; attentional, social, and emotional, with most factor loadings above 0.4. However, taken together these

Table 4–2. Quality criteria for evaluating questionnaires.

Property	Technique	Quality Criteria
Validity	Content validity	The items in the questionnaires are a correct and comprehensive reflection of the populations/constructs that the questionnaires are intended to measure.
	Structure validity	The items in the questionnaire adequately reflect the underlying unidimensional construct (e.g., sensitivity to sound) or multidimensional construct (i.e., composite measures) being measured. Explaining at least 50% of the variance and factor loadings >0.4. Factor analysis conducted on adequate sample size ≥100.
	Construct validity	The scores demonstrate expected correlations between similar measures (convergent validity) and expected differences between unrelated measures (discriminant validity) and these hypotheses should be defined *a priori.* Convergent — *r* — Discriminant Excellent — ≥ 0.60 — Inadequate Acceptable — 0.30–0.59 — Acceptable Inadequate — ≤ 0.30 — Excellent
Reliability	Internal consistency	The hyperacusis and misophonia questionnaires and any subscales assess different constructs, and all the items in a questionnaire or subscale measure the same construct. Internal consistency is poor if alpha is very low (indicates items in a subscale are not measuring the same construct) or very high (indicates some items in the subscale are redundant).

Table 4–2. *(continued)*

Property	Technique	Quality Criteria
	Reliability	People with hyperacusis and misophonia respectively can be distinguished from each other, despite measurement errors (relative measurement error).
	Agreement	Each of the respective hyperacusis and misophonia questionnaire scores for individuals tested on multiple occasions over a short time period (1 to 2 weeks) are close to each other (absolute measurement error).
Responsiveness	Responsive	The hyperacusis and misophonia questionnaires are able to detect clinically important change over time.
	Floor and ceiling effects	Few respondents (≤15%) achieve the lowest or highest possible score so that the hyperacusis and misophonia questionnaires do not compromise responsiveness, nor content validity and reliability.
Interpretation	Interpretability	It is possible to assign qualitative meanings to subgroups of scores providing a grading system, and to identify what change represents a minimal clinically important change for the patient group.

factors only accounted for 48% of the overall variance in the data; the unexplained variance implied measurement error associated with this structure (Terwee et al., 2007). There was also some cross loading of items in the social factor with the other two factors. Altogether, this set of findings called into question the independence of the subscales and validity of the proposed HQ structure.

An additional issue with the HQ relates to its initial validation in a general population, and not a population who reported decreased sound tolerance. In fact, the HQ has never been validated on a population whose primary complaint was decreased sound tolerance. Although Khalfa et al. (2002) were not explicit about the target population for the HQ, items that have been included could be confounding when presented to a tinnitus population. Item 1, for instance, asks, "Do you ever use earplugs or earmuffs to reduce your noise perception?" and while in a general population this might assess an attentional component of those with decreased sound tolerance, for a tinnitus population using ear protection in normal sound environments it is not encouraged, and so this item would not likely be endorsed. Fackrell, Fearnley, Hoare, and Sereda (2015) examined the validity and reliability of the HQ in a population of 264 adult research participants who had tinnitus. They found the HQ to have high internal consistency (Cronbach's alpha = 0.88) but Confirmatory Factor Analysis (which tests predefined questionnaire structure) showed that the originally proposed three-factor, and an alternative one-factor structure, were poor fits to the data. As a measurement tool the questionnaire did not perform well in this population. Four problematic items, including item 1 mentioned above, were identified and removed from the questionnaire. When an exploratory factor analysis was then performed on the remaining 10 items, a two-factor (attentional and social) structure emerged that provided a reasonably good fit. The authors concluded that this modified version of the questionnaire could reliably measure decreased sound tolerance in a tinnitus population; however, this analysis would need to be confirmed in a new study. Incidentally, Fackrell et al. (2015) also provided evidence of acceptable convergent and discriminant validity. Weak to moderate correlations ($r <$ 0.4) were observed between the (14 item) HQ and Tinnitus Handicap Questionnaire (THQ; Kuk, Tyler, Russell, & Jordan, 1990), the Beck Anxiety Inventory (BAI; Beck, Epstein, Brown, & Steer, 1988), and the Beck Depression Inventory (BDI; Beck, Steer, & Brown, 1996), suggesting the HQ measured a reasonably distinct construct. Furthermore, correlations > 0.5 were reported between the HQ and ULLs implying some commonality in what the two procedures measured. These correlations should be re-examined if and when the proposed 10-item HQ for tinnitus patients is tested.

In another interesting study, Wallén, Hasson, Theorell, and Canlon (2012) examined the validity of the HQ in patients with emotional exhaustion, comparing HQ scores with ULLs and different categories of emotional exhaustion derived from the emotional exhaustion-subscale of the Maslach burnout inventory general survey (MBI-GS; Maslach, Jackson, & Leiter, 1996). This study included 348 participants (140 men, 208 women) with low, intermediate, and high levels of emotional exhaustion, of which just four individuals (1.1%) were hyperacusic according to their HQ score (>28). The authors' exploratory factor analysis yielded three factors from the HQ that were reflective of those reported by Khalfa et al. (2002). However, in this case, the three factors accounted for 57.6% of the variance, and therefore less measurement error, despite most items loading onto one factor. Internal consistency was acceptable for both subscale and total scores (Cronbach's alpha = 0.65 to 0.86). HQ scores and ULLs were weakly correlated in those subjects with intermediate and high levels of emotional exhaustion ($r < 0.3$), but there was little to no correlation in those with low emotional exhaustion ($r < 0.1$). The authors concluded the need for clinicians to be vigilant to factors such as emotional exhaustion (e.g., due to long-term stress) when using the HQ.

The HQ has now been translated into several languages including Egyptian, Italian, and Japanese, and undergone further testing. Shabana, Selim, El Refaie, El Dessouky, and Soliman (2011) reported an assessment using the (3-factor) Egyptian version of the HQ in a population of 60 adults (aged 19 to 45) with and without tinnitus who complained of decreased sound tolerance, and a control group without complaint. The sample was not sufficient to perform factor analysis, but data were explored descriptively with some interesting observations. For example, it was noted that the emotional domain score was significantly higher in female patients, and the attentional domain score was significantly higher in males, and that scores on the social domain were highly correlated with age. Formal validation studies are indicated.

In validating the Italian version of the HQ, Fioretti et al. (2015) recruited 117 patients with tinnitus (64 male, 53 female, aged 14 to 88) and subjected them to a test battery including ULLs. They found the questionnaire to have high internal consistency (Cronbach's alpha = 0.89) and strong correlations between HQ scores and ULLs, once again indicating communality between constructs being measured. However, no predictions on expected correlations were made *a priori*. ROC analysis identified a cut-off score of just 16 points on the HQ as indicative of significant hyperacusis. This was in startling contrast to the score of 28 initially proposed and generally referred to. The original cut-off score of 28 was also questioned by Meeus, Spaepen, De Ridder, and Van de Heyning (2010), who found that most patients reporting lower tolerance for noise scored <28 on the HQ. There is a risk, therefore, of underestimating the presence of significant hyperacusis if the HQ is relied upon clinically.

Most recently, Oishi et al. (2017) examined the validity of a Japanese version of the HQ in a sample of 112 patients with a complaint of hyperacusis, and 103 patients with hearing loss and/or tinnitus but without hyperacusis. The groups were similar in age (average of 59.1 and 63.4 years, respectively). Overall internal consistency of the HQ was high (Cronbach's alpha = 0.92). Patients complaining of hyperacusis scored higher on the questionnaire (average = 11.8 points) compared to the other group (average = 5.7 points). Within the hyperacusis group, those who reported hyperacusis as their primary complaint scored higher (average = 18.1 points) than those for whom hyperacusis was no more or less a problem than tinnitus or hearing loss (average = 9.9 points). The authors concluded that a cut-off score of 16 was essential in selecting which individuals with hyperacusis require treatment.

Multiple-Activity Scale for Hyperacusis (MASH)

The Multiple-Activity Scale for Hyperacusis (MASH) was developed in France by Dauman and Bouscau-Faure (2005). It was designed to (1) account for diverse situations that can be hindered by noise discomfort, (2) separate noise annoyance from noise-induced deterioration of speech understanding, and (3) quantify the severity of hyperacusis over time (Dauman & Bouscau-Faure, 2005). It is a clinician-led questionnaire describing 15 activities, including "driving a car," "pottering about," and "other." Patients provide a score from 0 to 10 to indicate their level of annoyance relative to that activity. The questionnaire allows for irrelevant items to be deleted, for example, if a person is simply not interested in live music events, and does not attend them, then that item would not have to be scored. Cinema and TV activities are grouped within the questionnaire with one score representing both; if a patient scores the two activities differently, then the highest individual score is taken as the score for both. A mean MASH score is calculated by dividing the total score by the number of activities, giving a possible range of 0 to 10.

The development procedure of the MASH is not documented. No information was provided on how or why the activities were chosen or the number of items that could be deleted and still have a valid overall score. Dauman and Bouscau-Faure (2005) reported acceptable convergent validity with strong correlations between the mean MASH scores and scores on an overall annoyance 10-point Likert scale in a tinnitus population. Correspondingly, Meeus et al. (2010) also found that MASH scores strongly correlated with HQ scores in a tinnitus population; indicating that similar underlying constructs were being measured. However, Meeus et al. (2010) found that MASH scores showed similar correlations with the Tinnitus Questionnaire (TQ; Hallam, Jakes, & Hinchcliffe, 1988; Hiller & Goebel, 1992) scores. Therefore, the common construct may be one of annoyance as opposed to some hyperacusis-specific construct. Furthermore, given that patients can delete items, the underlying structure needs to be further examined. It would be interesting to determine whether all the items were related to an underlying construct of annoyance and whether this relation changed depending on the number of items. Patient-generated measures, such as the MASH, on which patients can choose to add or delete items (activities in this case), are believed to be more relevant and meaningful to patients. However, although appealing for individual assessment, they are liable to cloud comparisons across individuals as the composite scores would be difficult to interpret. It is unlikely to be a suitable measure of effect of treatment in a clinical trial, for example (Patel, Veenstra, & Patrick, 2003).

German Questionnaire on Hypersensitivity to Sound (Geräuschüberempfindlichkeit: GÜF)

The German Questionnaire on Hypersensitivity to Sound (GÜF) is a 27-item questionnaire developed by Nelting, Reinhoff, Hesse, and Lam (2002) who described its purpose as providing a brief tool to inform treatment needs (identify urgency) and treatment planning. It was developed by a team in Germany which included physicians, psychologists, and therapists. Based on clinical experience and what patients had reported within group therapy sessions, the team generated an initial set of 85 items that was later distilled to 27 items the team considered representative of the behaviors of interest, for example, "because of sensitivity to sound I am nervous and irritable." The possible responses to each item were "not true," "sometimes true," "often," or "always true," scored 0 to 3, respectively, with greater total scores indicating a bigger problem. The initial validation work involved 226 patients (94 female, 132 male, aged 15 to 76) who complained of both hyperacusis and tinnitus. The study team used principal components analysis and identified a three-factor solution explaining 50.6% of the variance in the data. The factors were named cognitive responses to the hyperacusis, actional/somatic behavior, and emotional response to external noise source. Based on results of the factor analysis and internal consistency analysis, the number of items was again reduced to the final 15 items included in the questionnaire, to yield a total score of 0–45. Initial validation of the GÜF showed evidence of high internal consistency, good reliability within the factors, and acceptable convergent validity with a strong correlation (r = 0.8) between the GÜF and therapeutic expert assessment of hyperacusis (Nelting et al., 2002). However, the authors also reported strong correlations between the GÜF and the TQ, in particular with the TQ hearing problem subscale indicating that the GÜF was potentially measuring aspects of tinnitus-related hearing problems.

Bläsing, Goebel, Flötzinger, Berthold, and Kröner-Herwig (2010) further validated the GÜF in a sample of 91 inpatients (55 males, 36 females, aged between 15 and 76 years) who also had both tinnitus and hyperacusis. They found the questionnaire to have good internal consistency (Cronbach's alpha = 0.92), and while their explorative principal components factor analysis produced a three-factor solution to their data, the factors did not concur with the factor structure identified by Netling et al. (2002).

The GÜF has been translated into Spanish (Test Hypersensitivity to Sound; THS; Herráiz, de los Santos, Diges, Díez, & Aparicio, 2006) and its use examined in a study involving 40 patients (age range = 27 to 68) referred to clinic because of hyperacusis. Thirty-six of those participants also had tinnitus. Face validity of the questionnaire was assessed; 97% of participants rated it as simple, clear, and easy to understand. Internal consistency was high (Cronbach's alpha = 0.90). The team found that higher THS scores correlated with higher self-rating of severity of hyperacusis. Based on this small sample they concluded that the THS could be reliably used in clinical practice to measure the impact of hyperacusis on a patient's quality of life. Further work is required to evaluate the factor structure and responsiveness to change in patient complaint of this version of the questionnaire.

An English translation of the GÜF is also available (Noise Avoidance Questionnaire: NAQ; Bläsing & Kroener-Herwig, 2012); however, this version has not been subject to validation studies and has not yet been used in the clinics or research.

Sound Sensitive Tinnitus Index

The Sound Sensitive Tinnitus Index (SSTI; Greenberg, Walsh, & Carlos, 2016) is a questionnaire specifically developed to measure sound tolerance in patients with tinnitus. As sound tolerance problems are often co-morbid with tinnitus, this is a welcome addition to the clinician toolkit. The SSTI is a 33-item questionnaire developed using items identified through literature review, including items from the HQ and MASH. The first validation study of the SSTI was conducted online and involved 277 adults with tinnitus from 32 different countries (primarily the United States). For inclusion participants had to report that loud sounds at least sometimes exacerbated tinnitus. Further detail on the questionnaire has yet to be published and analysis of this data is ongoing; both will be important additions to the literature.

Misophonia Questionnaire

The Misophonia Questionnaire (MQ) was developed by Wu, Lewin, Murphy, and Storch (2014). Questionnaire items were derived from a search of research literature, reviewed by psychologists and psychiatrists with clinical experience related to misophonia, and checked for clarity and readability by two patients with misophonia in an outpatient clinic for obsessive compulsive disorder. A preliminary psychometrics evaluation was then conducted on a general population of 483 undergraduate students (79 males: 404 females, mean age 21.4 years). Using exploratory factor analysis, a three-factor solution was determined and used to define 3 MQ subscales. The "Misophonia Symptom Scale" included items that specify sound sensitivities (e.g., dislike of eating or tapping sounds). The "Misophonia Emotions and Behaviors Scale" measured emotional and behavioral reactions to misophonia symptoms (e.g., leaving the environment where a particular sound was heard). Items in both these scales were rated on a 0 (not at all true) to 4 (always true) scale, and summed to give a total score from 0 to 68. The third subscale, the "Misophonia Severity Scale," was an adaptation of the National Institute of Mental Health Global Obsessive-Compulsive Scale (NIMH GOCS; Murphy, Pickar, & Alterman, 1982). On this scale patients rated their sound sensitivity on a 15-point scale ("minimal" to "very severe") with a score of 7 indicating sound sensitivities that caused a substantial problem. Internal consistency of the three subscales was adequate (α = 0.86, 0.86, and 0.89, respectively). The MQ total score showed moderate convergent validity; correlation with the Adult Sensory Questionnaire (ASQ; Kinnealey & Oliver, 2002) sound sensitivity question was moderate ($r = 0.05$). Discriminant validity was high; correlation between the MQ total score and the ASQ visual, olfactory, and tactile sensitivities were low ($r = 0.33$, 0.28, and 0.34, respectively).

To date the MQ has also been used for reporting pre- and post-treatment effects; McGuire, Wu, and Storch (2015) reported cases of two girls, ages 17 and 11 years, who underwent cognitive behavior therapy for misophonia. Whereas the 17-year-old girl completed the MQ independently, the 11-year-old girl completed it with the guidance of her mother. After treatment both girls showed a reduction in total MQ score which was reported as a large reduction in misophonia symptoms. The MQ's validity for these different ages and for different methods of completion is yet to be confirmed. A clinically-meaningful change in MQ score must be determined before measurement recommendations can be made.

Other Misophonia Tools

Many other questionnaire measures of misophonia have recently been developed and used in reporting but have yet to undergo psychometric evaluation. The Amsterdam Misophonia Scale (A-MISO-S; Schröder, Vulink, & Denys, 2013) is an adapted version of the Yale-Brown Obsessive-Compulsive Scale (Y-BOCS; Goodman et al., 1989) developed to measure the severity of misophonia symptoms. The scale contains 6 items asking patients about (1) time they spent thinking about misophonia; (2) interference with social functioning; (3) level of anger; (4) resistance against the impulse; (5) control they had over their thoughts and anger; and (6) time they spent avoiding misophonic situations. Each item is scored on a scale from 0 to 4 giving a total score ranging from 0 to 24. Schröder et al. (2013) also offered an interpretation of total scores whereby scores 0 to 4 indicated subclinical, 5 to 9 indicated mild, 10 to 14 indicated moderate, 15 to 19 indicated severe, and 20 to 24 indicated extreme misophonic symptoms. In their study, A-MISO-S scores in 42 adults with misophonia were compared to their scores on standard psychiatric questionnaires. The authors concluded that misophonia should be delineated as a separate psychiatric disorder.

Some of the multi-item misophonia questionnaires reported by Dozier (2015a, 2015b) appear to have evolved in clinical practice and have yet to be validated. These include the Misophonia Assessment Questionnaire (MAQ) and the Misophonia Coping Responses (MCR) surveys which Dozier attributed to Marsha Johnson, and the authors' own questionnaire, the Misophonia Emotional Response (MER) survey.

The MAQ consists of 21 items that ask about the negative impact misophonia has on a person's activities, thoughts, and feelings (e.g., *My sound issues have recently created problems for me in groups*, or *My sound issues are classified as "crazy"*). Items are rated from 0 (not at all) to 3 (almost all the time) giving a maximum questionnaire score of 63. Johnson (2014) provided an interpretation of the total score as mild (scoring 0 to 21), moderate (scoring 22 to 42), or severe (scoring 43 to 63) misophonia. The MCR uses the same 4-point scale as the MAQ to rate the frequency of certain behaviors that are elicited by misophonia trigger sounds (e.g., *Put on headphones*, or *Walk away from the person making the sound*). The MER uses a 4-point scale to rate the frequency of emotions that are elicited by misophonia trigger sounds (e.g., *You wish you were deaf*, or *You want to physically assault the person making the noise*), providing important information to support treatment planning. However, both surveys' value would increase upon determination of their psychometric properties.

Conclusion

There is general agreement in the literature that ULL estimates of decreased sound tolerance provide a valid clinical measure of the "threshold of discomfort" for sound, although several studies have commented upon the unsatisfactory variability of this and similar procedures. ULLs can be affected by factors such as the choice of stimulus or the set of instructions used; consistency of methodology is key to reliable repeated measures. Some research studies also confirm overlap in the health construct that is measured by ULLs and clinical questionnaire measures of decreased sound tolerance, suggesting the two procedures should be complementary when used clinically (Meeus et al., 2012; Wallén et al., 2012). ULLs are particularly indicated when the clinical questionnaire has not been formally validated for use or there is no robust method of interpreting the scores. Based on the evidence identified for this chapter, results obtained from all existing questionnaires would benefit from further psychometric evaluation.

Problems of decreased sound tolerance are commonly co-morbid with tinnitus. In an analysis of the Tinnitus Research Initiative patient database, Schecklmann et al. (2014) found that of 1713 tinnitus patients 935 responded "yes" to the single question "Do sounds cause you pain or physical discomfort?" when completing the Tinnitus Sample Case History Questionnaire (TSCHQ; Landgrebe et al., 2010). Variables significantly associated with reporting both tinnitus and decreased sound tolerance were younger age, higher tinnitus-related distress, and higher ratings of pain (headache, neck pain) or vertigo. It is not surprising therefore that the development and validation studies of hyperacusis questionnaires reviewed here have largely been based on populations reporting tinnitus over and above hyperacusis. This affects the utility, reliability, and validity of the questionnaires. Items must be representative of the construct they measure, such that the aims and objectives of the questionnaire are relevant to the population of interest. Item selection and reduction based on the responses from one specific population may not represent the complaints or beliefs of a different population. Overall, this would influence other aspects of the questionnaire's psychometric properties and clinical utility, that is, the factor structure and reliability of their use over time. The accuracy with which the current hyperacusis questionnaires measure sound tolerance specifically in patients with both hyperacusis and tinnitus is questionable (Fackrell et al., 2015). Indeed, in general, and for both hyperacusis and misophonia, the current lack of psychometrically validated instruments suggests there is still much to know about (1) how well the questionnaires currently available measure the construct of interest, (2) how scores can be meaningfully interpreted in their target populations and in prevalent clinical subgroups, and then (3) whether new methods of interpreting scores are needed for particular subgroups, and (4) whether new clinical questionnaires need to be systematically developed.

References

Anari, M., Axelsson, A., Eliasson, A., & Magnusson, L. (1999). Hypersensitivity to sound: Questionnaire data, audiometry and classification. *Scandinavian Audiology*, *28*, 219–230.

Baguley, D. M., & Andersson, G. (2008). *Hyperacusis: Mechanisms, diagnosis, and therapies*. San Diego, CA: Plural.

Beck, A. T., Steer, R. A., & Brown, G. K. (1996). Beck depression inventory-II. San Antonio, TX.

Beck, A. T., Epstein, N., Brown, G., & Steer, R. A. (1988). An inventory for measuring clinical anxiety: Psychometric properties. *Journal of Consulting and Clinical Psychology*, *56*, 893.

Beattie, R. C., Svihovec, D. A., Carmen, R. E., & Kunkel, H. A. (1980). Loudness discomfort level for speech: comparison of two instructional sets for saturation sound pressure level selection. *Ear and Hearing*, *1*, 197–205.

Beattie, R. C., & Boyd, R. L. (1986). Relationship between pure-tone and speech loudness discomfort levels among hearing-impaired subjects. *Journal of Speech and Hearing Disorders, 51*, 120–125.

Bläsing, L., & Kroener-Herwig, B. (2012). Self-reported and behavioral sound avoidance in tinnitus and hyperacusis subjects, and association with anxiety ratings. *International Journal of Audiology, 51*, 611–617.

Bläsing, L., Goebel, G., Flötzinger, U., Berthold, A., & Kröner-Herwig, B. (2010). Hypersensitivity to sound in tinnitus patients: an analysis of a construct based on questionnaire and audiological data. *International Journal of Audiology, 49*, 518–526.

Bornstein, S. P., & Musick, F. E. (1993). Loudness discomfort level and reliability as a function of instructional set. *Scandinavian Audiology, 22*, 125–131.

Brännström, K. J., Olsen, S. Ø., Holm, L., Kastberg, T., & Ibertsson, T. (2014). The effect of repeated measurements and working memory on the most comfortable level in the ANL test. *International journal of Audiology, 53*(11), 787–795.

British Society of Audiology. (2011). Recommended Procedure: Determination of Uncomfortable Loudness Levels. Available from www.thebsa.org.uk/. Last accessed January 6, 2017.

Coren, S. (1994). Most comfortable listening level as a function of age. *Ergonomics, 37*, 1269–1274.

Dauman, R., & Bouscau-Faure, F. (2005). Assessment and amelioration of hyperacusis in tinnitus patients. *Acta Oto-Laryngologica, 125*, 503–509.

Dozier, T. H. (2015a). Counterconditioning treatment for misophonia. *Clinical Case Studies, 14*, 374–387.

Dozier, T. H. (2015b). Treating the initial physical reflex of misophonia with the neural repatterning technique: A counterconditioning procedure. *Psychological Thought, 8*, 189–210.

Elberling, C., & Nielsen, C. (1993). The dynamics of speech and the auditory dynamic range in sensorineural hearing impairment. In J. Beilin and G. R. Jensen (Eds.). *Recent developments in hearing instrument technology* (pp. 99–134). Denmark: Danavox Jubilee Foundation.

Elberling, C. (1999). Loudness scaling revisited. *Journal of the American Academy of Audiology, 10*, 248–260.

Fackrell, K., Fearnley, C., Hoare, D. J., & Sereda, M. (2015). Hyperacusis questionnaire as a tool for measuring hypersensitivity to sound in a tinnitus research population. *BioMed Research International*, Article ID 290425.

Fioretti, A., Tortorella, F., Masedu, F., Valenti, M., Fusetti, M., & Pavaci, S. (2015). Validity of the Italian version of Khalfa's Questionnaire on hyperacusis. *Acta Otorhinolaryngologica Italica, 35*, 110.

Filion, P., & Margolis, R. (1992). Comparison of clinical and real-life judgments of loudness discomfort. *Journal of the American Academy of Audiology, 3*, 193–199.

Goldstein, B., & Shulman, A. (1996). Tinnitus-hyperacusis and the loudness discomfort level test—A preliminary report. *The International Tinnitus Journal, 2*, 83–89.

Goodman, W K., Price, L. H., Rasmussen, S. A., Mazure, C., Fleischmann, R. L. et al. (1989). The Yale-Brown Obsessive Compulsive Scale. I. Development, use, and reliability. *Archives of General Psychiatry, 46*, 1006–1011.

Greenberg, B., Walsh, B., & Carlos, M. (2016). Assessing the impact of sound sensitivity in tinnitus: Preliminary data from the Sound Sensitive Tinnitus Index. *Proceeding of the American Auditory Society*.

Hallam, R. S., Jakes, S. C., & Hinchcliffe, R. (1988). Cognitive variables in tinnitus annoyance. *British Journal of Clinical Psychology*, 27, 213–222.

Hawkins, D. B. (1980). Loudness discomfort levels. A clinical procedure for hearing aid evaluations. *Journal of Speech and Hearing Disorders, 45*, 3–15.

Hawkins, D. B., Walden, B. E., Montgomery, A., & Prosek, R. A. (1987). Description and validation of an LDL procedure designed to select SSPLSO. *Ear and Hearing, 8*, 162–169.

Hellman, R. P., & Meiselman, C. H. (1990). Loudness relations for individuals and groups in normal and impaired hearing. *Journal of the Acoustical Society of America, 88*, 2596–2606.

Herráiz, C., De los Santos, G., Diges, I., Díez, R., & Aparicio, J. M. (2006). Evaluación de la hiperacusia: Test de hipersensibilidad al sonido. *Acta Otorrinolaringológica Española, 57*, 303–306.

Hiller, W., & Goebel, G. (1992). A psychometric study of complaints in chronic tinnitus. *Journal of Psychosomatic Research, 36*, 337–348.

Johnson, M. (1999). A tool for measuring hyperacusis. *The Hearing Journal, 52*, 34–35.

Johnson, M. (2014). 50 cases of misophonia using the MMP. *Proceedings of the Misophonia Conference of the Tinnitus Practitioners Association*, Atlanta, GA.

Jüris, L., Andersson, G., Larsen, H. C., & Ekselius, L. (2014). Cognitive behaviour therapy for hyperacusis: A randomized controlled trial. *Behaviour Research and Therapy, 54*, 30–37.

Kamm, C., Dirks, D. D., & Mickey, M. R. (1978). Effect of sensorineural hearing loss on loudness discomfort level and most comfortable loudness judgments. *Journal of Speech, Language, and Hearing Research, 21*, 668–681.

Khalfa, S., Dubal, S., Veuillet, E., Perez-Diaz, F., Jouvent, R., & Collet, L. (2002). Psychometric normalization of a hyperacusis questionnaire. *ORL, 64*, 436–442.

Kinnealey, M., & Oliver, B. (2002). *Adult sensory questionnaire*. Philadelphia, PA: Temple University, College of Allied Health Professionals.

Kopra, L. L., & Blosser, D. (1968). Effects of method of measurement on most comfortable loudness level for speech. *Journal of Speech, Language, and Hearing Research, 11*, 497–508.

Kuk, F. K., Tyler, R. S., Russell, D., & Jordan, H. (1990). The psychometric properties of a tinnitus handicap questionnaire. *Ear and Hearing, 11*, 434–445.

Landgrebe, M., Zeman, F., Koller, M., Eberl, Y., Mohr, M., et al. (2010). The Tinnitus Research Initiative (TRI) database: A new approach for delineation of tinnitus subtypes and generation of predictors for treatment outcome. *BMC Medical Informatics and Decision Making, 10*, 42.

Liu, T. C., & Chen, Y. S. (2000). Loudness discomfort levels in patients with conductive and mixed hearing loss. *Auris Nasus Larynx, 27*, 101–104.

Maslach C., Jackson S. E., & Leiter M. P. (1996). *Maslach burnout inventory manual*. Palo Alto, CA: Consulting Psychologists Press.

McGuire, J. F., Wu, M. S., & Storch, E. A. (2015). Cognitive-behavioral therapy for 2 youths with misophonia. *The Journal of Clinical Psychiatry, 76*, 573–574.

Meeus, O. M., Spaepen, M., De Ridder, D., & Van de Heyning, P. H. (2010). Correlation between hyperacusis measurements in daily ENT practice. *International Journal of Audiology, 49*, 7–13.

Mertens, G., De Bodt, M., & Van de Heyning, P. (2016). Cochlear implantation as a long-term treatment for ipsilateral incapacitating tinnitus in subjects with unilateral hearing loss up to 10 years. *Hearing Research, 331*, 1–6.

Morgan, D. E., Wilson, R. H., & Dirks, D. D. (1974). Loudness discomfort level: selected methods and stimuli. *The Journal of the Acoustical Society of America, 56*, 577–581.

Morgan, D. E., Dirks, D. D., Bower, D., & Kamm, C. A. (1979). Loudness discomfort level and acoustic reflex threshold for speech stimuli. *Journal of Speech, Language, and Hearing Research, 22*, 849–861.

Murphy, D. L., Pickar, D., & Alterman, I. S. (1982). Methods for the quantitative assessment of depressive and manic behavior. In E. I. Burdock, A. Sudilovsku, & S. Gershon (Eds.), *The behaviour of psychiatric patients: Quantitative techniques for evaluation* (pp. 335–392). New York, NY: Marcel Dekker.

Nelting, M., Rienhoff, N. K., Hesse, G., & Lamparter, U. (2002). Die Erfassung des subjektiven Leidens unter Hyperakusis mit einem Selbstbeurteilungsbogen zur Geräuschüberempfindlichkeit (GÜF). *Laryngo-Rhino-Otologie, 81*, 327–334.

Oishi, N., Yamada, H., Kanzaki, S., Kurita, A., Takiguchi, Y., Yugę, I., . . . & Ogawa, K. (2017). Assessment of hyperacusis with a newly produced Japanese version of the Khalfa hyperacusis questionnaire. *Acta Oto-Laryngologica*, 1–5.

Patel, K. K., Veenstra, D. L., & Patrick, D. L. (2003). A review of selected patient-generated outcome measures and their application in clinical trials. *Value in Health, 6*, 595–603.

Pienkowski, M., Tyler, R. S., Roncancio, E. R., Jun, H. J., Brozoski, T., Dauman, N., . . . & Martin, N. (2014). A review of hyperacusis and future directions: Part II. Measurement, mechanisms, and treatment. *American Journal of Audiology, 23,* 420–436.

Sammeth, C. A., Birman, M., & Hecox, K. E. (1989). Variability of most comfortable and uncomfortable loudness levels to speech stimuli in the hearing impaired. *Ear and Hearing, 10,* 94–100.

Schecklmann, M., Landgrebe, M., Langguth, B., & TRI Database Study Group. (2014). Phenotypic characteristics of hyperacusis in tinnitus. *PLoS One, 9,* e86944.

Shabana, M. I., Selim, M. H., El Refaie, A., El Dessouky, T. M., & Soliman, R. Y. (2011). Assessment of hyperacusis in Egyptian patients: Evaluation of the Arabic version of the Khalfa questionnaire. *Audiological Medicine, 9,* 127–134.

Sheldrake, J., Diehl, P. U., & Schaette, R. (2015). Audiometric characteristics of hyperacusis patients. *Frontiers in Neurology, 6,* 105.

Schröder, A., Vulink N., & Denys, D. (2013). Misophonia: Diagnostic criteria for a new psychiatric disorder. *PLoS ONE, 8,* e54706.

Sherlock, L. P., & Formby, C. (2005). Estimates of loudness, loudness discomfort, and the auditory dynamic range: Normative estimates, comparison of procedures, and test-retest reliability. *Journal of the American Academy of Audiology, 16,* 85–100.

Stephens, S. D. G., Blegvad, B., & Krogh, H. J. (1977). The value of some suprathreshold auditory measures. *Scandinavian Audiology, 6,* 213–221.

Terwee, C. B., Bot, S. D., de Boer, M. R., van der Windt, D. A., Knol, D. L., Dekker, J., . . . & de Vet, H. C. (2007). Quality criteria were proposed for measurement properties of health status questionnaires. *Journal of Clinical Epidemiology, 60,* 34–42.

Tyler, R. S., Pienkowski, M., Roncancio, E. R., Jun, H. J., Brozoski, T., Dauman, N., . . . & Martin, N. (2014). A review of hyperacusis and future directions: part I. Definitions and manifestations. *American Journal of Audiology, 23,* 402–419.

Wallén, M. B., Hasson, D., Theorell, T., & Canlon, B. (2012). The correlation between the hyperacusis questionnaire and uncomfortable loudness levels is dependent on emotional exhaustion. *International Journal of Audiology, 51,* 722–729.

Walker, G., Dillon, H., Byrne, D., & Christen, R. (1984). The use of loudness discomfort levels for selecting the maximum output of hearing aids. *Australian Journal of Audiology, 6,* 23–32.

Wu, M. S., Lewin, A. B., Murphy, T. K., & Storch, E. A. (2014). Misophonia: Incidence, phenomenology, and clinical correlates in an undergraduate student sample. *Journal of Clinical Psychology, 70,* 994–1007.

SECTION II

Mechanisms

5

Peripheral Mechanisms of Decreased Sound Tolerance

Roland Schaette

Decreased sound tolerance (DST) is a relatively widespread phenomenon. The estimates for its prevalence differ widely in the literature; values of 2% (Sammeth et al., 2000), 8.6% (Andersson et al., 2002), or even 15.2% (Fabijanska, 1999) of the adult population have been reported. A large-scale questionnaire-based study from Sweden revealed a prevalence of 2.2% for physician-diagnosed hyperacusis, and 10.5% for self-reported hyperacusis (Paulin et al., 2016). For children, the estimates for the prevalence of DST range from 3.2 to 17.1%. (Rosing et al., 2016). One of the reasons for the wide range of estimates might be that different surveys have used different definitions of what constitutes decreased sound tolerance. However, even the most conservative estimates of around 2% indicate that decreased sound tolerance could affect millions.

Changes in loudness perception with DST have been characterized by measuring loudness discomfort levels (LDLs) and loudness growth functions. On average, the LDLs of affected patients were 15 to 20 dB (Anari et al., 1999; Formby et al., 2007; Sheldrake et al., 2015) lower than those of normal-hearing listeners (Sherlock and Formby, 2005). In some cases, however, LDLs were as low as 30 to 40 dB HL (Sheldrake et al., 2015). Perceived loudness measured through categorical loudness scaling (Cox et al., 1997) or similar rating procedures showed a rapid growth of loudness with sound intensity in hyperacusis patients, and they rated sounds as "too loud" at lower levels than control subjects (Brandy and Lynn, 1995; Norena and Chery-Croze, 2007). Interestingly, the pattern of decreased sound tolerance does not seem to show a distinct frequency dependence, as there was a consistent reduction of LDLs across all tested frequencies from 125 Hz to 8 kHz (Sheldrake et al., 2015). Categorical loudness scaling measurements also showed that loudness growth functions measured at different frequencies in hearing-impaired patients converged at high sound intensities, even though the functions differed considerably at low sound intensities due to hearing threshold differences (Norena and Chery-Croze, 2007).

Unfortunately, measurements of perceived loudness, and especially LDL data, likely yield an incomplete characterization of symptoms when introducing the phenotype of DST. First, LDLs are not sensitive or specific enough when used in isolation to diagnose hyperacusis (Sheldrake et al., 2015). A study that investigated LDLs and subjective reports of sound tolerance problems in daily life found only weak correlations between LDLs (measured for pure tones and speech) and subjective ratings for sound tolerance (Zaugg et al., 2016). Measurements of loudness might thus not accurately reflect the difficulties experienced in daily life by patients. In particular, the experience of pain from sounds might be insufficiently captured by LDL measurements. The threshold for experiencing pain from sound is between 120 and 140 dB SPL in normal-hearing listeners (Plutchik, 1963; American Institute of Physics and Gray, 1972), but in patients with DST, the level can be substantially reduced. For obvious reasons, there is no systematic data in the literature on the auditory pain threshold in hyperacusis patients, although in a study of 100 patients with sound sensitivity problems, 88 reported experiencing pain from sound (Anari et al., 1999). In a recent questionnaire study on members of a hyperacusis Facebook group, we found that 51 out of 58 responders (88%) reported that they experienced pain from loud sounds (Jeraj & Schaette, unpublished). Similarly, a recent survey conducted by the CORDAS (Coordination of Rare Diseases at Sanford) Registry showed that 95% of the respondents with hyperacusis experienced auditory pain at least occasionally, and 66% continuously or daily (Pollard, 2017, unpublished), with the ear pain triggered by loud sounds. The experience of pain from sound might thus be a major or even the defining component of DST.

The main features of DST are therefore changes in the perception of the loudness of sounds, in that sounds are perceived as too loud despite being judged as tolerable by normal-hearing listeners, and the experience of pain from sound at sound intensities that normally do not elicit a pain sensation. It is currently not known whether the same mechanisms that alter loudness perception and decrease the LDLs are also responsible for lowering the threshold for triggering the experience of pain from sound. Moreover, it is even conceivable that fear of experiencing auditory pain might influence LDL measurements, causing patients to abort the test early, and the expectation of pain could also change the evaluation of sounds in the brain, thereby altering loudness perception.

In the following, I will review and evaluate potential mechanisms of how altered loudness perception and pain from sound might be generated, focusing on the auditory periphery. As the relation between the two phenomena is unclear, I will treat alterations of loudness perception separate from auditory pain. For simplicity, I will use the term "pain hyperacusis" (Tyler et al., 2014) for the symptom of a decreased threshold for experiencing pain from sound, and the term "loudness hyperacusis" for increased loudness perception. Please bear in mind that these two symptoms are not mutually exclusive, and that patients with DST frequently suffer from a combination of both.

A Potential Peripheral Mechanism for Pain from Sound

One of the most distressing aspects of hyperacusis is the experience of pain from sound at levels that do not cause a pain sensation in normal-hearing subjects. The pain threshold for normal-hearing listeners is stated to be between 120 and 140 dB SPL (Plutchik, 1963; American Institute of Physics and Gray, 1972). The auditory pain threshold is thus in the intensity range at which even relatively brief exposures can cause cochlear damage leading to permanent hearing loss. Such sound levels would thus be well suited to trigger a behavioral response intended to prevent further damage to the sensitive structures of the inner ear, thereby supporting a role for auditory pain as a signal for risk of tissue damage. Up until relatively recently, however, it was unknown which cells and fibers detected tissue damage in the ear and created a pain signal. In 2015, two studies were published that provided evidence for a role of the type II auditory nerve fibers (ANFs), first as detectors of tissue damage in the ear (Liu et al., 2015), and second as a pathway to convey a damage signal to the brain (Flores et al., 2015). Based on these reports, the type II fibers would be prime candidates for a role as pain fibers of the ear.

There are two types of ANFs, type I and type II fibers. Type I fibers constitute about 90 to 95% of the auditory nerve fibers, and are often colloquially referred to simply as auditory nerve fibers. They are thick and myelinated, and synapse onto the inner hair cells (IHCs). Each type I fiber contacts only a single IHC, and each IHC is contacted by around 10 to 15 fibers (Ryugo, 1992). The type I fibers are activated by sound and they are essential for hearing, as they convey the information about the auditory signal received by the ear to the brain. Type II fibers, in contrast, are less numerous, as only 5 to 10% of the AN fiber population are type II. These fibers are thin and unmyelinated, and they contact the outer hair cells (OHCs) of the cochlea. Each type II fiber contacts approximately 7 OHCs (Weisz et al., 2012). Type II ANFs receive glutamatergic synaptic excitation from OHCs, but the synapses between OHCs and type II fibers are weak (Weisz et al., 2009); the lesser magnitude of synaptic drive received by the type II fibers indicates that they play a fundamentally different role in auditory signaling from that of type I afferents. It has been estimated that many of the presynaptic OHCs would need to release a neurotransmitter in order to make a type II fiber generate an action potential (Weisz et al., 2009, 2012), which might only happen for sounds at very high sound intensities.

A recent demonstration by Liu and co-workers (2015) indicated that type II ANFs can sense tissue damage in the cochlea. In an in-vitro preparation, they obtained patch-clamp recordings from type II fibers in excised cochleas. When they mechanically destroyed an OHC that had a synaptic contact with the fiber from which they were recording, action potentials were observed in response. On the other hand, destruction of adjacent, but unconnected, OHCs did not activate the fiber. The type II fibers thus do sense and report to higher centers damage to OHCs in a very specific fashion; this action makes them prime candidates for serving as the pain sensors or pain fibers of the ear. Interestingly, the damage response of the type II fibers could be completely blocked through the bath application of retigabine, suggesting that a "painkiller for the ear" might be a possibility.

Direct mechanical destruction of OHCs might not correspond to the situation that is created inside the inner ear in vivo by loud sounds. Flores and colleagues (2015) demonstrated that the type II fiber pathway could also be activated by acoustic stimuli delivered at intensities high enough to cause tissue damage in the inner ear. To differentiate activation of the type II fiber pathway from sound-evoked neural activity of the type I fiber pathways, they used mice that had been genetically modified to render the type I fibers inactive. In these mice, sounds presented at 120 dB SPL (which caused major damage to the OHCs) activated cells in those regions of the cochlear nucleus that receive projections from type II fibers. In contrast, a lower sound intensity of 80 dB SPL, which did not damage OHCs, did not generate neural activity in the cochlear nucleus. This study thus demonstrated that damaging sound levels activated the type II fiber pathway, and that this pathway conveyed a signal about the OHC damage to the cochlear nucleus, the first central processing stage of the auditory system. How this signal is processed further, and which other brain regions in the ascending auditory pathway are involved in this process, remains to be determined.

This discovery of an auditory pain pathway is a major breakthrough for research on pain hyperacusis, as it provides a target for research and therapies. However, the mechanism responsible for the activation of this pathway at much lower sound intensities, as would be required to generate the symptoms observed in patients with pain hyperacusis, remains to be determined. One possible scenario could involve cross-talk between type I and type II ANFs, which might happen, for example, when the myelin sheath around type I ANFs is damaged, as has been observed after acoustic trauma (Tagoe et al., 2014) and cisplatin administration (van Ruijven et al., 2004).

Loudness Perception

Before we can start investigating potential peripheral mechanisms of loudness hyperacusis, we first must establish what is currently known about the relation between peripheral auditory processing and normal loudness perception. Our understanding of the relation between the intensity of auditory stimuli and the sensation of loudness caused by them is based on theoretical models. The standard models of loudness can account for all major aspects of normal loudness perception, even though they are entirely based on the outer and inner ear, and do not take central auditory processing in the brain into account.

The most commonly used loudness models are based on cochlear filter bank models used to simulate the cochlear excitation pattern (Moore, 2014), that is, the distribution and magnitude of sound-evoked vibration along the basilar membrane (BM). Predictions about the loudness of a given sound are then derived from the cochlear excitation pattern. Narrow-band sounds at low intensities only excite a relatively small, restricted patch of the BM. Increasing sound intensity results not only in a larger BM vibration amplitude, but also in a spread of excitation to neighboring regions of the cochlea. It is especially important to note that this spread of excitation is asymmetric, spreading more in the basal direction to basilar membrane locations with higher characteristic frequencies, and much less in the apical direction to BM locations with lower characteristic frequencies (illustrated for ANF activity in Figure 5–1A). With the use of an appropriate basilar membrane model, the area under the cochlear excitation pattern is directly proportional to the perceived loudness measured on the sone scale (Chen et al., 2011). Moreover, when a more detailed physiological model of cochlea and auditory nerve is used, it can also be demonstrated that loudness is directly proportional to the overall activity of type I ANFs (Figure 5–1B) (Diehl & Schaette, 2015). The model simulations also show that the spread of excitation at high sound intensities can be so extreme that even low-frequency sounds (e.g., <500 Hz) can excite the cochlea up to the basal end when presented at sufficient volume, and thus provide excitation to the "high-frequency channels" of auditory processing.

For the assessment of potential peripheral mechanisms of loudness hyperacusis, the most important conclusion from the existing models is that perceived loudness is determined to a first approximation by the magnitude of the auditory nerve signal. It is currently unknown where in the brain this signal is then evaluated to generate the loudness percept. Potentially, the site of loudness perception is located at a relatively high level of auditory processing, at which signals from both ears are pooled and

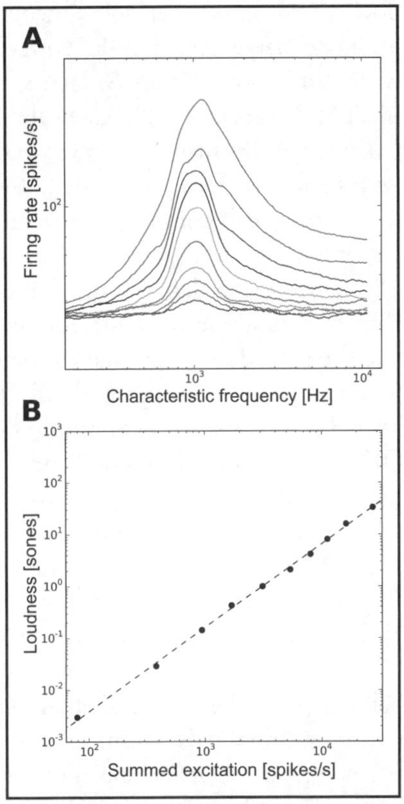

Figure 5–1. Illustration of a loudness model based on simulations of basilar membrane and auditory nerve responses. **A.** Simulated activity pattern of a population of ANFs with characteristic frequencies from 40 Hz to 13 kHz in response to brief 1-kHz tones from 0 to 90 dB SPL. The simulations were obtained using a modified version of the MAP model (Meddis et al., 2013). At high sound intensities, the spread of excitation is very pronounced, as the 1-kHz tones also strongly excite ANFs with the highest characteristic frequencies. **B.** Relation between the summed activity of all model ANFs (summed excitation) and the perceived loudness in sones according to ANSI S3.4-2007. The dashed line shows a fitted power-law function with a slope of 1.1, illustrating that perceived loudness is proportional to the overall sound-evoked activity in the auditory nerve. To view this image in full color visit the Plural Publishing website for the book at http://plural publishing.com/publication_hdsi.htm.

evaluated together (Munro et al., 2014). To cause the perception of increased loudness and steeper loudness growth, there are then two possibilities. First, through some pathological change, the output of the cochlea, that is, the summed activity of all type I ANFs, might be increased and thus provide a "louder" signal to the brain. Second, there might be changes in the central auditory system, either pathological amplification—for example, through increased excitation or disinhibition—of the signal in the first stages of auditory processing before it reaches the brain area that evaluates loudness, or changes in the "loudness evaluation circuit" itself could result in an auditory nerve signal of low magnitude being evaluated as too loud. The first scenario would constitute a direct peripheral effect, whereas the latter scenario represents changes in the central auditory system that might nevertheless be triggered by a peripheral event such as hearing loss. Both scenarios will be investigated in the following paragraphs.

Review of Potential Peripheral Mechanisms for Loudness Hyperacusis

A peripheral mechanism for loudness hyperacusis would need to influence cochlear processing such that the overall activity of the type I ANF population would be increased. There are two putative scenarios for how the output of the cochlea could be pathologically increased. The increase could either be directly caused as a side-effect of cochlear damage, or it might be due to changes in the efferent feedback that the cochlea receives. The following offers a review of the evidence for and against both scenarios. Please note that for simplicity, "ANF" always means "type I ANF" in the following.

Effect of Different Types of Cochlear Damage on the Activity of Type I ANFs

Damage to the cochlea can be caused by a variety of factors, with noise-induced and age-related damage probably the most common. The main effects of noise exposure on the inner ear are damage to the stereocilia of cochlear hair cells (Liberman & Dodds, 1984a; Liberman & Kiang, 1984; Kaltenbach et al., 1992), loss of synaptic ribbons (synaptopathy) (Kujawa & Liberman, 2009; Liberman et al., 2015; Song et al., 2016), degeneration of ANFs (neuropathy) (Kujawa & Liberman, 2009), and loss of outer as well as inner hair cells (Liberman & Dodds, 1984a; Kaltenbach et al., 1992; Chen & Fechter, 2003). Aging also damages hair cell stereocilia, triggers apoptosis of cochlear hair cells (Soucek et al., 1986; Francis et al., 2003), and produces degeneration of ANFs (Makary et al., 2011; Sergeyenko et al., 2013), as well as atrophy of the stria vascularis (Gates & Mills, 2005).

Damage to hair cell stereocilia affects activity of ANFs primarily by increasing their response thresholds (Liberman, 1984; Liberman & Dodds, 1984a). Moreover, while the spontaneous discharge rates of ANFs may be reduced as a consequence of stereocilia damage (Liberman & Dodds, 1984b), the maximum firing rates evoked by high-intensity sounds reportedly remain comparable to those from control ANFs (Liberman & Kiang, 1984).

The main function of the OHCs is to provide amplification of basilar membrane motion at low sound intensities, and compression at medium to high levels. Loss of OHCs thus increases the response thresholds of ANFs (Dallos & Harris, 1978), and the loss of compression might be reflected in a steepening of the rate-level functions of ANFs (Schmiedt & Zwislocki, 1980). Neither spontaneous nor maximum discharge rates of ANFs, however, are altered by OHC loss (Dallos & Harris, 1978; Schmiedt & Zwislocki, 1980). After OHC loss, the activity of ANFs may thus grow more rapidly with signal level for suprathreshold sounds, but their activity will not increase beyond rates normally produced by high-level sounds.

Both stereocilia damage and OHC loss can thus potentially lead to a steeper growth of perceived loudness for sounds that are above the increased hearing threshold. When considered with impaired hearing thresholds, the OHC loss reduces the dynamic range, although the output of the cochlea would not exceed normal levels at high sound intensities (Figure 5–2). This "catch-up-behavior" would be consistent with recruitment (Cox et al., 1997), but not with loudness hyperacusis.

While hyperacusis patients may present with all degrees of hearing loss, about a third have hearing thresholds within the normal range (Anari et al., 1999; Sheldrake et al., 2015). However, a normal audiogram does not necessarily indicate the absence of cochlear damage; a substantial degree of cochlear synaptopathy (Kujawa and Liberman, 2009), neuropathy (Makary et al., 2011), or even loss of IHCs (Lobarinas et al., 2013) may co-occur with normal hearing thresholds. Interestingly, a recent study in mice has indicated that synaptopathy could lead to behavioral signs consistent with loudness hyperacusis (Hickox & Liberman, 2014).

Loss of inner hair cells through noise- or age-related damage will remove the input signal from all type I ANFs that contact these hair cells, thereby rendering them unresponsive to sound. Therefore, if IHC loss is scattered along the length of the cochlea, then it will lead to a reduction of the overall auditory nerve signal in proportion to the degree of IHC loss (Schaette & Kempter, 2006). In a chinchilla model, selective loss of IHCs through carboplatin administration has been shown to be scattered

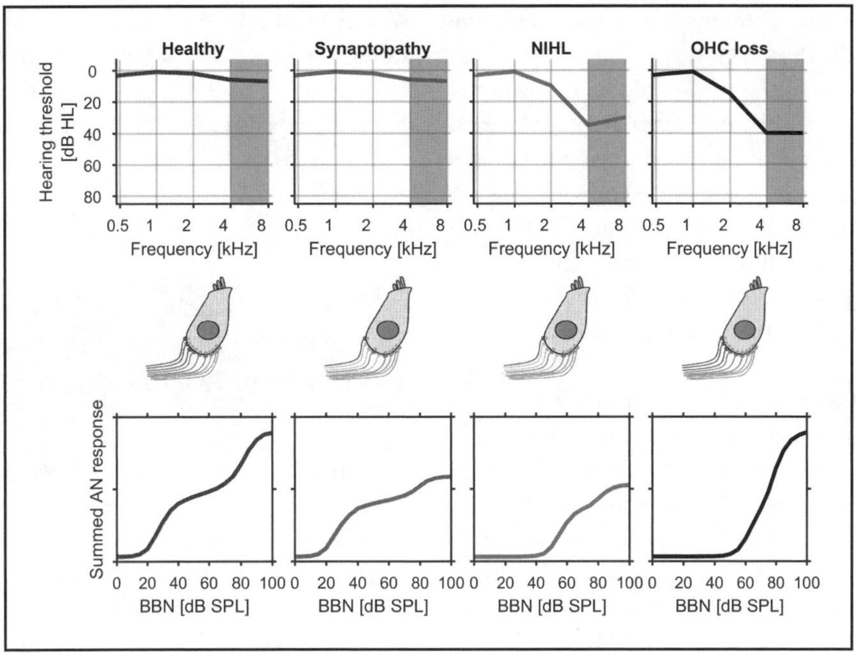

Figure 5–2. Simulation of the effects of different types of damage to or loss of cochlear hair cells on ANF responses. (Top row) Generic audiograms for noise-induced cochlear synaptopathy (hidden hearing loss), noise-induced hearing loss (NIHL), and outer hair cell (OHC) loss. (Middle row) Schematic picture of an IHC with type I ANFs, to illustrate the degree of cochlear synaptopathy, which renders the affected fibers unresponsive to sound (gray fibers). (Bottom row) Simulated AN population responses for AN fibers with characteristic frequencies of 4 to 8 kHz (indicated by shaded area in the top row). The MAP model (Meddis et al., 2013) has been used to simulate AN responses to short bursts of broadband noise for an AN fiber population comprising low-, medium-, and high-threshold AN fibers, with the extent of hearing loss corresponding to the audiograms in the top row. For NIHL, a combination of stereocilia damage, synaptopathy, and hair cell loss was assumed. The simulations demonstrate that the different kinds of damage to cochlear hair cells all reduce overall AN responses, indicating that damage to cochlear hair cells is unlikely to produce a neural correlate of loudness hyperacusis at the level of the AN. To view this image in full color visit the Plural Publishing website for the book at http://pluralpublishing.com/publication_hdsi.htm.

along the cochlea and to reduce the compound action potential of the auditory nerve in proportion to the degree of hair cell loss (Wang et al., 1997). Complete loss of IHCs along a stretch of the basilar membrane creates what is called a cochlear dead region (Moore, 2004), and might make certain frequency ranges completely inaudible. As for scattered IHC loss, the subsequent cochlear dead regions will reduce auditory nerve responses to sounds when such responses are compared to the output from a healthy cochlea. The magnitude of this effect will differ considerably for sounds within and outside the dead region.

Noise- and age-related damage can cause cochlear synaptopathy, that is, a permanent loss of synaptic ribbons at the synapse between inner hair cells and type I ANFs (Kujawa & Liberman, 2009; Sergeyenko et al., 2013). In mice, more than 50% loss of synaptic ribbons has been observed in the high-frequency parts of the cochlea after noise exposures that only caused a temporary increase of the hearing thresholds (Kujawa & Liberman, 2009). This loss of an essential part of the presynaptic machinery of the synapse has a strong effect on the responses of type I ANFs to sound, which can be observed in a proportional reduction in the amplitude of wave I of the auditory brainstem response (Kujawa & Liberman, 2009; Furman et al., 2013; Hesse et al., 2016), indicating that the affected auditory nerve fibers become less responsive to sound, if they respond at all. Over time, synaptopathy is followed by neuropathy, that is, degeneration of type I ANFs (Kujawa & Liberman, 2009; Makary et al., 2011; Sergeyenko et al., 2013; Fernandez et al., 2015), which might further reduce the number of ANFs that respond to sound. The overall effect of cochlear synaptopathy and neuropathy will therefore be a reduction of the magnitude of the signal transmitted by the auditory nerve to the brain (Figure 5–2). Synaptopathy and neuropathy thus generate the opposite form of peripheral change required to create a correlate of loudness hyperacusis at the level of the auditory nerve.

In summary, one can conclude that the overall effect for noise-induced or age-related damage to cochlear hair cells is a reduction of AN activity, and therefore they are highly unlikely to produce pathological increases in the activity of type I ANFs that would be required as a peripheral mechanism for loudness hyperacusis. This is matched by audiometric findings that reveal neither a "typical" shape of the audiogram in hyperacusis patients (Anari et al., 1999; Sheldrake et al., 2015), nor a relation between the pattern or degree of hearing loss and the degree of LDL reduction or the shape of the LDL curve (Sheldrake et al., 2015).

Failure of Efferent Feedback Could Potentially Increase ANF Responses to Loud Sounds

Both the middle ear and the inner ear receive efferent innervation. One of the functions of the efferent feedback to the auditory periphery is to regulate the responses of the inner ear to loud sounds. Feedback to the middle ear triggers the acoustic reflex, which reduces the efficiency of energy transfer to the cochlea. The inner ear receives efferent feedback through two distinct pathways, the medial and the lateral olivocochlear bundle. The fibers of the medial olivocochlear (MOC) bundle project onto the OHCs, and the fibers of the lateral olivocochlear (LOC) bundle contact type I ANFs just behind the synaptic contact between type I fibers and IHCs. MOC feedback to OHCs reduces the effect of the cochlear amplifier (Guinan, 2006). Moreover, efferent feedback has a protective effect on the inner ear (Lendvai et al., 2011; Maison et al., 2013; Liberman et al., 2014), and it has been shown that efferent innervation of the ear may undergo plastic remodeling with aging and after noise trauma (Nouvian et al., 2015). It is thus conceivable that a disruption of efferent feedback could contribute to hyperacusis, because malfunction of the efferent system might lead to abnormal auditory nerve responses to a wide range of sound levels, potentially decreasing sound tolerance.

The acoustic or so-called middle ear reflex is a brainstem reflex that involves the bilateral contraction of the middle ear muscles in response to a high sound level presented to either ear (Borg, 1973). The contraction of the stapedius muscle in the middle ear stiffens the ossicular chain, thereby reducing the transmission of primarily low-frequency sound energy to the inner ear by approximately 15 dB. The threshold for eliciting the acoustic reflex is usually between 70 and 100 dB HL, depending on stimulus frequency and bandwidth (Munro et al., 2014). A reduction of the strength of the acoustic reflex, or even a complete absence, could thus increase the stimulus intensity received by the inner ear, theoretically resulting in a higher cochlear output that could contribute to DST. However, the ARTs of hyperacusis patients have been reported to be in the normal range (Brandy & Lynn, 1995; Anari et al., 1999), and it is thus unlikely that malfunction of the acoustic reflex contributes to hyperacusis.

The main effect of MOC feedback to the inner ear is to reduce the amplification provided by the OHCs (Cooper & Guinan, 2006; Guinan, 2006), which shifts the response functions of type I ANFs to higher sound intensities (Guinan & Gifford, 1988). MOC feedback is elicited by sound in a level-dependent fashion (Smalt et al., 2014), with time constants on the order of hundreds of milliseconds (Backus & Guinan, 2006). While a malfunction of this mechanism could in principle increase type I ANF responses to loud sounds, the effect might actually be most pronounced at moderate sound intensities, in the compressive range of the OHC contribution to the basilar membrane response. At very high sound intensities, the basilar membrane response becomes linear again and is not governed by the OHCs, and thus the effects of MOC feedback (and lack thereof) might be limited in this intensity range (compare also the depiction of the effects of OHC loss on ANF activity in Figure 5–2). In human patients, removal of MOC feedback to the cochlea can occur, for example, when the vestibular nerve is sectioned to improve the symptoms of Meniere's disease. Thus far, the effects of this intervention have only been investigated for tinnitus, where it did not have a consistent effect (Baguley et al., 2002). Whether the vestibular nerve section alters loudness perception and hyperacusis remains to be investigated.

The LOC feedback system utilizes a variety of neurotransmitters, especially acetylcholine, GABA, and dopamine (Elgoyhen, 2010), suggesting a modulatory or even inhibitory function. One of the potential functions of the LOC feedback system is to fine-tune auditory nerve responses to balance interaural sensitivity (Darrow et al., 2006). After removal or blocking of LOC feedback to the cochlea, both increases (Darrow et al., 2007) and decreases (Le Prell et al., 2005) of auditory nerve responses, quantified through measurements of ABR wave I magnitude, have been observed. It is thus unclear whether malfunction of the LOC feedback would increase or decrease sound sensitivity.

Complete removal of both MOC and LOC feedback to the cochlea has been investigated in a rat model. Following chronic cochlear de-efferentation produced by sectioning the olivocochlear bundle, type I ANFs showed increased sound-evoked activity and decreased dynamic range of their rate-level functions, more pronounced responses to sound onsets, and decreased thresholds in the tails of their tuning curves (Zheng et al., 1999). These effects were most pronounced in ANFs with high characteristic frequencies (2 to 8 kHz), and would be consistent with loudness hyperacusis.

In conclusion, changes in efferent feedback to the cochlea could enhance auditory nerve responses to loud sounds, which could make loud environments uncomfortable and would be consistent with loudness hyperacusis. Whether efferent malfunctions are actually present in patients with decreased sound tolerance remains to be determined.

Indications for Peripheral Processes as a Trigger for Central Changes that Might Underlie Loudness Hyperacusis

Thus far, I have only considered how changes in the auditory periphery could directly create decreased sound tolerance (DST) and pain from sound. However, when we consider peripheral mechanisms of sound sensitivity, we also must consider the case in which DST might be triggered through a peripheral event, for example, cochlear damage, even when the pathological changes that underlie the sound sensitivity problems occur in the central auditory system. It is now well established that cochlear damage can trigger neuronal plasticity in the central auditory system (Roberts et al., 2010), and it has been proposed that neuroplastic changes might underlie the development of hyperacusis (Auerbach et al., 2014).

A recent neuroimaging study reported increases in sound-evoked neuronal responses in the auditory midbrain, thalamus, and cortex of subjects with DST (Gu et al., 2010). As fMRI, the imaging technique used in this study, could not measure auditory nerve activity, it has remained unclear whether the enhanced activation seen throughout the central auditory system might be generated by increased input from the auditory nerve, or through amplification of the auditory nerve signal along the auditory pathway through pathological changes within the central auditory system. A theoretical study postulated that hyperacusis might be due to an abnormal increase in neuronal gain in the central auditory system (Zeng, 2013). Specifically, it was hypothesized that hyperacusis might be due to an increase in a nonlinear gain mechanism. This hypothesis was investigated in more detail by Diehl and Schaette (2015), who concluded that the decreased LDLs of hyperacusis patients were best accounted for by a generalized, frequency-independent increase in nonlinear gain in the central auditory system. In the model, gain was applied to suprathreshold responses only, that is, after subtracting the spontaneous activity of the auditory nerve, thereby differentiating "hyperacusis gain" from gain mechanisms postulated to underlie the development of tinnitus (Schaette & Kempter, 2006). Considering the research findings summarized above, these modeling studies, and any theories about an increase in neuronal gain in the central auditory system as a mechanism of hyperacusis, should probably be considered as models for loudness hyperacusis only.

Peripheral damage or hearing loss might trigger changes in the central auditory system related to loudness hyperacusis. Many studies investigated the effects of simulating a conductive hearing loss on the auditory system by letting normal-hearing volunteers wear earplugs for a few days. This relatively mild form of auditory deprivation triggered a variety of changes in the central auditory system in the absence of any peripheral damage. First, wearing an earplug for several days in one or both ears increased perceived loudness (Formby et al., 2003; Munro et al., 2014). Changes in perceived loudness developed over days, and reverted back to pre-occlusion ratings within 24 hours after earplug removal (Munro et al., 2014). Interestingly, when only one ear was plugged, perceived loudness was increased in both ears (Munro et al., 2014), indicating that the changes in loudness might be due to plasticity at a relatively high level of the auditory processing chain, where input from both ears is integrated and evaluated. In parallel with changes in perceived loudness, changes in acoustic reflex thresholds (elicited via a brainstem reflex arc) were observed, but here the changes went in opposite directions in the plugged and the open ear (Munro & Blount, 2009; Munro et al., 2014). Plasticity of loudness works in both directions, as additional stimulation through noise generators (Formby et al., 2003) or low-gain hearing aids (Munro & Merrett, 2013) decreased perceived loudness when measured in the same manner as in the plugged ears. These studies indicated that the auditory system adapted to changes in the input it received from the periphery, and that loudness perception was modulated consequently. The observed changes in loudness and acoustic reflex threshold were interpreted as changes in neuronal gain in the auditory system, and it was proposed that such gain changes might underlie abnormal loudness perception in hyperacusis (Brotherton et al., 2015). LDL measurements in hyperacusis patients generally show a flat, frequency-independent pattern of LDL decreases (Anari et al., 1999; Sheldrake et al., 2015). Theoretical modeling showed that similar decreases in LDLs could be generated by gain mechanisms operating in a frequency-specific manner or across frequencies (Diehl & Schaette, 2015). It remains unclear whether plasticity of loudness might occur in a frequency-specific manner, for example, driven by the amount of input deprivation or additional stimulation at each frequency, or whether it occurs in an unspecific manner through a generalized increase in sensitivity that affects all frequencies.

In the earplug experiments, adult volunteers wore the ear plugs for a maximum duration of 14 days (Formby et al., 2003), and changes in loudness perception were fully reversible within hours to days after earplug removal. However, animal studies provided indications that periods of conductive hearing loss may have long-lasting effects, especially when they occur early in life. When conductive hearing loss was induced by damaging the tympanic membrane in young rats, the animals showed enhanced acoustic startle responses, and even an increased susceptibility to audiogenic seizures. These changes persisted for months even after the hearing loss recovered (Sun et al., 2011). It was also demonstrated that temporary conductive hearing loss caused lasting changes in the brain, with increased neuronal gain upstream of the cochlear nucleus and synaptic changes in the cochlear nucleus (Clarkson et al., 2016). The gain increase would be consistent with hypotheses on loudness hyperacusis. However, the interpretation of animal results remains hampered by the lack of an animal model of hyperacusis. Many studies have relied on measuring the amplitude of the acoustic startle reflex, with increases in amplitude interpreted as a sign of hyperacusis. However, a recent study in humans showed that while elevated startle responses were related to reductions in LDLs, they did not correlate with the patients' self-reports of hyperacusis, as assessed via questionnaires (Knudson and Melcher, 2016).

Conclusions

Recent results have delivered compelling evidence that type II ANFs might act as the pain sensors of the ear (Flores et al., 2015; Liu et al., 2015). While we do not yet understand why the threshold for experiencing pain from sound is decreased in hyperacusis patients, investigations of pathological changes in this system at a peripheral level would be a logical starting point to uncover the mechanisms. For loudness hyperacusis, the evaluation of potential peripheral mechanisms indicated that malfunction of efferent feedback might produce changes to the activity of type I ANFs that would be consistent with decreased LDLs and increased loudness growth. However, if we consider that many patients with DST experience pain from sound, a change in the evaluation of sounds in the central auditory system must also be considered. Offending sound exposures could modify a patient's perception of loudness as a secondary effect of the experience of pain from sound, thereby initiating changes in behavior. We have seen that reducing the input signal to the central auditory system through wearing an earplug can increases loudness perception after the plug is removed (Formby et al., 2003; Munro et al., 2014), and sound avoidance out of fear of pain might have a similar effect. A treatment that reduces the likelihood of experiencing pain from sound might thus also help to renormalize loudness perception.

In the future, a better understanding of the physiology of type II ANFs, especially regarding their activation in patients who experience sound-induced pain, might facilitate development of new treatments for hyperacusis. However, a better understanding of the physiology, and the development of new drugs, requires an animal model of pain hyperacusis, which is unfortunately not available yet. Nevertheless, the finding that retigabine can block the damage response of type II AN fibers (Liu et al., 2015) provides a promising start for the development of pharmacological interventions, as this drug is already approved for human use. Moreover, if the induction of auditory pain in hyperacusis is at the periphery, then the side-effects of retigabine (and those of any other potential new drug) could be minimized if delivered locally through systems for drug administration to the inner ear, and we might thus see some progress toward clinical trials in the not too distant future.

References

American Institute of Physics & Gray, D. E. (1972). *American Institute of Physics Handbook* (3rd ed.). Section editors: B. H. Billings [and others]. Coordinating editor: D. E. Gray. New York, NY: McGraw-Hill.

Anari, M., Axelsson, A., Eliasson, A., & Magnusson, L. (1999). Hypersensitivity to sound—questionnaire data, audiometry and classification. *Scand. Audiol.*, *28*, 219–230.

Andersson, G., Lindvall, N., Hursti, T., & Carlbring, P. (2002). Hypersensitivity to sound (hyperacusis): A prevalence study conducted via the Internet and post. *Int. J. Audiol.*, 41, 545–554.

Auerbach, B. D., Rodrigues, P. V., & Salvi, R. J. (2014). Central gain control in tinnitus and hyperacusis. *Front. Neurol.*, *5*, 206.

Backus, B. C., & Guinan, J. J., Jr. (2006). Time-course of the human medial olivocochlear reflex. *J. Acoust. Soc. Am.*, *119*, 2889–2904.

Baguley, D. M., Axon, P., Winter, I. M., & Moffat, D. A. (2002). The effect of vestibular nerve section upon tinnitus. *Clin. Otolaryngol. Allied Sci.*, *27*, 219–226.

Borg, E. (1973). On the neuronal organization of the acoustic middle ear reflex. A physiological and anatomical study. *Brain Res.*, *49*, 101–123.

Brandy, W. T., & Lynn, J. M. (1995). Audiologic findings in hyperacusic and nonhyperacusic subjects. *Am. J. Audiol.*, *4*, 46–51.

Brotherton, H., Plack, C. J., Maslin, M., Schaette, R., & Munro, K. J. (2015) Pump up the volume: Could excessive neural gain explain tinnitus and hyperacusis? *Audiol. Neurootol.*, *20*, 273–282.

Chen, G. D., & Fechter, L. D. (2003). The relationship between noise-induced hearing loss and hair cell loss in rats. *Hear Res.*, *177*, 81–90.

Chen, Z., Hu, G., Glasberg, B. R., & Moore, B. C. (2011). A new method of calculating auditory excitation patterns and loudness for steady sounds. *Hear Res.*, *282*, 204–215.

Clarkson, C., Antunes, F. M., & Rubio, M. E. (2016). Conductive hearing loss has long-lasting structural and molecular effects on presynaptic and postsynaptic structures of auditory nerve synapses in the cochlear nucleus. *J. Neurosci.*, 36, 10214–10227.

Cooper, N. P., & Guinan, J. J., Jr. (2006). Efferent-mediated control of basilar membrane motion. *J. Physiol.*, *576*, 49–54.

Cox, R. M., Alexander, G. C., Taylor, I. M., & Gray, G. A. (1997). The contour test of loudness perception. *Ear Hear.*, *18*, 388–400.

Dallos, P., & Harris, D. (1978). Properties of auditory nerve responses in absence of outer hair cells. *J. Neurophysiol.*, *41*, 365–383.

Darrow, K. N., Maison, S. F., & Liberman, M. C. (2006). Cochlear efferent feedback balances interaural sensitivity. *Nat. Neurosci.*, *9*, 1474–1476.

Darrow, K. N., Maison, S. F., & Liberman, M. C. (2007). Selective removal of lateral olivocochlear efferents increases vulnerability to acute acoustic injury. *J. Neurophysiol.*, *97*, 1775–1785.

Diehl, P. U., & Schaette, R. (2015). Abnormal auditory gain in hyperacusis: Investigation with a computational model. *Front. Neurol.*, *6*, 157.

Elgoyhen, A. B. F. P. A. (2010). Efferent innervation and function. In: Fuchs, P. A. (Ed.), *Oxford Handbook of Auditory Science: The Ear* (pp. 283–306). Oxford, U.K.: Oxford University Press.

Fabijanska, A., Rogowski, M., Bartnik, G., & Skarzynski, H. (1999). Epidemiology of tinnitus and hyperacusis in Poland. In: *Sixth International Tinnitus Seminar* (pp. 569–571). London, U.K.: The Tinnitus and Hyperacusis Centre.

Fernandez, K. A., Jeffers, P. W., Lall, K., Liberman, M. C., & Kujawa, S. G. (2015). Aging after noise exposure: Acceleration of cochlear synaptopathy in "recovered" ears. *J. Neurosci.*, *35*, 7509–7520.

Flores, E. N., Duggan, A., Madathany, T., Hogan, A. K., Marquez, F. G., Kumar, G., Seal, R. P., Edwards, R. H., Liberman, M. C., & Garcia-Anoveros, J. (2015) A non-canonical pathway from cochlea to brain signals tissue-damaging noise. *Curr. Biol.*, *25*, 606–612.

Formby, C., Sherlock, L. P., & Gold, S. L. (2003). Adaptive plasticity of loudness induced by chronic attenuation and enhancement of the acoustic background. *J. Acoust. Soc. Am.*, *114*, 55–58.

Formby, C., Gold, S. L., Keaser, M. L., Block, K. L., & Hawley, M. L. (2007). Secondary benefits from tinnitus retraining therapy: Clinically significant increases in loudness discomfort level and expansion of the auditory dynamic range. *Seminars in Hearing*, *28*, 227–260.

Francis, H. W., Ryugo, D. K., Gorelikow, M. J., Prosen, C. A., & May, B. J. (2003). The functional age of hearing loss in a mouse model of presbycusis. II. Neuroanatomical correlates. *Hear. Res.*, *183*, 29–36.

Furman, A. C., Kujawa, S. G., & Liberman, M. C. (2013). Noise-induced cochlear neuropathy is selective for fibers with low spontaneous rates. *J. Neurophysiol.*, *110*, 577–586.

Gates, G. A., & Mills, J. H. (2005). Presbycusis. *Lancet*, *366*, 1111–1120.

Gu, J. W., Halpin, C. F., Nam, E. C., Levine, R. A., & Melcher, J. R. (2010). Tinnitus, diminished sound-level tolerance, and elevated auditory activity in humans with clinically normal hearing sensitivity. *J. Neurophysiol.*, *104*, 3361–3370.

Guinan, J. J., Jr. (2006). Olivocochlear efferents: Anatomy, physiology, function, and the measurement of efferent effects in humans. *Ear Hear.*, *27*, 589–607.

Guinan, J. J., Jr., & Gifford, M. L. (1988). Effects of electrical stimulation of efferent olivocochlear neurons on cat auditory-nerve fibers. I. Rate-level functions. *Hear Res.*, *33*, 97–113.

Hesse, L. L., Bakay, W. H., Anderson, L., Ong, H.- C., Ashmore, J., McAlpine, D., Linden, J. F., & Schaette, R. (2016). Non-monotonic relation between noise exposure severity and neuronal hyperactivity in the auditory midbrain. *Front. Neurol.*, *7*.

Hickox, A. E., & Liberman, M. C. (2014). Is noise-induced cochlear neuropathy key to the generation of hyperacusis or tinnitus? *J. Neurophysiol.*, *111*, 552–564.

Kaltenbach, J. A., Schmidt, R. N., & Kaplan, C. R. (1992). Tone-induced stereocilia lesions as a function of exposure level and duration in the hamster cochlea. *Hear. Res.*, *60*, 205–215.

Knudson, I. M., & Melcher, J. R. (2016). Elevated acoustic startle responses in humans: Relationship to reduced loudness discomfort level, but not self-report of hyperacusis. *J. Assoc. Res. Otolaryngol.*, *17*, 223–235.

Kujawa, S. G., & Liberman, M. C. (2009). Adding insult to injury: Cochlear nerve degeneration after "temporary" noise-induced hearing loss. *J. Neurosci.*, *29*, 14077–14085.

Le Prell, C. G., Halsey, K., Hughes, L. F., Dolan, D. F., & Bledsoe, S. C., Jr. (2005). Disruption of lateral olivocochlear neurons via a dopaminergic neurotoxin depresses sound-evoked auditory nerve activity. *J. Assoc. Res. Otolaryngol.*, *6*, 48–62.

Lendvai, B., Halmos, G. B., Polony, G., Kapocsi, J., Horvath, T., Aller, M., Sylvester Vizi, E., & Zelles, T. (2011). Chemical neuroprotection in the cochlea: The modulation of dopamine release from lateral olivocochlear efferents. *Neurochem. Int.*, *59*, 150–158.

Liberman, L. D., Suzuki, J., & Liberman, M. C. (2015). Dynamics of cochlear synaptopathy after acoustic overexposure. *J. Assoc. Res. Otolaryngol.*, *16*, 205–219.

Liberman, M. C. (1984). Single-neuron labeling and chronic cochlear pathology. I. Threshold shift and characteristic-frequency shift. *Hear. Res.*, *16*, 33–41.

Liberman, M. C., & Dodds, L. W. (1984a). Single-neuron labeling and chronic cochlear pathology. III. Stereocilia damage and alterations of threshold tuning curves. *Hear. Res.*, *16*, 55–74.

Liberman, M. C., & Dodds, L. W. (1984b). Single-neuron labeling and chronic cochlear pathology. II. Stereocilia damage and alterations of spontaneous discharge rates. *Hear. Res.*, *16*, 43–53.

Liberman, M. C., & Kiang, N. Y. (1984). Single-neuron labeling and chronic cochlear pathology. IV. Stereocilia damage and alterations in rate- and phase-level functions. *Hear. Res.*, 16, 75–90.

Liberman, M. C., Liberman, L. D., & Maison, S. F. (2014). Efferent feedback slows cochlear aging. *J. Neurosci.*, *34*, 4599–4607.

Liu, C., Glowatzki, E., & Fuchs, P. A. (2015). Unmyelinated type II afferent neurons report cochlear damage. *Proc. Natl. Acad. Sci. U.S.A.*, *112*, 14723–14727.

Lobarinas, E., Salvi, R., & Ding, D. (2013). Insensitivity of the audiogram to carboplatin induced inner hair cell loss in chinchillas. *Hearing Research*, *302*, 113–120.

Maison, S. F., Usubuchi, H., & Liberman, M. C. (2013). Efferent feedback minimizes cochlear neuropathy from moderate noise exposure. *J. Neurosci.*, *33*, 5542–5552.

Makary, C. A., Shin, J., Kujawa, S. G., Liberman, M. C., & Merchant, S. N. (2011). Age-related primary cochlear neuronal degeneration in human temporal bones. *J. Assoc. Res. Otolaryngol.*, *12*, 711–717.

Meddis, R., Lecluyse, W., Clark, N. R., Jurgens, T., Tan, C. M., Panda, M. R., & Brown, G. J. (2013). A computer model of the auditory periphery and its application to the study of hearing. *Adv. Exp. Med. Biol.*, *787*, 11–20.

Moore, B. C. (2004). Dead regions in the cochlea: conceptual foundations, diagnosis, and clinical applications. *Ear Hear.*, *25*, 98–116.

Munro, K. J., & Blount, J. (2009). Adaptive plasticity in brainstem of adult listeners following earplug-induced deprivation. *J. Acoust. Soc. Am.*, *126*, 568–571.

Munro, K. J., Merrett, J. F. (2013). Brainstem plasticity and modified loudness following short-term use of hearing aids. *J. Acoust. Soc. Am.*, *133*, 343–349.

Munro, K. J., Turtle, C., & Schaette, R. (2014). Sub-cortical plasticity and modified loudness following short-term unilateral deprivation: evidence of multiple neural gain mechanisms within the auditory system. To appear in *J. Acoust. Soc. Am.*

Norena, A. J., & Chery-Croze, S. (2007). Enriched acoustic environment rescales auditory sensitivity. *Neuroreport.*, *18*, 1251–1255.

Nouvian, R., Eybalin, M., & Puel, J. L. (2015). Cochlear efferents in developing adult and pathological conditions. *Cell Tissue Res.*, *361*, 301–309.

Paulin, J., Andersson, L., & Nordin, S. (2016). Characteristics of hyperacusis in the general population. *Noise Health*, *18*, 178–184.

Plutchik, R. (1963). Auditory pain thresholds for intermittent, "beat" and steady signals. *Percept. Mot. Skills*, *16*, 863–870.

Roberts, L. E., Eggermont, J. J., Caspary, D. M., Shore, S. E., Melcher, J. R., & Kaltenbach, J. A. (2010). Ringing ears: The neuroscience of tinnitus. *J. Neurosci.*, *30*, 14972–14979.

Rosing, S. N., Schmidt, J. H., Wedderkopp, N., & Baguley, D. M. (2016). Prevalence of tinnitus and hyperacusis in children and adolescents: a systematic review. *BMJ Open*, 6, e010596.

Ryugo, D. K. (1992). The auditory nerve: Peripheral innervation, cell body morphology, and central projections. In D. B. Webster, A. N. Popper, & R. R. Fay (Eds.), *The mammalian auditory pathway, neuroanatomy* (pp. 23–65). New York: Springer.

Sammeth, C. A., Preves, D. A., & Brandy, W. T. (2000). Hyperacusis: Case studies and evaluation of electronic loudness suppression devices as a treatment approach. *Scand. Audiol.*, *29*, 28–36.

Schaette, R., & Kempter, R. (2006). Development of tinnitus-related neuronal hyperactivity through homeostatic plasticity after hearing loss: A computational model. *Eur. J. Neurosci.*, *23*, 3124–3138.

Schmiedt, R. A., & Zwislocki, J. J. (1980). Effects of hair cell lesions on responses of cochlear nerve fibers. II. Single- and two-tone intensity functions in relation to tuning curves. *J. Neurophysiol.*, *43*, 1390–1405.

Sergeyenko, Y., Lall, K., Liberman, M. C., & Kujawa, S. G. (2013). Age-related cochlear synaptopathy: an early-onset contributor to auditory functional decline. *J. Neurosci.*, *33*, 13686–13694.

Sheldrake, J., Diehl, P. U., & Schaette, R. (2015). Audiometric characteristics of hyperacusis patients. *Front. Neurol.*, *6*, 105.

Sherlock, L. P., Formby, C. (2005). Estimates of loudness, loudness discomfort, and the auditory dynamic range: Normative estimates, comparison of procedures, and test-retest reliability. *J. Am. Acad. Audiol.*, *16*, 85–100.

Smalt, C. J., Heinz, M. G., Strickland, E. A. (2014). Modeling the time-varying and level-dependent effects of the medial olivocochlear reflex in auditory nerve responses. *J. Assoc. Res. Otolaryngol.*, *15*, 159–173.

Song, Q., Shen, P., Li, X., Shi, L., Liu, L., Wang, J., . . . Wang, J. (2016). Coding deficits in hidden hearing loss induced by noise: The nature and impacts. *Sci. Rep.*, *6*, 25200.

Soucek, S., Michaels, L., & Frohlich, A. (1986). Evidence for hair cell degeneration as the primary lesion in hearing loss of the elderly. *J. Otolaryngol.*, *15*, 175–183.

Sun, W., Manohar, S., Jayaram, A., Kumaraguru, A., Fu, Q., Li, J., & Allman, B. (2011). Early age conductive hearing loss causes audiogenic seizure and hyperacusis behavior. *Hear Res.*, *282*, 178–183.

Tagoe, T., Barker, M., Jones, A., Allcock, N., & Hamann, M. (2014). Auditory nerve perinodal dysmyelination in noise-induced hearing loss. *J. Neurosci.*, *34*, 2684–2688.

Tyler, R. S., Pienkowski, M., Roncancio, E. R., Jun, H. J., Brozoski, T., Dauman, N., . . . Moore, B. C. (2014). A review of hyperacusis and future directions: Part I. Definitions and manifestations. *Am. J. Audiol.*, *23*, 402–419.

van Ruijven, M. W., de Groot, J. C., & Smoorenburg, G. F. (2004). Time sequence of degeneration pattern in the guinea pig cochlea during cisplatin administration. A quantitative histological study. *Hear Res.*, *197*, 44–54.

Wang, J., Powers, N. L., Hofstetter, P., Trautwein, P., Ding, D., & Salvi, R. (1997) Effects of selective inner hair cell loss on auditory nerve fiber threshold, tuning and spontaneous and driven discharge rate. *Hear Res.*, *107*, 67–82.

Weisz, C., Glowatzki, E., & Fuchs, P. (2009). The postsynaptic function of type II cochlear afferents. *Nature*, *461*, 1126–1129.

Weisz, C. J., Lehar, M., Hiel, H., Glowatzki, E., & Fuchs, P. A. (2012). Synaptic transfer from outer hair cells to type II afferent fibers in the rat cochlea. *J. Neurosci.*, *32*, 9528–9536.

Zaugg, T. L., Thielman, E. J., Griest, S., Henry, J. A. (2016). Subjective reports of trouble tolerating sound in daily life versus loudness discomfort levels. *Am. J. Audiol.*, *25*, 359–363.

Zeng, F. G. (2013). An active loudness model suggesting tinnitus as increased central noise and hyperacusis as increased nonlinear gain. *Hear Res.*, *295*, 172–179.

Zheng, X. Y., Henderson, D., McFadden, S. L., Ding, D. L., Salvi, R. J. (1999). Auditory nerve fiber responses following chronic cochlear de-efferentation. *J. Comp. Neurol.*, *406*, 72–86.

6

Tinnitus and Hyperacusis: Relationship, Mechanisms, and Initiating Conditions

Larry E. Roberts, Tanit Ganz Sanchez, and Ian C. Bruce

A university student contacted our laboratory asking whether we might be able to suppress his tinnitus. He had experienced tinnitus for about 10 years following a sports-related concussion but it had worsened and was now affecting his studies. His audiogram measured in the laboratory showed hearing thresholds below 5 dB HL at frequencies to 16 kHz except for a small but notable notch peaking at 20 dB HL centered at 10 kHz. Tinnitus loudness measured by matching to a 1 kHz sound (where hearing thresholds were 0 dB HL or better) was 50.5 dB SPL. His tinnitus spectrum stepped up at 3 kHz and plateaued in the range of 6 to 12 kHz, which is typical of young subjects measured in our laboratory who have clinically normal hearing thresholds. Our subject also experienced a modest residual inhibition to band-limited noise maskers with center frequencies in this frequency region. Although he consulted our laboratory for tinnitus, reduced sound level tolerance also appeared to be a problem. Upon follow-up about a year later his parents indicated that increased sound sensitivity had led their son to avoid public places, especially shopping malls which were intolerable and made his tinnitus worse. We were able to contact our subject 7 years after his initial laboratory session. He reported then that while he still experienced tinnitus, its intrusiveness and his sensitivity to sound had diminished to the point that quality of life was no longer affected.

Introduction

While tinnitus (chronic ringing of the ears) and hyperacusis (where ordinary environmental sounds are perceived to be intolerably loud) are frequently co-morbid conditions, the nature of their relationship is increasingly a topic of discussion (Nelson & Chen, 2004; Sheldrake, Diehl, & Schaette, 2015; Pienkowski et al., 2014). Population surveys suggest that tinnitus is the more prevalent condition affecting approximately 15% of adults (Shargorodsky, Curhan, & Farwell et al., 2010), which is about twice that of hyperacusis (Andersson, Lindvall, Hursti, & Carlbring, 2002). Consistent with these statistics, it has been observed that 86% of individuals with hyperacusis report tinnitus but only about 40% of tinnitus patients report hyperacusis (Baguley, 2003). A limiting factor, however, is that the two phenomena likely have different thresholds for self-reporting. Chronic tinnitus is a continuous phantom percept that intrudes on consciousness while hyperacusis requires the presence of sound for its expression and may not be noticed in quiet environments but only when moderate to high level environmental sounds are present.

The possibility of a different threshold for reporting hyperacusis suggests that more objective psychoacoustic measurements are needed to establish its presence in a tinnitus patient. One such measure is to determine the level of a sound at which a subject reports discomfort and a preference not to be presented with still louder sounds (loudness discomfort level, LDL). Another method is to measure the slope of functions relating the perceived loudness of a sound to the physical intensity of that sound (loudness growth functions, LGF). Both measures require norms based on population data gathered using standardized clinical procedures for their interpretation in individual cases. While such data are presently limited, Sherlock and Formby (2005) concluded from their study of 59 normal hearing adults that LDL provides a simple and valid measure of the threshold for discomfort that may be useful in assessing sound level tolerance (SLT) in clinical populations. LDLs have been found to be about 15 dB lower in hyperacusis sufferers compared to controls (Sheldrake, Diehl, & Schaette, 2015), and the slope of LGFs is similarly steeper in hyperacusis patients (Noreña & Chery-Croze, 2007). LDL also correlates with cortical metabolic blood oxygenation level dependent (BOLD) responses evoked by a 95-dB noise burst (Gu et al., 2010) and with the amplitude of the acoustic startle response (ASR), an involuntary eye blink that increases with physical sound intensity (Knudsen & Melcher, 2016). However, while these results support the utility of LDL, LGF slope, and ASR as measures of loudness perception, neither measure uniquely identifies individuals seeking treatment for hyperacusis in an otolaryngology clinic ("clinical" hyperacusis). Sheldrake, Diehl, and Schaette (2015) found that an LDL of ~90 dB SPL was sufficient to identify 90% of individuals within a group of hyperacusis patients, but at a cost of about 50% of false positive errors; a more stringent LDL of ~70 dB SPL identified ~30% of hyperacusis patients with no false positives, but at a cost of ~70% false negative errors. The relationship of LDL and the ASR to hyperacusis assessed by questionnaires is also inconsistent (Knudsen & Melcher, 2016; Gu et al., 2010). These results suggest that while LDL, LGF slope, and the ASR are sensitive to loudness perception, abnormal loudness perception may not be the only factor that brings an individual to seek clinical help for hyperacusis. Psychological factors such as fear of sound and the impact of reduced SLT on quality of life may modulate auditory perceptual responses in quiet environments and increase the likelihood of ascertainment by a clinic. In this chapter we will focus on hyperacusis defined as reduced SLT measured by LDLs, LGFs, ASRs, and similar psychoacoustic methods, recognizing that these measures may not capture all aspects of clinical hyperacusis.

A further distinction is between hyperacusis so defined and recruitment. In recruitment, perceived loudness grows rapidly above the threshold of hearing, which is typically in the audiometric hearing loss range. Subsequently the LGF plateaus follow a near-normal course at higher sound intensities. In hyperacusis, on the other hand, perceived sound intensity exceeds that associated with normal hearing at higher sound intensities, although at lower intensities loudness perception may be more or less normal. Another difference is that while recruitment is accompanied by audiometric hearing loss, hyperacusis can be observed with or without hearing impairment expressed in the clinical audiogram. Examples of the difference between hyperacusis and recruitment in LGFs measured in hyperacusis patients can be found in Noreña and Chéry-Croze (2007, their Figure 1).

In this chapter we distinguish recruitment from hyperacusis because its mechanism is debated and may be different from that of hyperacusis. It has been suggested that recruitment is caused by a loss of compressive nonlinearity on the basilar membrane owing to OHC damage or by the spread of excitation from cochlear dead regions to adjacent regions with increasing sound intensity (Joris, 2009). These hypotheses imply that recruitment reflects pathology in the cochlear transduction mechanism and thus should be expressed in the behavior of auditory nerve fibers (ANFs), but studies have failed to consistently find such evidence (Joris, 2009; Heinz & Young, 2004). Alternatively, recruitment may be caused by increases in the gain (input/output response) of neurons in central auditory structures that occur following cochlear injuries (Cai, Ma, & Young, 2009; Noreña, 2011). In this alternate explanation, recruitment could be considered to arise from a degree of central gain increase that is commensurate with the amount of audiometric threshold shift and roughly normalizes loudness at higher sound levels, whereas hyperacusis is generated by excessive central gain increases, disproportionate with the audiogram. Furthermore, numerous studies have suggested that central gain increases triggered by cochlear pathology may also lead to aberrant spontaneous neural activity that is perceived as tinnitus. Based on these observations, Zeng (2013) proposed a conceptual framework whereby central gain changes could lead to tinnitus and/or recruitment or hyperacusis, depending on the location(s) and degree(s) of the gain changes. However, Zeng (2013) did not discuss in detail the neural mechanisms potentially involved in tinnitus and hyperacusis or changes in central gain.

In the following we first consider the relationship between hyperacusis and tinnitus by examining the time course of their development, and whether they share a common initiating condition, which could be cochlear pathology that may or may not be hidden from the audiogram. We then discuss the neural changes that appear to underlie tinnitus and hyperacusis from the cochlear nucleus to the auditory cortex, and the implications of the findings for the treatment of both conditions.

The Time Course of Hyperacusis and Tinnitus Development

One approach to understanding the relationship of tinnitus and hyperacusis (defined as reduced SLT) is to compare their development over time in a cohort of participants selected for neither condition. Sanchez et al. (2016) studied the prevalence of both phenomena in a sample of 170 adolescents in a private school, first by a detailed questionnaire that assessed their risky listening habits and prior experience of tinnitus in the natural environment, and then by psychoacoustic measurements in a sound chamber. The audiogram (to 16 kHz), transient evoked and distortion product otoacoustic emissions at several frequencies, and LDL at four frequencies, were measured for all subjects. When tinnitus was heard in the sound booth, its pitch and loudness were determined by audiometric methods. Three groups were distinguished, consisting of (1) adolescents who reported a history of tinnitus on questionnaire and heard it in the sound booth (Group Q+B+, 46/170 or 27.1% of the sample), (2) adolescents reporting tinnitus by questionnaire but did not hear it in the booth (Group Q+B-, 47/170 cases or 27.6% of the sample), or (3) adolescents who reported no experience of tinnitus at all (Group Q-B-, 74/170 cases, 43.5% of the sample). Hearing thresholds and otoacoustic emissions were normal and did not discriminate among the three groups (Figure 6–1, A–C), but LDL did so, being reduced by 11.3 dB ($p < 0.0001$) only for Group Q+B+ where tinnitus was reported by both assessment methods (Figure 6–1D). The tinnitus percepts of these adolescents (loudness and pitch matching) were congruent with those of adult chronic tinnitus sufferers. These findings suggest that tinnitus and reduced SLT follow a similar course of development over time. It should also be noticed that LDL was reduced for all frequencies tested (0.5 to 4 kHz), unlike tinnitus frequencies measured in the sound booth which were concentrated above 3 kHz in accordance with other published data (Henry, Roberts, Ellingson, & Thielman 2013; Roberts et al., 2008; Schaette & McAlpine, 2011). LGFs measured in hyperacusis patients (Noreña & Chery-Croze, 2007) and in tinnitus sufferers with normal audiograms (Hébert, Fournier, & Noreña, 2013) are also steepened across frequencies, in agreement with these LDL data.

Tinnitus verified by questionnaire and psychoacoustic measurement (Group Q+B+, 27.1% of the sample) likely reflects an upper estimate of the prevalence of verified tinnitus in adolescents because new cases of tinnitus can subside over time (Roberts, 2016). It is noteworthy that the adolescents in Group Q+B+ did not appear to have been exposed to more or higher levels of recreational sound than other teens, since risky listening habits were almost universal in the sample. On the contrary, the affected adolescents reported significant tendencies to listen at lower volume levels and to attend parties and raves for a shorter period of time than their unaffected classmates, suggesting that they tended to be comparatively more protective of their hearing. Fifty-four of the 170 subjects tested by Sanchez et al. (2016) were available for retest one year later. On retest 8/54 (14%) of teens qualified as Q+B+ cases, and 6/54 of these cases (11%) were repeat Q+B+ cases. The latter percentage (11%) may be a conservative estimate of prevalence of persistent tinnitus in adolescents that takes into account the possibility that in the absence of continued excessive sound exposure tinnitus may resolve. However, the LDLs of the affected teens were again reduced compared to other teens by an amount (17.2 dB, $p < 0.0002$) that was similar to Group Q+B+ in the initial test (see Figure 6–1D), while their audiograms and otoacoustic emissions (not shown) remained normal and were highly repeatable. A further result was that, while a clear group difference was observed in the averaged LDL data of Figure 6–1D, approximately half of the adolescents in Group Q+B+ at both tests expressed LDLs > 90 dB SPL which overlapped those of adolescents without tinnitus. Thus, reduced LDL and tinnitus while related in the group data were not inextricably linked, in agreement with the results reported in the introductory section of this chapter.

Further information on the time course of tinnitus and reduced SLT came from studies in which input to auditory pathways was attenuated in normal hearing volunteers who wore ear plugs for 1 to 2 weeks. These studies found that auditory deprivation could modulate SLT and the threshold of the middle ear stapedius reflex in normal hearing humans (Formby, Sherlock, & Gold, 2003; Munro, Turtle, & Schaette, 2014; see Brotherton et al., 2015 for a review). In one study, loudness perception at several levels of an LGF decreased

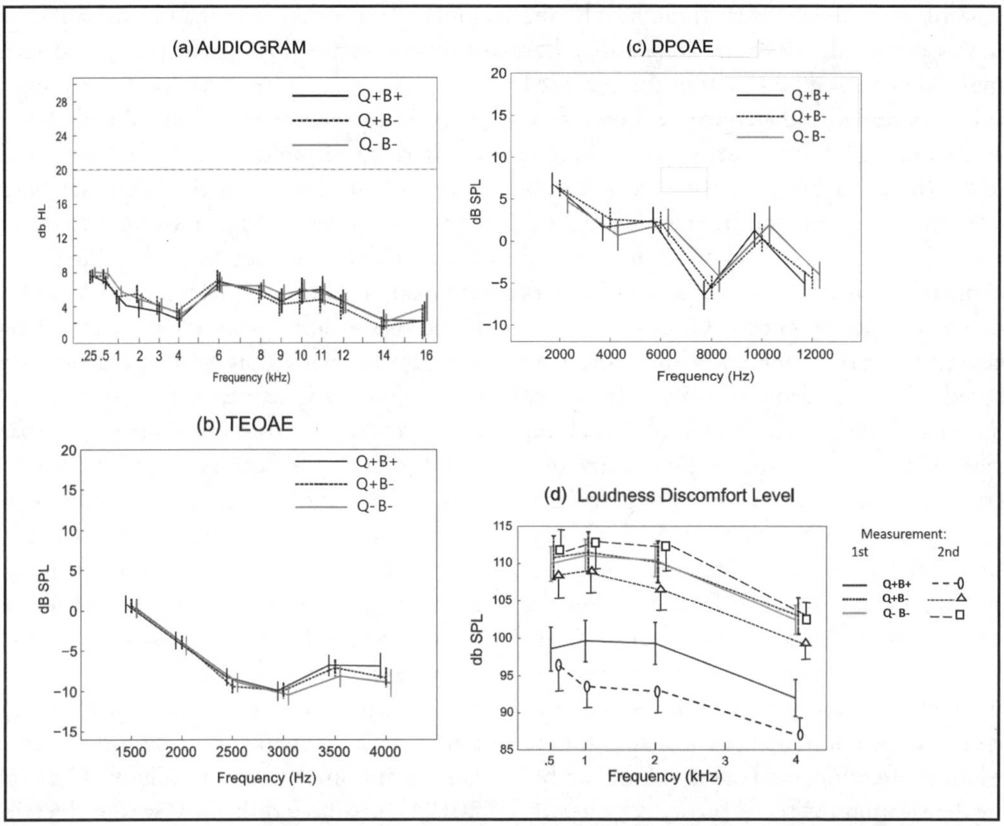

Figure 6–1. Audiometric, otoacoustic, and loudness discomfort level measurements in 170 adolescents. Tinnitus was assessed by questionnaire and by psychoacoustic measurements in a sound booth. Three groups are shown: Q+B+ history of tinnitus reported on questionnaire and verified by psychoacoustic testing in the sound booth (46/170 adolescents); Q+B- history of tinnitus reported by questionnaire but not heard during psychoacoustic testing (47/170 adolescents); Q-B- no history or experience of tinnitus (74/170 adolescents). **A.** Audiogram measured from 0.25–16 kHz. **B.** Transient otoacoustic measurements at six frequencies. **C.** Distortion product otoacoustic emissions at six frequencies. **D.** Loudness discomfort levels measured at four frequencies. Of the original sample of 170 subjects, 54 subjects returned for a second measurement one year later (8/54 Q+B+, 20/54 Q+B-, 26/54 Q-B-). Their data are identified by the symbols and bold broken lines. Their audiograms and otoacoustic emissions were unchanged from the first measurement (data not shown). The bars are ±1 SE (for clarity, only one direction is shown for subjects retested at one year). See text for details. *Source*: A–C. From Sanchez et al. (2016). D. Data are from the study of Sanchez et al. (2016), with new results reported for the follow up.

by ~7 dB in both ears even though only one ear was occluded, while the stapedius reflex threshold decreased by ~3 dB in the occluded ear but increased in the control ear by a similar amount (Munro, Turtle, & Schaette, 2014). These changes were observed at 2 kHz where sound attenuation by the ear plug was maximal (~25 dB) but also at 0.5 kHz where attenuation was less (~8 dB), suggesting frequency nonspecific effects. Opposing effects between the ears on the reflex threshold may be explained by evidence (Darrow, Maison, & Liberman, 2006) that lateral olivocochlear efferents tend to balance neural activation between the two ears over a long integration window, which may aid spatial localization for transient sounds based on interaural level differences. This mechanism would be expected to yield equivalent loudness judgments between the occluded and unoccluded ear which was observed; nonetheless a stimulus of given physical intensity was perceived to be louder after unilateral deprivation than before deprivation (Munro, Turtle, & Schaette, 2014). Munro et al. interpreted their results to suggest that multiple gain mechanisms may be triggered by auditory occlusion. In an animal study, unilateral ear plugging upregulated excitatory glutamatergic receptors on fusiform and bushy cells in the cochlear nucleus within 24 hours ipsilaterally as well as contralaterally, and downregulated inhibitory glycinergic synapses on fusiform cells ipsilaterally, which are further mechanisms that could affect gain in central auditory pathways (Whiting, Moiseff, & Rubio, 2009).

Noting that normal hearing subjects often report phantom sounds after confinement in an anechoic chamber, Schaette, Turtle, and Munro (2012) investigated the effects of ear plugging on tinnitus. Eighteen volunteers with normal hearing wore a silicone ear plug for 1 week, which provided an attenuation of <10 dB at 0.25 kHz and >30 dB at 3 and 4 kHz emulating a mild sensorineural hearing loss. At the end of week 11, participants reported a stable bilateral tinnitus with a measured high-pitched frequency spectrum aligning with that reported by chronic tinnitus sufferers with (Roberts et al., 2008; Noreña, Micheyl, Chery-Croze, & Collet, 2002) or without (Sanchez et al., 2016; Schaette & McAlpine, 2010; Gu, Herrman, Levine, & Melcher, 2012) audiometric hearing loss. Tinnitus resolved when the ear plug was removed, indicating that auditory deprivation was its cause.

The results of studies employing artificial sound attenuation techniques are important because they indicate that the development of tinnitus and reduced SLT follow a similar time course. Rescaling of neural input/output functions (increased central gain) commences at low levels of sound attenuation, which might explain why the audiograms of hyperacusis patients do not necessarily exhibit substantial high frequency hearing loss which is more common in tinnitus patients. Gu et al. (2010) noted how difficult it was to find tinnitus patients with measured normal SLT; cases of reduced SLT without tinnitus were easier to recruit. However, studies of artificial sound attenuation also show that tinnitus and reduced SLT can be induced when the cochlea is intact. We can thus conclude that cochlear pathology is not necessary for either phenomenon, although some level of sound attenuation may be necessary. On the other side of the equation, there are many individuals, particularly among senior citizens, who have permanent high-frequency hearing loss expressed in the audiogram but do not have tinnitus (Roberts et al., 2008; Eggermont, 2012). This may apply to hyperacusis as well, although psychoacoustic data on the topic are lacking. This suggests that cochlear hearing damage alone may not be sufficient for tinnitus or hyperacusis, either.

Yet the three conditions are undeniably related, given the high prevalence of audiometric hearing loss observed in tinnitus and hyperacusis patients compared to the general population. It has been suggested that disparities between hearing loss and tinnitus may reflect a causal role for extracochlear mechanisms in generating chronic tinnitus. Proposed mechanisms include individual differences in the access of tinnitus-related neural activity to brain networks for conscious awareness (De Ridder, Elgoyhen, Romo, & Langguth, 2011) or deficiencies in a proposed noise cancellation system in the subcallosal brain region that modulates an inhibitory feedback loop engaging the reticular nucleus of the thalamus (Rauschecker, Leaver, & Mühlau, 2010). These hypotheses are based on functional imaging evidence for brain changes in these regions in tinnitus (Rauschecker, Leaver, & Mühlau, 2010; Mühlau et al., 2006). However, the evidence is not consistent (Melcher, Knudsen, & Levine, 2013), and the role of the brain changes in modulating or generating tinnitus percepts is debated (Eggermont & Roberts, 2015). Alternatively, we discuss in the following section whether evidence of a role for hidden hearing loss in tinnitus may clarify the relationship of hearing loss to tinnitus and hyperacusis.

Hearing Loss Is an Initiating Condition

Normal hearing requires a healthy cochlear transduction mechanism (outer and inner hair cells and the physical structures that support them) and intact ANFs that connect the inner hair cells to the brain. The audiograms and otoacoustic emissions observed in the young adolescents of Figure 6–1 expressing persistent tinnitus and reduced LDL (Group Q+B+) were robust and not discriminably different from those of adolescents not experiencing these conditions, which suggests that the cochlear transduction mechanism was intact in these young individuals. However, the possibility of hidden injuries to ANFs resulting from the adolescents' near universal exposure to recreational sound cannot be ruled out. ANFs are connected to inner hair cells (IHCs) through synapses containing ribbon-like structures that govern the release of neural transmitters when the IHC is stimulated by sound. ANFs contacting the pillar side of the IHC discharge at very low levels of sound (low threshold fibers, LT ANFs) and therefore determine the threshold of hearing as measured by the audiogram. ANFs contacting the modiolar side of the IHC, on the other hand, are high-threshold fibers (HT ANFs) that discharge only to sounds exceeding ~50 dB SPL. ANFs differing in threshold are one mechanism by which the auditory system codes sound intensity varying over orders of magnitude using neurons that have a limited dynamic range. Several studies have now shown that ribbon synapses on HT ANFs are especially vulnerable to damage by noise exposure (Kujawa & Liberman, 2009; Lin, Furman, Kujawa, & Liberman, 2011; Furman, Kujawa, & Liberman, 2013). This is particularly true for HT ANFs with high frequency tuning, which notably is where tinnitus frequencies typically reside. Kujawa and Liberman (2009) found that ~40% of synaptic ribbons innervating these ANFs in their mouse model were permanently lost following exposure to an octave-band noise for 2 hours at 100 dB that produced a temporary threshold shift (TTS) in the auditory brainstem response (ABR) audiogram but did not permanently elevate audiometric thresholds. In this model, synaptic loss was followed by a delayed loss of 50% of spiral ganglion neurons after 2 years compared to unexposed control animals. Notably, the same level of noise trauma did not affect ribbon synapses on LT ANFs or lead to persisting structural damage to cochlear hair cells or their stereocilia. Thus, permanent cochlear injury induced by noise trauma did not involve the cochlear transduction mechanism but was preferential for ANFs with high firing thresholds and high-frequency tuning (Furman, Kujawa, & Liberman, 2013). Subsequent research in a guinea pig model (Shi et al., 2013) revealed losses of synaptic ribbons of similar magnitude after TTS induced by a 105-dB noise exposure, with greater losses occurring in higher (60 to 70%) compared to lower (10 to 30%) cochleotopic frequency regions in agreement with the frequency profile of Kujawa and Liberman (2009) for the mouse. Similar to the mouse, none of these losses gave a permanent threshold shift (PTS) in the guinea pig model, suggesting that synapses on HT ANFs were predominately affected. However, synapse counts in the guinea pig model showed a more robust recovery than in the mouse, returning to control levels in the low frequency cochleotopic region and recovering to about 80% of control levels in the high frequency region 1 month after noise exposure (Shi et al., 2016a). Nonetheless, persisting ribbon loss in the high frequency cochleotopic region (20%) was sufficient to reduce the compound action potential evoked by suprathreshold sounds and to impair temporal processing ability assessed by a forward masking procedure (Shi et al., 2013). Thus, while much remains to be learned about the effects of noise exposure on ANF synapses and dendrites in different species and how injury is expressed in peripheral and central auditory processing (Shi et al., 2016a,b), it is apparent that not all forms of cochlear injury affect hearing thresholds. Hearing loss arising from HT ANF synaptopathy has been called "hidden hearing loss" because it will not appear in the clinical audiogram (Kujawa & Liberman 2009).

Hidden hearing loss does, however, lead to changes in central auditory pathways that are expressed as hyperacusis-like behavior in animals and humans. Hickox and Liberman (2014) assessed the effect synaptopathic noise trauma in mice on behavioral startle responses (whole body movement sensed by an accelerometer) evoked by tone bursts of increasing level, presented either in quiet or the presence of background noise. Behavioral startle responses are mediated by auditory nerve afferents that project to the pontine reticular formation, ventral cochlear nucleus (VCN), and dorsal cochlea nucleus (DCN), interfacing ultimately with spinal motor neurons evoking whole body movement. All of these structures become hyperactive after noise exposure (Kaltenbach, 2011; Eggermont & Roberts, 2015). In the study of Hickox and Liberman (2014), noise-exposed mice with normal hearing thresholds but verified synaptopathy (hidden hearing loss) exhibited startle responses that were comparable to those of control mice when startle responses were evoked in quiet, but were larger than controls when startle responses were evoked in background noise. Because in the presence of background noise LT but not HT ANFs would have reached saturation, the results revealed changes in central auditory structures innervated by HT ANFs (e.g., the small cap region of the anterior VCN) as the source of increased behavioral excitability. Consistent with this observation, wave I amplitude of the ABR reflecting the output of the cochlea was *reduced* in synaptopathic mice compared to controls when evoked by suprathreshold sounds; however, wave V amplitude which is generated by sources in the auditory midbrain was *increased* in exposed compared to control animals when evoked by sounds of increasing intensity (Hickox & Liberman, 2014). Similar findings have been reported for tinnitus patients with clinically normal audiograms (Schaette & McAlpine, 2011; Gu, Herrman, Levine, & Melcher, 2012). In these studies, ABR wave 1 evoked by clicks >80 dB SPL was reduced in the patients while wave V was normal or enhanced compared to non-tinnitus controls, although Guest et al. (2016) could not confirm a reduced Wave I in tinnitus subjects in their study. Mechanisms of homeostatic and/or Hebbian plasticity are believed to underlie these effects which reflect increased "central gain" in auditory pathways. The association of tinnitus and hyperacusis with reduced LDLs, stapedius reflex thresholds, and steepened LGFs reported above for subjects with normal audiograms is also consistent with increased central gain following hidden hearing loss. Extrapolating to the results of Figure 6–1, tinnitus experienced by the adolescents with reduced LDLs could similarly signal hidden damage to HT ANFs, particularly when these effects persisted during retest 1 year later. Reversible transient injury to the cochlear transduction mechanism insufficient to elevate hearing thresholds or individual differences in synaptic repair could apply to cases in which tinnitus and altered LDL resolved prior to retest.

While hidden loss affecting HT ANFs appears to be present in tinnitus and hyperacusis without threshold shifts, reduced LT ANF activity is likely also a factor, given that high frequency hearing loss is prevalent in these clinical populations. Synaptopathy affecting LT ANFs can also be hidden from the audiogram, since hearing thresholds do not appear to be elevated as long as at least ~20% of IHCs remain intact (Lobarinas, Salvi, & Ding, 2016). Paul, Bruce, and Roberts (2017) applied cochlear modeling using a well-established model of the auditory periphery to investigate the putative contribution of both fiber types to individual differences in temporal processing ability in young adults with and without tinnitus, all of whom had normal audiometric hearing. Subjects were first required to detect the presence of amplitude modulation (AM) in a 5-kHz tone embedded in background noise intended to degrade the contribution of LT fibers, such that AM coding was preferentially reliant on HT fibers. The frequency of 5 kHz was chosen because this frequency was in the tinnitus frequency region of the tinnitus subjects. Subsequently neural coding in the auditory midbrain was measured using the "envelope following response" (EFR), a response recorded by electroencephalography (EEG) that has been shown to correlate with temporal processing skills in normal hearing listeners (Bharadwaj et al., 2015) and to be sensitive to noise-induced ANF synaptopathy in animals (Shaheen, Valero, & Liberman, 2015). EFRs were measured in background noise where HT fibers were expected to be required to encode the AM, and also in quiet where both LT and HT ANFs were expected to contribute to AM coding. Paul et al. found that subjects without tinnitus whose EFRs were comparatively resistant to the addition of background noise had better AM detection thresholds in background noise than subjects whose EFRs were more affected by noise. Simulated auditory nerve responses using the peripheral model suggested that synaptic losses affecting HT ANFs alone were sufficient to explain the EFR results of non-tinnitus subjects with poor AM coding. In comparison, tinnitus subjects had worse AM detection thresholds and exhibited reduced EFRs overall compared to controls, even though thresholds for the test stimuli averaged <2 dB HL in both groups. Simulated auditory nerve responses found that in addition to severe HT fiber loss, a degree of LT fiber loss that would not be expected to affect audiometric thresholds was needed to explain the results of the tinnitus subjects. Thus, while HT synaptic loss appeared to degrade temporal coding ability, additional LT fiber losses hidden from the audiogram were necessary to explain tinnitus (Paul, Bruce, & Roberts, 2017).

These observations do not rule out a role for extracochlear mechanisms in cases of tinnitus and hyperacusis without audiometric hearing loss, or of hearing loss without either condition. However, they suggest that hidden hearing losses could in principle be sufficient to explain many such cases. LT fiber synaptopathy appears to be especially important, in part because loss of these fibers is likely accompanied by damage to the more vulnerable HT fibers. However, an important functional difference between LT and HT fibers is that LT ANFs exhibit much higher rates of spontaneous activity in quiet than do HT fibers. Accordingly, LT fibers are often referred to as high-spontaneous rate (HSR) fibers in the literature, although the designation HSR/LT fibers would be more accurate. Injury to HSR/LT fibers appears to add a tinnitus deficit to impaired temporal processing in individuals where hearing thresholds are normal. In the next section we review evidence regarding how hearing loss (hidden or otherwise) may lead to tinnitus and hyperacusis. Because tinnitus and hyperacusis have different frequency profiles, their mechanisms must to some extent be distinguishable although they are likely to interact by virtue of sharing a common initiating condition.

Distinguishable Mechanisms for Tinnitus and Hyperacusis

Experiments on ear plugging discussed above indicate that reducing input to auditory pathways by as little as 20 dB SPL can be sufficient to trigger an increase in central gain and decrease SLT in humans and animal models, even when the cochlea is intact. This indicates that when the initiating condition of cochlear injuries sufficient to reduce auditory nerve activity is present, changes in central gain will occur and thus be present not only in hyperacusis but also overlap those involved in tinnitus, although for the reasons discussed above the degree of ANF impairment required for a clinically-significant tinnitus may be greater than that needed for hyperacusis-like behavior. In the following we first consider the mechanisms that may lead to tinnitus and its distinctive frequency profile, and then shift the focus to hyperacusis. Events occurring in subcortical auditory structures converge on the thalamus and cortex, which can be expected to play a role in both phenomena.

Spotlight on Tinnitus

Neural changes associated with tinnitus have been studied by exposing animals to putative tinnitus-inducing procedures such as salicylate administration or to noise trauma which can be scaled to give TTS or PTS (Hickox & Liberman, 2014; Kujawa & Liberman, 2009). The presence of tinnitus has subsequently been evaluated by methods such as gap detection (a silent gap inserted in a sound delivered prior to an acoustic startle stimulus will suppress a startle response, unless tinnitus fills the gap) or by making a tinnitus-like sound a cue for a behavioral response (responding in quiet after a tinnitus-inducing manipulation signals tinnitus). Noise exposure producing TTS or PTS can also enhance sound-driven behavioral responses suggesting hyperacusis (Hickox & Liberman, 2014) although to date the emphasis has been on studying tinnitus. Aside from enabling physiological investigations, an advantage of these models is that animals can be divided into those expressing evidence of tinnitus and those that do not, when their preceding experience has been the same.

It has long been known that noise trauma sufficient to damage the cochlear transduction mechanism or auditory nerve synapses reduces the spontaneous and driven activity in the auditory nerve (Eggermont & Roberts, 2004). In response to reduced input from the auditory nerve, neurons in central auditory structures tend to become hyperactive, reflecting changes in central gain that restore the responsiveness of neurons in central auditory pathways to their remaining inputs. Hyperactivity is expressed as an increase in the spontaneous firing rates (SFRs) of auditory neurons and in their sound-evoked responses, both of which have been recorded at all levels of the auditory pathway in animals subjected to traumatizing noise or to ototoxic drugs that selectively destroy IHCs (reviewed by Kaltenbach, 2011; Eggermont & Roberts, 2015; Shore, Roberts, & Langguth, 2016; Salvi et al., 2017; Hesse et al., 2016). Increased driven responses are likely to relate to hyperacusis, while increases in the SFRs of auditory neurons are likely to relate to tinnitus as it is a persisting phantom percept. Supporting this view, SFRs and driven responses have been found to increase in animals that express behavioral evidence of tinnitus compared to animals that do not, implicating these phenomena as part of the tinnitus phenotype. Increased SFRs specific to tinnitus animals have been reported in the ventral (Volger, Robertson, & Mulders, 2011) and dorsal (Koehler & Shore, 2013) cochlear nucleus, the inferior colliculus (IC) (Middleton et al. 2011), and in the auditory cortex (Basura, Kohler, & Shore, 2015), reflecting propagation of increased SFRs up the auditory pathway or mechanisms operating locally in these structures.

A further neural correlate observed in animals expressing tinnitus behavior compared to animals that do not is an increase in the cross-correlated (*synchronous*) activity of neurons within the DCN and higher auditory structures. In DCN increased synchrony following noise-induced TTS was seen among neurons connected primarily by short physical and tonotopic distances but also by longer distances, giving tinnitus a spectral profile situated about 1 octave above the exposure band which is where TTS was most strongly expressed (Wu, Martel, & Shore, 2016). While SFRs also increased in this frequency region, SFRs have been observed to increase below the exposure frequencies as well (Dehmel et al., 2012), suggesting a difference in the frequency profile of tinnitus-related synchrony compared to that of SFRs. These results concur with those reported in an early study of cats with hearing loss induced by noise exposure (tinnitus was not tested). In this research, SFRs increased across the tonotopic frequency map of primary auditory cortex below as well as in the hearing loss frequencies, while increased synchrony was confined to the hearing loss region (Noreña & Eggermont, 2003). Because human tinnitus percepts may similarly localize to the hearing loss frequencies (Noreña, Micheyl, Chery-Croze, & Collet, 2002; Roberts et al., 2008), aberrant neural synchrony has been proposed by several authors as the proximal neural correlate of tinnitus. A neural synchrony code for phantom sound is also consistent with the principle that synchronous firing among a group of neurons may be used by the brain to detect an acoustic event in the environment using neural elements (ANFs) that are inherently spontaneously active (Eggermont, 1990).

One unanswered question is how increased synchrony and SFRs associated with tinnitus develop following noise-induced TTS and PTS. Wu, Martel, and Shore (2016) observed that while SFR and synchrony were increased in their tinnitus animals, changes in synchrony and SFRs were poorly correlated in the data, in part because synchrony between long-distance unit pairs with low cross-correlation strengths were increased specifically in the tinnitus animals and corresponded more closely with their tinnitus frequencies. One factor affecting synchronous activity in a tonotopic map could be down regulation of glycinergic inhibition, which has been observed in the DCN of tinnitus animals (Wang et al., 2009) as well as after cochlear ablation in the guinea pig (Potashner, Suneja, & Benson, 2000). In this respect, it may be instructive to consider what the functional role of this inhibition might be in the DCN, and how its loss might generate tinnitus-like behavior after PTS or TTS.

Fusiform cells in the DCN are the first site of cross-modal auditory and somatosensory integration in auditory pathways (Oertel &

Young, 2004; Zeng et al., 2009). Inputs from the auditory nerve contact the basal dendrites of fusiform cells, which are then targeted after one synaptic delay by strong feed-forward inhibition from glycinergic vertical cells contacted by the same ANF (Sedlacek & Brenowitz, 2014). In contrast, somatosensory information from the head and neck region is conveyed by parallel fibers to the apical dendrites of fusiform cells, which are similarly targeted by feed-forward inhibition on their cell bodies (from cartwheel cells driven by parallel fibers in this case) after one synaptic delay (Roberts & Trussell, 2010; Mancilla & Manis, 2009). Koehler & Shore (2013) found that the timing rules of spike-timing dependent plasticity (STDP) induced by paired bimodal auditory-somatosensory stimulation were changed in animals giving behavioral evidence of tinnitus, such that potentiation dominated over suppression for a wider range of bimodal intervals on parallel fiber synapses (Wu, Martel, & Shore, 2016). One mechanism leading to this change could be a loss of feedforward inhibition from ANFs via vertical cells onto fusiform cells, which may in the intact brain gate STDP on the parallel fibers protecting synapses that convey temporally convergent auditory and somatosensory inputs to the neuron from down-regulation while other synapses are weakened. If feedforward inhibition driven from the auditory pathway is diminished or lost owing to deafferentation, STDP could be unleashed on synapses connecting parallel fibers to fusiform apical dendrites, leading to increased synchronous activity among fusiform cells and to tinnitus. Diminished feedforward inhibition (Ma & Young, 2009) does not necessarily require a downregulation in inhibitory neurotransmitter but may simply be caused by reduced input from ANFs to the DCN neural circuitry following deafferentation (Zheng et al., 2009). Integration among multiple somatosensory inputs gated by feedforward inhibition from cartwheel cells would continue unchecked in this scenario, since cartwheel cells are driven by parallel fiber and not ANF activity. Plasticity unleashed on parallel fibers may explain why glutamate transporters in somatosensory pathways are upregulated when the auditory nerve is cut (Zeng et al., 2009) and why up to 80% of chronic tinnitus sufferers are able to modulate their tinnitus by clenching their jaws and similar movements of the head and neck region (Levine, Abel, & Cheng, 2003; Sanchez et al., 2002).

If the mechanism just described is one contributing to hypersynchrony in the DCN, loss of LT ANF inputs would be especially patholytic. This is because in normal hearing the high rates of spontaneous firing of these robust ANFs may be sufficient to constrain STDP on parallel fiber synapses preventing maladaptive plasticity. In contrast, HT ANFs exhibit lower rates of spontaneous activity such that their loss would have a smaller effect, although these ANFs are important for coding suprathreshold sounds (Paul, Bruce, & Roberts, 2107; Bharadwaj et al., 2014). Consistent with a role for LT ANFs in hypersynchrony, behavioral evidence of tinnitus in animals has been found to correlate with the magnitude of PTS (Bauer, Brozoski, & Myers, 2007) with a similar trend ($r = 0.539$, $p = 0.10$) following TTS (Wu, Martel, & Shore, 2016) although the findings are not consistent on this point (Li, Kalappa, & Tzounopoulos, 2015).

It is recognized, however, that other mechanisms could be at work in the DCN or elsewhere in addition to (or instead of) this process. Altered GABAergic inhibition has been demonstrated in tissue slices taken from the DCN of mice giving behavioral evidence of tinnitus, although the role of this form of inhibition in tinnitus behavior is not known (Middleton et al., 2011). The DCN is targeted by a dense serotonergic input that increases the probability of spikes evoked in fusiform cells by parallel fiber stimulation but not by stimulation of the auditory nerve (Tang &Trussell,

2015, 2017). Cholinergic neuromodulators are also known to act via endocannabinoid signaling to convert long-term potentiation (LTP) to long-term depression (LTD) at DCN parallel fiber synapses (Zhao & Tzounopoulos, 2011). Blockade of cholinergic muscarinic receptors by atropine infused into the fusiform cell layer of the DCN decreased the spontaneous firing rates of fusiform cells and increased their synchrony (Stefanescu & Shore, 2017), revealing effects of cholinergic modulation that altered the rules of STDP in the direction of those seen in tinnitus animals. Changes in intrinsic membrane conductance are a further consideration and have been reported in the fusiform cells of mice giving behavioral evidence of tinnitus (Li, Choi, & Tzounopoulos, 2013). Overall, it seems likely that neural correlates of tinnitus are generated by multiple processes involving reduced inhibition (Wang et al., 2009; Middleton et al., 2011), altered synaptic plasticity (Koehler & Shore, 2013), changes in central gain (Noreña, 2011), and alterations in intrinsic ion channels (Li, Choi, & Tzounopoulos, 2013) that occur consequent on deafferentation of auditory pathways.

Finally, the feedforward circuitry seen in the DCN is observed at other levels of the brain including the primary auditory cortex and the cerebellum, where changes could be generated independently or in parallel with subcortical mechanisms. Tinnitus-related activation has been reported in these structures in electrophysiological recordings and functional imaging of tinnitus in animal models (Yang et al., 2011; Basura, Koehler, & Shore, 2013; Bauer, Wisner, Sybert, & Brozoski, 2013) and human tinnitus patients (Gu et al., 2010; Lanting, Woźniak, van Dijk, & Langers, 2016). Computational studies have shown how changes in the auditory cortex due to homeostatic plasticity (HSP) following deafferentation could generate synchronous activity and map reorganization in this structure (Dominguez, Becker, Bruce, & Read, 2006; Chrostowski et al., 2011) both of which have been reported in tinnitus patients (Weisz et al., 2007; Wienbruch et al., 2006). One important aspect of cortical and subcortical HSP is how it interacts with Hebbian plasticity such as STDP. When the model of Chrostowski et al. (2011) was extended in Chrostowski (2012) to include STDP, it was found that changes in cortical connectivity initiated by HSP after deafferentation became consolidated and magnified through STDP. Another possible interaction between HSP and STDP can occur due to the *failure* of HSP to appropriately regulate STDP, one of HSP's main functions in addition to setting overall levels of activity (Turrigiano & Nelson, 2008). In the study of Rüttiger et al. (2013), sound-exposed rats were more likely to develop behavioral evidence of tinnitus if they exhibited substantial ANF deafferentation *and* reduced expression of Arc, a gene involved in HSP. If HSP fails, then unconstrained STDP could lead to destabilization of cortical networks and increased spontaneous synchrony. We discuss the role of thalamocortical pathways in tinnitus and hyperacusis further, in a later section below.

Spotlight on Hyperacusis

While STDP occurring after TTS/PTS and its effects conveyed to the auditory cortex may give tinnitus its distinctive frequency profile, other changes taking place in auditory pathways following hearing impairment may relate more closely to hyperacusis. In principle, interrelated mechanisms are likely to contribute.

One mechanism involves forms of HSP that adjust the input/output functions (gain) of neurons in central auditory pathways to maintain neuron firing rates within their dynamic ranges in different acoustic environments or when acoustic input is diminished by hearing injuries (Pozo & Goda, 2010). In one example, Qui, Salvi, Ding, and Burkard et al. (2000) recorded the response evoked by a sound in the auditory nerve, the IC, and auditory cortex, of chinchillas in which ~30% of IHCs had been destroyed by an ototoxic drug (carboplatin). Input/output functions were reduced for the auditory nerve response (compound action potential) reflecting suprathreshold hearing impairment, but were near-normal in the IC and normal or supranormal in the auditory cortex, revealing an increase in gain as the recording site ascended the auditory pathway (also see Syka, Rybalko, & Popelář, 1994). HSP could increase gain by increasing presynaptic neural transmitter release, modifying receptors in the post-synaptic membrane of the affected neurons, or by modifying the intrinsic response of the neuron to its inputs, or all three mechanisms (Noreña & Farley, 2013). Whiting, Moiseff, and Rubio (2009) found that synapses on bushy cell somata in the VCN and the basal dendrites of fusiform cells in DCN upregulated their excitatory AMPA receptor subunits while inhibitory synapses reduced their expression of glycine subunits within 24 hours after monaural ear-plugging. Synapses on the apical dendrites of fusiform cells were not affected, which distinguishes these plastic modifications from those produced by STDP in animals expressing behavioral evidence of tinnitus. The modifications appeared to reflect a mechanism that balances the response of auditory pathways to asymmetric inputs from the ear to support sound localization based on interaural level differences. In contrast, other changes in the VCN described by Cai, Ma, and Young (2009) may be more closely related to hyperacusis. Non-primary like neurons in this structure (those exhibiting chopper response profiles) showed steepened rate-level functions and elevated discharge rates at high sound intensities after noise trauma. Notably, the frequency response of the affected neurons was also broadened at high sound intensities. Output from these VCN neurons distributes up the auditory pathway and may alter rate-level functions seen in higher auditory structures. Interestingly, primary-like neurons in VCN showed opposite effects suggesting that neural changes related to hyperacusis may be selective for specific neuron types. Steepened rate-level functions have also been recorded from the DCN of guinea pigs 2 weeks after a TTS induced by noise exposure (Dehmel et al., 2012). Although the neuron types contributing to this effect were not specified, slope was steepened over a wide frequency range and were steeper compared to unexposed controls in neurons with center frequencies below as well as in the range where tinnitus behavior was expressed in the animals (Dehmel et al., 2012). These observations suggest that the mechanisms underlying increased central gain may be distinguishable from those underlying tinnitus on the basis of their frequency profile.

In addition to its expression in many levels of the auditory pathway, gain enhancement occurs at different time scales and even in structures outside of classical auditory pathways (Auerbach, Rodrigues, & Salvi, 2014). Computational studies suggest that a homeostatic mechanism that maintains the average rate of firing in a network of neurons can increase the spontaneous activity of the network as well as restore driven responses of the network (Schaette & Kempter, 2006; Dominguez et al., 2006; Schaette & McAlpine, 2011; Chrostowski et al., 2011). However, supranormal driven responses are needed for hyperacusis. Descending projections from the auditory cortex and other structures are a further factor that can modulate rate-level functions underlying hyperacusis (Popelár, Nwabueze-Ogbo, & Syka et al., 2003). Asokan, Williamson, and Polley (2017) found that feedback from cortico-collicular neurons to the IC scaled with sound intensity and increased above baseline following TTS, revealing hyperacusis-like behavior in both structures. Neuromodulators (Coomber et al., 2015) and interactions with glial cells (Stellwagen & Malenka, 2006) are also involved in HSP and might spread the bandwidth of its effects. Overall one can say that while HSP is a key process in hyperacusis, many questions remain as to its specific mechanisms and multiple sites of action.

If HSP is involved in the development of hyperacusis, it must by definition fail to produce correct neural activity levels for moderate to high level sounds. One possibility is that HSP tries to correctly increase central gain to compensate for deafferentation but subsequently enables STDP to create increased neural connectivity and too much overall gain (Chrostowski, 2012). Another potential mechanism is that HSP works to normalize neural activity for low level sounds but in doing so applies too much gain for moderate to high level sounds. A hint that this could be occurring in some hyperacusis patients is the fact that some individuals experience a reduction in hyperacusis through the use of a low-level sound generator. This and other sound therapies for hyperacusis will be discussed further in a later section of this chapter. An alternative explanation for hyperacusis development in some individuals may be a *failure* of HSP to regulate STDP, which has been demonstrated to also produce tinnitus in an animal model (Rüttiger et al., 2013). If this mechanism is widespread in the human hyperacusis patient population, it might explain why tinnitus is so prevalent in this population, whereas there are multiple mechanisms described earlier that could lead to abnormal spontaneous and synchronous activity (tinnitus) without abnormal sound-driven activity (hyperacusis).

Notwithstanding these possibilities, it should be noted that loss of input from deafferentation could yield a net decrease in inhibition in cortical networks without plasticity necessarily being involved. Although its mechanism is unclear, reduced GABAergic inhibition has been observed in VCN (Godfrey et al., 2015), DCN (Wang et al., 2009), IC (Middleton et al., 2011), and auditory cortex (Llano, Turner, & Caspary, 2012; Salvi et al., 2017) of animals exhibiting TTS or PTS after noise trauma, and at the level of the auditory cortex in human tinnitus sufferers (Sedley et al., 2015a). In the study by Llano et al. (2012) noise-exposed mice showed a 68% increase in the amplitude of the cortical response evoked by electrical stimulation of thalamocortical afferents compared to controls, which correlated with behavioral evidence of tinnitus. Tinnitus animals also exhibited reduced sensitivity to GABAergic blockade revealing diminished inhibitory tone, consistent with increased driven responses. Notably, the decrease in GABA sensitivity was greater at cortical sites distant from the site of stimulation, suggesting that inhibition conveyed by cortico-cortical projections was affected. Similarly, Chen, Radziwon, Auerbach, and Salvi (2017) observed increased rate/level functions (hyperacusis) in the auditory cortex of noise-exposed rats at tonotopic frequencies below the noise exposure band (16 to 20 kHz) revealing hyperactivity in this region but shallow functions suggesting hypoactivity at high frequencies. This pattern of hyper- and hypo-responsiveness resembles responses evoked from primary auditory cortex in human tinnitus sufferers (Roberts et al. 2015). In this study the auditory steady-state response evoked in the primary auditory cortex of tinnitus subjects by 5 kHz 40-Hz AM sound (5 kHz in the tinnitus and hearing loss region of the subjects) was smaller than that observed in hearing-level-matched controls suggesting hypoactivity and reduced temporal coding in the 5 kHz region of the tinnitus subjects. However, the results were reversed when the responses were evoked at 500 Hz, suggesting hyperactivity in the 500 Hz region of the tinnitus group. One explanation of these findings could be that hypoactivity in the tinnitus region caused by hearing loss reduced lateral inhibition of distant frequencies in the cortical tonotopic map, such that neurons tuned to more distant frequencies became hypersensitive.

A mechanism of this type could account for the steepened LGFs seen below the audiometric cut-off frequency seen in the hyperacusis patients of Noreña and Chery-Croze (2007). It should be noted that overall hypoactivity in a frequency band reflecting peripheral cochlear impairment is not necessarily incompatible with localized synchronous activity giving a tinnitus percept in that band. Alternatively, disinhibition of cortical networks may involve distinctive events in the thalamus that have been associated with tinnitus and hyperacusis.

Convergence in the Thalamus and Cortex

One might expect that decreased inhibition consequent on decreased auditory nerve activity would be transmitted to the medial geniculate body (MGB) of the thalamus through the cochlear nucleus (VCN/DCN) and IC. At the level of the MGB, however, there is little evidence of tinnitus-related decreases in GABAergic neurotransmission. Instead, Sametsky et al. (2015) observed an *increase* in tonic GABAergic inhibition in a subset of thalamic projection neurons that was specific to animals showing behavioral evidence of tinnitus. This effect requires an initiating condition, which could be tinnitus-related neural synchrony inherited from subcortical pathways. Hyperpolarization also switched the affected MGB neurons into a burst firing mode and enhanced their driven responses, the latter of which may potentially relate to hyperacusis (Langers, van Dijk, Schoenmaker, & Backes, 2007). The tonic inhibition producing these effects was mediated by extra-synaptic $GABA_A$ receptors, which is consistent with a role for this inhibition in exerting a nonspecific modulatory effect on cortical processing (Brickley & Mody, 2012). Caspary and Llano (2016) and others (Weisz et al., 2007) have proposed that the switch to bursting activity in MGB neurons could be responsible for generating low-frequency (<4 Hz) delta and theta oscillations which have been recorded from the auditory cortex and several other brain regions from indwelling electrodes in a tinnitus patient (Sedley et al., 2015b) and may reflect disinhibited interlaminar processing and synaptic rescaling in the affected regions (Carracedo et al., 2013). There is evidence that increased slow wave activity is associated with high frequency oscillations in primary auditory cortex that appear to relate to tinnitus percepts (Llinas et al., 2005). High frequency oscillations of cortical origin in the gamma range (~40 to 70 Hz) have been found to correlate with tinnitus perception in tinnitus sufferers (Weisz et al., 2007), although in the study of Sedley et al. (2015b) gamma activity while present in the primary auditory cortex of their patient appeared to be more closely related to tinnitus suppression by forward masking than to the tinnitus percept itself. It was suggested that gamma activity is generated by neural networks as they update current sensory state in accordance with predictive coding models of tinnitus (Sedley et al., 2016; Roberts, Husain, & Eggermont, 2013; De Ridder, Vanneste, & Freeman, 2014) and auditory perception (Winkler, Denham, & Nelkin, 2009).

Overall, current evidence suggests that slow-wave activity generated by deafferentation of MGB neurons disinhibits processing over wide cortical areas potentially contributing to hyperacusis and broadening its frequency profile (Caspary & Llano, 2016). Faster gamma oscillations recorded from the tinnitus region of the primary auditory cortex appear to reflect the processing of tinnitus-related neural activity occurring there. Similar oscillatory changes (described as thalamocortical dysrhythmia by Llinás et al., 2005) have been observed in other disconnection syndromes and may thus seem pathological, but this may not necessarily be the case. In normal functioning, low frequency bursting activity distributed to the brain by thalamic neurons could be a teaching signal that integrates information in sensory pathways with that represented in brain regions underlying memory, emotion, and consciousness in order to support adaptive behavior. If this hypothesis is correct, the oscillatory dynamics and brain network activity seen in tinnitus (Sedley et al., 2015b; Husain & Schmidt, 2014) could be a prolongation of dynamics that occur during normal information processing on a much shorter time scale. In tinnitus the dynamics are prolonged, although possibly at an adapted level, because they are driven by persisting maladaptive changes that occur in auditory pathways following deafferentation.

Implications for Treating Hyperacusis and Tinnitus

Growing knowledge about the neural correlates of tinnitus and hyperacusis and the role of neural plasticity provide a rationale for sound therapies aimed at these conditions (see Chapters 14 and 15 for further discussion of this topic). We briefly consider two approaches, one using passive or attended exposure to engineered environmental sounds to suppress to tinnitus and hyperacusis neural activity, and another that exploits the timing rules of auditory-somatosensory STDP to suppress this activity.

Exposure to Environmental Sound

While in principle experience with low frequency sounds might be expected to distribute lateral inhibition into the tinnitus frequency region, such sounds give poor or no residual inhibition (RI) (Roberts et al., 2008) indicating little interaction with neural activity occurring in the tinnitus region. This may explain why in one study of sound therapy a group that received low frequency sounds did not experience suppression of their tinnitus (Tass et al., 2012). In contrast, sounds covering the tinnitus frequencies (3 to 12 kHz) do interact with tinnitus neural activity inducing a degree of RI (Roberts et al., 2008; Terry, Jones, Davis, & Slater, 1983) particularly when bandwidth of the frequency match is close (Sedley et al., 2015b). Sound therapies utilizing sounds in the tinnitus frequency range have been motivated by various principles. One approach presents the constituent frequencies of complex sounds at variable time delays, aiming to fragment the oscillatory neural activities believed to underlie tinnitus by resetting their phases (Tass et al., 2012). Other methods have engineered music to conform to the measured tinnitus spectrum (Li, Bao, & Chrostowski, 2016) or the audiograms (Davis, Wilde, Steed, & Hanley, 2008), or to distribute lateral inhibition into the tinnitus region by notching sounds closely around the dominant tinnitus pitch (Stracke, Okamoto, & Pantev, 2010). Patients typically receive these treatments on the order of an hour or two per day over a treatment period of a few weeks. Modest reductions in tinnitus loudness (measured by visual analog scales) and improved quality of life (assessed by questionnaires) have been reported, with ~20 to 30% of patients achieving improvements deemed to be clinically meaningful in some studies. However, no particular method has presented strong evidence for improvement in a majority of patients using these acute treatment methods, particularly in relation to control groups (for reviews of tinnitus see Hobson, Chisholm, & El Refaie, 2010; Roberts & Bosnyak, 2010; Hoare, Kowalkowski, Kang, & Hall, 2011; for a review of SLT, see Fournier, Schönwiesner, & Hébert, 2014).

There is evidence, however, that *long-term* exposure to low-level, complex sounds covering the tinnitus frequency region can be beneficial for tinnitus and hyperacusis. Noreña and Eggermont (2005, 2006) found that rearing cats in complex background sound 24 hours per day for several weeks after a single noise trauma prevented tonotopic map reorganization and suppressed putative neural correlates of tinnitus otherwise induced by acoustic trauma. These benefits were observed when the background environment covered the hearing loss frequencies but not when sounds were presented below these frequencies. Because improvement was also seen in the ABR audiogram, the therapeutic environment appeared to have supported repair of the cochlear transduction mechanism. Other findings suggest that potential benefits may not be limited to the auditory periphery. Passive exposure to complex low-level sound profoundly suppressed the responsivity of cortical neurons to the exposure frequencies when delivered to normal hearing cats 24 hours per day over weeks and months (Noreña, Gourévitch, Aizawa, & Eggermont, 2006; Pienkowski & Eggermont, 2011). Concurrently, responsivity increased outside of the exposed frequency band reflecting reduced lateral inhibition delivered from the exposed region. Roberts et al. (2015) reported similar on- and off-frequency effects in EEG responses evoked from primary auditory cortex in human tinnitus sufferers, when the tinnitus subjects experienced deep RI after exposure to a masker overlapping their tinnitus percepts. These and other results (Galazuk, Voytenko, & Longenecker 2017) suggest that forward suppression of neural responses underlying tinnitus may scale over an extraordinarily wide range of exposure durations (from seconds to several weeks), engaging mechanisms that could be beneficial for tinnitus. Although to date this has not been attempted for tinnitus, it has been attempted for hyperacusis. Noreña and Chery-Croze (2007) found that listening for 15 weeks to a just-audible complex high frequency sound for a few hours a day improved SLT by as much as ~15 dB in hyperacusis patients. SLT was improved for sounds below as well as above the cut-off frequency in the audiogram, consistent with the broad frequency profile often observed in hyperacusis patients. Improvement persisted for 1 month after the end of therapy and exhibited a gradual return to baseline subsequently. The mechanisms underlying suppression of neural responsiveness over such a wide range of exposure durations are presently not well understood (Malmierca, Anderson, & Antunes, 2014; Wehr & Zador, 2005). Forms of HSP or stimulus-specific habituation are believed to be involved.

Bimodal Auditory-Somatosensory Treatments for Tinnitus

A different and more recent approach has been to use combined auditory-somatosensory stimulation in an attempt to suppress tinnitus. Initially this approach was motivated by evidence that somatosensory, auditory, and visual pathways interact in multisensory regions of the brain (Hamilton et al., 2016; Oertel & Young, 2004) and by a belief that modulation of deep brain structures by multimodal stimulation might alter the neural substrate of tinnitus (Offutt, Ryan, Konop, & Lim, 2014). More recently, the studies of STDP in the DCN described above have established a scientific foundation for this approach (Tzounopoulos, Rubio, Keen, & Trussell, 2007; Zhao & Tzounopoulos, 2011; Dehmel et al., 2012; Koehler & Shore, 2013; Wu, Martel, & Shore, 2016). Although the timing rules of STDP induced by paired auditory-somatosensory stimulation are altered in animals expressing neural correlates of tinnitus, some bimodal timing orders and intervals depress these correlates, presumably by inducing LTD. Marks et al. (2018) found that auditory and somatosensory stimulation paired at one such interval for 20 minutes daily for 25 sessions suppressed neural and behavioral evidence of tinnitus in their animal model while three control procedures (auditory alone, somatosensory alone, or no stimulation) did not. Remarkably, the same bimodal therapy applied to tinnitus patients (30 min/day) in a blinded cross-over design (four weeks of bimodal treatment followed by auditory alone or vice versa, separated by wash-out of the same duration) progressively reduced tinnitus measured by psychoacoustic loudness-matching (Marks et al., 2018). Tinnitus loudness decreased after bimodal but not unimodal treatment to an extent (12.2 dB) that gave tinnitus elimination in two patients. Tinnitus distress assessed by questionnaire also decreased significantly but only when preceded by a bimodal treatment series. During bimodal treatment somatosensory stimulation was presented at a level that was generally imperceptible, which suggests that auditory stimulation alone was an effective control procedure for non-specific treatment effects. Because tinnitus reduction accumulated gradually over four weeks it must have persisted on the order of days, although tinnitus loudness returned to baseline within the first week of the wash-out period.

Further investigations will be needed to confirm the present findings, assess their predicted dependence on specific bimodal intervals, and determine whether additional exposure will prolong its benefits. At present it is not known whether bimodal therapy will modify SLT, which may involve additional pathways and different plasticity mechanisms.

Summary and Conclusion

We have discussed evidence suggesting that tinnitus and hyperacusis measured as reduced SLT follow a similar time course of development and share a common initiating condition, which is cochlear hearing impairment that may or may not be hidden from the clinical audiogram. Injury to ANFs exhibiting low thresholds and high rates of spontaneous firing may be particularly important for tinnitus, which can develop even when the extent of damage to such fibers is not sufficient to affect hearing thresholds. If the high spontaneous activity of these ANFs is sufficiently diminished or lost, maladaptive hypersynchronous neural activity driven by STDP or enabled by HSP mechanisms may be unleashed in the affected frequency regions of central auditory structures generating tinnitus and giving it its distinctive frequency profile. Tinnitus-related neural activity also appears to hyperpolarize a subset of neurons in the thalamic medial geniculate nucleus, switching these neurons into a burst firing mode and generating low-frequency oscillations that have been recorded over wide brain areas in tinnitus patients. Burst firing and slow oscillations may serve under normal conditions to integrate auditory information with information contained in other brain regions to support adaptive behavior. However, in tinnitus (and other disconnection syndromes) low frequency oscillations may persist at some level of strength, driven by aberrant signals inherited from subcortical pathways.

These neural changes may also occur in hyperacusis patients, most of whom experience tinnitus. However, the frequency profile of hyperacusis is broader than that of tinnitus, appearing at frequencies where tinnitus is experienced but also well below this frequency range implying that some of its mechanisms are different. HSP mechanisms activated by deafferentation are believed to amplify the input/output functions of the affected neurons in order to maintain their responding and support auditory functions such as sound localization based on interaural level differences. However, in so doing these mechanisms may also amplify driven responses to moderate and higher-level sounds, giving rise to hyperacusis. The broadened frequency range of hyperacusis may be a consequence of several possible mechanisms including the frequency-nonspecific effects of altered HSP on central gain and STDP, neuromodulators released by tinnitus neural activity, reduced lateral inhibition conveyed from the tinnitus region, or disinhibition of cortical networks by low-frequency bursting activity in thalamic neurons. Areas outside of the cortical tonotopic tinnitus frequency region appear to be disinhibited by these or other mechanisms, which may implicate cortical processing as one source of a broadened frequency profile for hyperacusis.

Novel treatments are being evaluated to suppress or renormalize the maladaptive neuroplastic changes believed to underlie tinnitus and hyperacusis. One approach involves exposure to background sounds covering the region of hearing impairment to suppress these changes, while another delivers paired auditory-somatosensory stimulation using an order and timing interval believed to induce LTD in auditory pathways. Because cochlear pathology is likely a triggering factor in tinnitus and hyperacusis, periodic retraining may be required to prevent the recurrence of maladaptive plasticity in central auditory structures. A challenge for the future is to determine whether these procedures (which potentially draw on different plasticity mechanisms) can aid individuals such as the young tinnitus and hyperacusis sufferer whose history prefaced this chapter. Of course, a preferable solution would be to prevent hearing injuries altogether, or at least detect them early in order to avoid accelerating age-related declines in hearing (Roberts, Martin, & Bosnyak, 2010). The presence of persisting tinnitus and reduced SLT affecting more than 14% of the adolescents in the study of Sanchez et al. (2016) is a potential early warning sign of cochlear injuries that may be hidden from the audiogram (Harrison, 2008; Shargorodsky, Curhan, Curhan, & Eavey, 2010). However, it is notable that the majority of adolescents examined by Sanchez et al. (2016) did not experience tinnitus or altered SLT during psychoacoustic assessment, even though their listening habits appeared to be as risky as those of the adolescents who were affected. Why this was so is another important area for study. Individual differences in the responsivity of olivocochlear efferents is one factor that could modulate driven responses in the auditory pathway (Kujawa & Liberman, 1999), potentially explaining why some adolescents with persistent tinnitus reported LDLs similar to those of adolescents without tinnitus during psychoacoustic testing. Prior exposure to levels of background sound that are not synaptopathic have also been reported to reduce cochlear injuries arising from subsequent noise trauma in animal models (Canlon, Borg, & Flock, 1988; Canlon & Fransson 1995; Roy et al., 2016). The relationship of noise exposure history to tinnitus and hyperacusis appears to be complex and modulated by individual difference factors that are not well understood.

Abbreviations

ABR	Auditory brainstem response
AM	Amplitude modulation
ANF	Auditory nerve fiber
ASR	Acoustic startle response
BOLD	Blood oxygenation level dependent (fMRI imaging)
CN	Cochlear nucleus (VCN+DCN)
DCN	Dorsal cochlear nucleus
DPOAE	Distortion product otoacoustic emissions
EEG	Electroencephalography
EFR	Envelope following response
HT	High threshold
HSP	Homeostatic plasticity
HSR	High spontaneous rate

IC	Inferior colliculus
LDL	Loudness discomfort level
LGF	Loudness growth function
LTD	Long-term depression
LTP	Long-term potentiation
MGB	Medial geniculate body
PTS	Permanent threshold shift
RI	Residual inhibition
SLT	Sound level tolerance
SFR	Spontaneous firing rate
STDP	Spike-timing-dependent plasticity
TEOAE	Transient otoacoustic emissions
TTS	Temporary threshold shift
VCN	Ventral cochlear nucleus

Acknowledgments. The authors acknowledge the following institutions for financial and in-kind support. In Canada (LER, ICB): The Natural Sciences and Engineering Research Council of Canada. In Brazil (TGS): Fundação de Amparo à Pesquisa do Estado de São Paulo, Aché, Biosom, Sancout Electronic Technology, and Fundação Companhia Energética de São Paulo.

References

Andersson, G., Lindvall, N., Hursti, T., & Carlbring P. (2002). Hypersensitivity to sound (hyperacusis): A prevalence study conducted via the Internet and post. *International Journal of Audiology*.

Asokan, M., Williamson, R. S., & Polley, D. B. (2017). Changes in corticocollicular feedback following cochlear synaptopathy. Presented at the Annual Meeting of the Association for Research in Otolaryngology, Baltimore, MD (PS 631).

Atencio, C. A., & Schreiner, C. E. (2010). Columnar connectivity and laminar processing in cat primary auditory cortex. *PLoS ONE*, *5*(3). https://doi.org/10.1371/journal.pone.0009521.

Auerbach, B. D., Rodrigues, P. V., & Salvi, R. J. (2014). Central gain control in tinnitus and hyperacusis. *Frontiers in Neurology*, *5*(October), 206. https://doi.org/10.3389/fneur.2014.00206.

Baguley, D. M. (2003). Hyperacusis. *Journal of the Royal Society of Medicine*, *96*(December), 582–585. https://doi.org/10.1258/jrsm.96.12.582.

Basura, G. J., Koehler, S. D., & Shore, S. E. (2015). Bimodal stimulus timing dependent plasticity in primary auditory cortex is altered after noise exposure with and without tinnitus. *Journal of Neurophysiology*, jn.00319.2015. https://doi.org/10.1152/jn.00319.2015.

Bauer, C. A., Brozoski, T. J., & Myers, K. (2007). Primary afferent dendrite degeneration as a cause of tinnitus. *Journal of Neuroscience Research*, *85*, 1489–1498.

Bauer, C. A., Wisner, K. W., Baizer, J. S., & Brozoski, T. J. (2013). Tinnitus, unipolar brush cells, and cerebellar glutamatergic function in an animal model. *PLoS ONE*, *8*(6). https://doi.org/10.1371/journal.pone.0064726.

Bharadwaj, H. M., Masud, S., Mehraei, G., Verhulst, S., & Shinn-Cunningham, B. G. (2015). Individual differences reveal correlates of hidden hearing deficits. *Journal of Neuroscience*, *35*(5), 2161–2172. https://doi.org/10.1523/JNEUROSCI.3915-14.2015.

Brickley, S. G., & Mody, I. (2012). Extrasynaptic GABA A receptors: Their function in the CNS and implications for disease. *Neuron*, *73*(1), 23–34. https://doi.org/10.1016/j.neuron.2011.12.012.

Brotherton, H., Plack, C. J., Maslin, M., Schaette, R., & Munro, K. J. (2015). Pump up the volume: Could excessive neural gain explain tinnitus and hyperacusis? *Audiology and Neurotology*, *20*(4), 273–282. https://doi.org/10.1159/000430459.

Cai, S., Ma, W. L. D., & Young, E. D. (2009). Encoding intensity in ventral cochlear nucleus following acoustic trauma: Implications for loudness recruitment. *JARO—Journal of the Association for Research in Otolaryngology*, *10*(1), 5–22. https://doi.org/10.1007/s10162-008-0142-y.

Canlon, B., Borg, E., & Flock, Å. (1988). Protection against noise trauma by pre-exposure to a low level acoustic stimulus. *Hearing Research*, *34*(2), 197–200. https://doi.org/10.1016/0378-5955(88)90107-4.

Canlon, B., & Fransson, A. (1995). Morphological and functional preservation of the outer hair cells from noise trauma by sound conditioning. *Hearing Research, 84*, 112–124.

Carracedo, L. M., Kjeldsen, H., Cunnington, L., Jenkins, A., Schofield, I., Cunningham, M. O., . . . Whittington, M. A. (2013). A neocortical delta rhythm facilitates reciprocal interlaminar interactions via nested theta rhythms. *Journal of Neuroscience, 33*(26), 10750–10761. https://doi.org/10.1523/JNEUROSCI.0735-13.2013.

Caspary, D. M., & Llano, D. A. (2016). Auditory thalamic circuits and GABAA receptor function: Putative mechanisms in tinnitus pathology. *Hearing Research.* https://doi.org/10.1016/j.heares.2016.08.009.

Chen, G.-D., Radziwon, K., Auerbach, B. D., & Salvi, R. (2017). Noise-induced hyperacusis/recruitment in rats and the underlying hyperactivity in the central auditory areas. Presented at the Annual Meeting of the Association for Research in Otolaryngology, Baltimore, MD (PD 23).

Chrostowski, M. (2012). Cortical Plasticity and Tinnitus. Ph.D. thesis, McMaster University. http://hdl.handle.net/11375/12585.

Chrostowski, M., Yang, L., Wilson, H. R., Bruce, I. C., & Becker, S. (2011). Can homeostatic plasticity in deafferented primary auditory cortex lead to travelling waves of excitation? *Journal of Computational Neuroscience, 30*(2), 279–299. https://doi.org/10.1007/s10827-010-0256-1.

Coomber, B., Kowalkowski, V. L., Berger, J. I., Palmer, A. R., & Wallace, M. N. (2015). Modulating central gain in tinnitus: Changes in nitric oxide synthase in the ventral cochlear nucleus. *Frontiers in Neurology, 6*(MAR). https://doi.org/10.3389/fneur.2015.00053.

Darrow, K. N., Maison, S. F., & Liberman, M. C. (2006). Cochlear efferent feedback balances interaural sensitivity. *Nature Neuroscience, 9*(12), 1474–1476. https://doi.org/10.1038/nn1807.

Davis, P. B., Wilde, R. A., Steed, L. G., & Hanley, P. J. (2008). Treatment of tinnitus with a customized acoustic neural stimulus: A controlled clinical study. *Ear, Nose and Throat Journal, 87*, 330–339.

Dehmel, S., Pradhan, S., Koehler, S., Bledsoe, S., & Shore, S. (2012). Noise overexposure alters long-term somatosensory-auditory processing in the dorsal cochlear nucleus—Possible basis for tinnitus-related hyperactivity? *Journal of Neuroscience, 32*(5), 1660–1671. https://doi.org/10.1523/JNEUROSCI.4608-11.2012.

De Ridder, D., Elgoyhen, A. B., Romo, R., & Langguth, B. (2011). Phantom percepts: Tinnitus and pain as persisting aversive memory networks. *Proc. Natl Acad. Sci. U.S.A. 108*, 8075–8080.

De Ridder, D., Vanneste, S., & Freeman, W. (2014). The Bayesian brain: Phantom percepts resolve sensory uncertainty. *Neuroscience and Biobehavioral Reviews 44*, 4–15.

Diehl, P. U., & Schaette, R. (2015). Abnormal auditory gain in hyperacusis: Investigation with a computational model. *Frontiers in Neurology, 6*(JUN), 1–14. https://doi.org/10.3389/fneur.2015.00157.

Dominguez, M., Becker, S., Bruce, I., & Read, H. (2006). A spiking neuron model of cortical correlates of sensorineural hearing loss: Spontaneous firing, synchrony, and tinnitus. *Neural Computation, 18*(12), 2942–2958. https://doi.org/10.1162/neco.2006.18.12.2942.

Eggermont, J. J. (1990). On the pathophysiology of tinnitus: A review and a peripheral model. *Hearing Research, 48*, 111–124.

Eggermont, J. J. (2012). *The neuroscience of tinnitus.* Oxford, U.K.: Oxford University Press.

Eggermont, J. J., & Roberts, L. E. (2004). The neuroscience of tinnitus. *Trends in Neurosciences, 7*(11), 676–682. https://doi.org/10.1016/j.tins.2004.08.010.

Eggermont, J. J., & Roberts, L. E. (2015). Tinnitus: Animal models and findings in humans. *Cell and Tissue Research, 361*(1), 311–336. https://doi.org/10.1007/s00441-014-1992-8.

Formby, C., Sherlock, L. P., & Gold, S. L. (2003). Adaptive plasticity of loudness induced by chronic attenuation and enhancement of the acoustic background. *Journal of the Acoustical Society of America, 114*(1), 55–58. https://doi.org/10.1121/1.1582860.

Fournier, P., Schönwiesner, M., & Hébert, S. (2014). Loudness modulation after transient and permanent hearing loss: Implications for tinnitus and hyperacusis. *Neuroscience, 283*, 64–77. https://doi.org/10.1016/j.neuroscience.2014.08.007.

Furman, A. C., Kujawa, S. G., & Liberman, M. C. (2013). Noise-induced cochlear neuropathy is selective for fibers with low spontaneous rates.

Journal of Neurophysiology, *110*(3), 577–86. https://doi.org/10.1152/jn.00164.2013.

Galazyuk, A. V., Voytenko, S. V., & Longenecker, R. J. (2017). Long-lasting forward suppression of spontaneous firing in auditory neurons: Implication to the residual inhibition of tinnitus. *Journal of the Association for Research in Otolaryngology*, *18*(2), 343–353. https://doi.org/10.1007/s10162-016-0601-9.

Godfrey, D. A., Chen, K., Godfrey, M. A., Lee, A. C., Crass, S. P., Shipp, D., . . . Robinson, K. T. (2015). Cochlear ablation effects on amino acid levels in the chinchilla cochlear nucleus. *Neuroscience*, *297*, 137–159. https://doi.org/10.1016/j.neuroscience.2015.03.055.

Gu, J. W., Halpin, C. F., Nam, E.-C., Levine, R. A., & Melcher, J. R. (2010). Tinnitus, diminished sound-level tolerance, and elevated auditory activity in humans with clinically normal hearing sensitivity. *Journal of Neurophysiology* (September 2010), jn.00226.2010. https://doi.org/10.1152/jn.00226.2010.

Gu, J. W., Herrmann, B. S., Levine, R. A., & Melcher, J. R. (2012). Brainstem auditory evoked potentials suggest a role for the ventral cochlear nucleus in tinnitus. *JARO—Journal of the Association for Research in Otolaryngology*, *13*(6), 819–833. https://doi.org/10.1007/s10162-012-0344-1.

Guest, H., Munro, K. J., Prendergast, G., Howe, S., & Plack, C. J. (2016). Tinnitus with a normal audiogram: Relation to noise exposure but no evidence for cochlear synaptopathy. *Hearing Research*. https://doi.org/10.1016/j.heares.2016.12.002.

Hamilton, C., D'Arcy, S., Pearlmutter, B. A., Crispino, G., Lalor, E. C., & Conlon, B. J. (2016). An investigation of feasibility and safety of bimodal stimulation for the treatment of tinnitus: An open-label pilot study. *Neuromodulation: Technology at the Neural Interface*, *19*(8), 832–837. https://doi.org/10.1111/ner.12452.

Harrison, R. (2008). Noise-induced hearing loss in children: A "less than silent" environmental danger. *Paediatric Child Health*, *13*(5), 377–382.

Hébert, S., Fournier, P., & Noreña, A. (2013). The auditory sensitivity is increased in tinnitus ears. *Journal of Neuroscience*, *33*(6), 2356–2364. https://doi.org/10.1523/JNEUROSCI.3461-12.2013.

Heinz, M. G., & Young, E. D. (2004). Response growth with sound level in auditory-nerve fibers after noise-induced hearing loss. *Journal of Neurophysiology*, *91*(2), 784–795. https://doi.org/10.1152/jn.00776.2003.

Henry, J. A., Roberts, L. E., Ellingson, R. M., & Thielman, E. J. (2013). Computer-automated tinnitus assessment: Noise-band matching, maskability, and residual inhibition. *Journal of the American Academy of Audiology*, *24*(6), 486–504. https://doi.org/10.3766/jaaa.24.6.5.

Hesse, L. L., Bakay, W., Ong, H. C., Anderson, L., Ashmore, J., McAlpine, D., . . . Schaette, R. (2016). Non-monotonic relation between noise exposure severity and neuronal hyperactivity in the auditory midbrain. *Frontiers in Neurology*, *7*(AUG), 1–13. https://doi.org/10.3389/fneur.2016.00133.

Hickox, A. E., & Liberman, M. C. (2014). Is noise-induced cochlear neuropathy key to the generation of hyperacusis or tinnitus? *Journal of Neurophysiology*, *111*(3), 552–564.

Hoare, D. J., Kowalkowski, V. L., Kang, S., & Hall, D. A. (2011). Systematic review and meta-analyses of randomized controlled trials examining tinnitus management. *Laryngoscope*, *121*(7), 1555–1564. https://doi.org/10.1002/lary.21825.

Hobson, J., Chisholm, E., & El Refaie, A. (2012). Sound therapy (masking) in the management of tinnitus in adults. *Cochrane Database of Systematic Reviews*, doi:10.1002/14651858.CD006371.pub3.

Husain, F.T., & Schmidt, S.A. (2014). Using resting state functional connectivity to unravel networks of tinnitus. *Hearing Research*, *307*, 153–162.

Joris, P. X. (2009). Recruitment of neurons and loudness: Commentary on "encoding intensity in ventral cochlear nucleus following acoustic trauma: Implications for loudness recruitment" by Cai et al. J. Assoc. Res. Otolaryngol. doi: 10.1007/s10162-008-0142-y. *JARO—Journal of the Association for Research in Otolaryngology*, *10*(1), 1–4. https://doi.org/10.1007/s10162-009-0156-0.

Kaltenbach, J. A. (2011). Tinnitus: Models and mechanisms. *Hearing Research*, *276*(1–2), 52–60. https://doi.org/10.1016/j.heares.2010.12.003.

Knudson, I. M., & Melcher, J. R. (2016). Elevated acoustic startle responses in humans: relationship to reduced loudness discomfort level, but not self-report of hyperacusis. *JARO—Journal of the Association for Research in Otolaryngology, 17*(3), 223–235. https://doi.org/10.1007/s10162-016-0555-y.

Koehler, S. D., & Shore, S. E. (2013). Stimulus timing-dependent plasticity in dorsal cochlear nucleus is altered in tinnitus. *Journal of Neuroscience, 33*(50), 19647–19656. https://doi.org/10.1523/JNEUROSCI.2788-13.2013.

Kujawa, S. G., & Liberman, M. C. (2009). Adding insult to injury: Cochlear nerve degeneration after "temporary" noise-induced hearing loss. *Journal of Neuroscience, 29*(45), 14077. https://doi.org/10.1523/JNEUROSCI.2845-09.2009.

Kujawa, S. G., & Liberman, M. C. (1999). Long-term sound conditioning enhances cochlear sensitivity. *Journal of Neurophysiology, 82*(2), 863–73. Retrieved from http://www.ncbi.nlm.nih.gov/pubmed/10444683.

Langers, D. R. M., van Dijk, P., Schoenmaker, E. S., & Backes, W. H. (2007). fMRI activation in relation to sound intensity and loudness. *NeuroImage, 35*(2), 709–718. https://doi.org/10.1016/j.neuroimage.2006.12.013.

Lanting, C., Woźniak, A., van Dijk, P., & Langers, D. R. (2016). Tinnitus- and task-related differences in resting-state networks. *Adv Exp Med Biol.* 894, 175–187. doi: 10.1007/978-3-319-25474-6_19.

Levine, R. A., Abel, M., & Cheng, H. (2003). CNS somatosensory–auditory interactions elicit or modulate tinnitus. *Exp. Brain Res. 153*, 643–648.

Li, S. A., Bao, L., & Chrostowski, M. (2016). Investigating the effects of a personalized, spectrally altered music-based sound therapy on treating tinnitus: A blinded, randomized controlled trial. *Audiology and Neurotology*, 296–304. https://doi.org/10.1159/000450745.

Li, S., Choi, V., & Tzounopoulos, T. (2013). Pathogenic plasticity of Kv7. 2/3 channel activity is essential for the induction of tinnitus. *Proceedings of the National Academy of Sciences USA, 110*, 9980–9985. https://doi.org/10.1073/pnas.1216671110/-/DCSupplemental.www.pnas.org/cgi/doi/10.1073/pnas.1302770110.

Li, S., Kalappa, B. I., & Tzounopoulo, T. (2015). Noise-induced plasticity of KCNQ2/3 and HCN channels underlies vulnerability and resilience to tinnitus. *eLife, 4*(August2015), 1–23. https://doi.org/10.7554/eLife.0724.

Lin, H. W., Furman, A. C., Kujawa, S. G., & Liberman, M. C. (2011). Primary neural degeneration in the guinea pig cochlea after reversible noise-induced threshold shift. *JARO—Journal of the Association for Research in Otolaryngology, 12*(5), 605–616. https://doi.org/10.1007/s10162-011-0277-0.

Llano, D. A., Turner, J., & Caspary, D. M. (2012). Diminished cortical inhibition in an aging mouse model of chronic tinnitus. *Journal of Neuroscience, 32*(46), 16141–16148. https://doi.org/10.1523/JNEUROSCI.2499-12.2012.

Llinas, R., Urbano, F. J., Leznik, E., Ramirez, R. R., & Van Marle, H. J. (2005). Rhythmic and dysrhythmic thalamocortical dynamics: GABA systems and the edge effect. *Trends in Neurosciences. 28*, 325–333.

Lobarinas, E., Salvi, R., & Ding, D. (2016). Selective inner hair cell dysfunction in chinchillas impairs hearing-in-noise in the absence of outer hair cell loss. *JARO—Journal of the Association for Research in Otolaryngology, 17*(2), 89–101. https://doi.org/10.1007/s10162-015-0550-8.

Ma, W. L. D., & Young, E. D. (2006). Dorsal cochlear nucleus response properties following acoustic trauma: Response maps and spontaneous activity. *Hearing Research, 216–217*, 176–188. https://doi.org/10.1016/j.heares.2006.03.011.

Malmierca, M. S., Anderson, L. A., & Antunes, F. M. (2015). The cortical modulation of stimulus-specific adaptation in the auditory midbrain and thalamus: A potential neuronal correlate for predictive coding. *Frontiers in Systems Neuroscience, 9*(March), 19. https://doi.org/10.3389/fnsys.2015.00019.

Mancilla, J. G., & Manis, P. B. (2009). Two distinct types of inhibition mediated by cartwheel cells in the dorsal cochlear nucleus. *Journal of Neurophysiology, 102*(May 2009), 1287–1295. https://doi.org/10.1152/jn.91272.2008.

Marks, K., Martel, D. T., Wu, C., Basura, G. J., Roberts, L. E., Schvartz-Leyzac, K. C., & Shore, S. E. (2018). Auditory-somatosensory bimodal stimulation desynchronizes brain circuitry to reduce tinnitus in guinea pigs and humans. *Science Translational Medicine*, 10, eaal3175.

Melcher, J. R., Knudson, I. M., & Levine, R. A. (2013). Subcallosal brain structure: Correlation with hearing threshold at supra-clinical frequencies (>8 kHz), but not with tinnitus. *Hearing Research*, *295*, 79–86. https://doi.org/10.1016/j.heares.2012.03.013.

Middleton, J. W., Kiritani, T., Pedersen, C., Turner, J. G., Shepherd, G. M. G., & Tzounopoulos, T. (2011). Mice with behavioral evidence of tinnitus exhibit dorsal cochlear nucleus hyperactivity because of decreased GABAergic inhibition. *Proceedings of the National Academy of Sciences of the United States of America*, *108*(18), 7601–7606. https://doi.org/10.1073/pnas.1100223108.

Mühlau, M., Rauschecker, J. P., Oestreicher, E., Gaser, C., Röttinger, M., Wohlschläger, A. M., . . . Sander, D. (2006). Structural brain changes in tinnitus. *Cerebral Cortex*, *16*(9), 1283–1288. https://doi.org/10.1093/cercor/bhj070.

Munro, K. J., Turtle, C., & Schaette, R. (2014). Plasticity and modified loudness following short-term unilateral deprivation: Evidence of multiple gain mechanisms within the auditory system. *Journal of the Acoustical Society of America*, *135*(1), 315–322. https://doi.org/10.1121/1.4835715.

Nelson, J. J., & Chen, K. (2004). The relationship of tinnitus, hyperacusis, and hearing loss. *Ear Nose and Throat Journal*, *83*, 472–476.

Noreña, A., Micheyl, C., Chery-Croze, S., & Collet, L. (2002). Psychoacoustic characterization of the tinnitus spectrum: Implications for the underlying mechanisms of tinnitus. *Audiology and Neurootology*, *7*, 358–369.

Noreña, A. J., & Eggermont, J. J. (2003). Changes in spontaneous neural activity immediately after an acoustic trauma: Implications for neural correlates of tinnitus. *Hearing Research*, *183* (1–2), 137–153. https://doi.org/10.1016/S0378-5955(03)00225-9.

Noreña, A. J. & Eggermont, J. J. (2005). Enriched acoustic environment after noise trauma reduces hearing loss and prevents cortical map reorganization. *Journal of Neuroscience*, *25*(3), 699–705. https://doi.org/10.1523/JNEUROSCI.2226-04.2005.

Noreña, A. J., & Eggermont, J. J. (2006). Enriched acoustic environment after noise trauma abolishes neural signs of tinnitus. *Neuroreport*, *17*(6), 559–563. https://doi.org/10.1097/00001756-200604240-00001.

Noreña, A. J., & Farley, B. J. (2013). Tinnitus-related neural activity: Theories of generation, propagation, and centralization. *Hearing Res.*, *295*, 161–171.

Noreña, A. J., Gourévitch, B., Aizawa, N., & Eggermont, J. J. (2006). Spectrally enhanced acoustic environment disrupts frequency representation in cat auditory cortex. *Nature Neuroscience*, *9*(7), 932–939. https://doi.org/10.1038/nn1720.

Noreña, A. J. (2011). An integrative model of tinnitus based on a central gain controlling neural sensitivity. *Neuroscience and Biobehavioral Reviews*, *35*(5), 1089–1109. https://doi.org/10.1016/j.neubiorev.2010.11.003.

Noreña, A. J., & Chery-Croze, S. (2007). Enriched acoustic environment rescales auditory sensitivity. *Neuroreport*, *18*(12), 1251–1255. https://doi.org/10.1097/WNR.0b013e3282202c35.

Oertel, D., & Young, E. D. (2004). What's a cerebellar circuit doing in the auditory system? *Trends in Neurosciences*, *27*(2), 104–110. https://doi.org/10.1016/j.tins.2003.12.001.

Offutt, S. J., Ryan, K. J., Konop, A. E., & Lim, H. H. (2014). Suppression and facilitation of auditory neurons through coordinated acoustic and midbrain stimulation: Investigating a deep brain stimulator for tinnitus. *Journal of Neural Engineering, Dec; 11*(6), 066001. doi: 10.1088/1741-2560/11/6/066001.

Paul, B. T., Bruce, I. C., & Roberts, L. E. (2017). Evidence that hidden hearing loss underlies amplitude modulation encoding deficits in individuals with and without tinnitus. *Hearing Research*, *344*, 170–182. https://doi.org/10.1016/j.heares.2016.11.010.

Pienkowski, M., & Eggermont, J. J. (2011). Cortical tonotopic map plasticity and behavior. *Neuroscience and Biobehavioral Reviews*, *35*(10), 2117–2128. https://doi.org/10.1016/j.neubiorev.2011.02.002

Pienkowski M., Tyler R. S., Roncancio, E. R., Jun, H. J., Brozoski, T., Dauman, N., Coelho C. B., Andersson, G., Keiner, A. J., Cacace, A. T.,

Martin, N., & Moore, B. C. J. (2014). A review of hyperacusis and future directions: Part II: Measurement, mechanisms, and treatment. *American Journal of Audiology*, *23*, 424–436.

Popelář, J., Nwabueze-Ogbo, F. C., & Syka, J. (2003). Changes in neuronal activity of the inferior colliculus in rat after temporal inactivation of the auditory cortex. *Physiological Research*, *52*(5), 615–628.

Potashner S. J., Suneja, S. K., & Benson, C. G. (2000). Altered glycinergic synaptic activities in guinea pig brain stem auditory nuclei after unilateral cochlear ablation. *Hearing Research* *147*(2000), 125–136.

Pozo, K., & Goda, Y. (2010). Unraveling mechanisms of homeostatic synaptic plasticity. *Neuron*, *66*(3), 337–351. https://doi.org/10.1016/j.neuron.2010.04.028.

Qiu, C., Salvi, R., Ding, D., & Burkard, R. (2000). Inner hair cell loss leads to enhanced response amplitudes in auditory cortex of unanesthetized chinchillas: Evidence for increased system gain. *Hearing Research*, *139*(1–2), 153–171. https://doi.org/10.1016/S0378-5955(99)00171-9.

Rauschecker, J. P., Leaver, A. M., & Mühlau, M. (2010). Tuning out the noise: Limbic-auditory interactions in tinnitus. *Neuron*, *66*(6), 819–826. https://doi.org/10.1016/j.neuron.2010.04.032.

Roberts, L. E., & Bosnyak, D. J. (2010). Auditory training in tinnitus. In Møller, A., Kleinjung, T., Langguth, B., and De Ridder, D. (Eds.). *Textbook of Tinnitus* (pp. 563–574). Humana-Springer.

Roberts, L. E., Martin, W. H., & Bosnyak, D. J. (2010). The prevention of tinnitus and noise-induced hearing loss. In Møller, A., Kleinjung, T., Langguth, B., and De Ridder, D. (Eds.). *Textbook of Tinnitus* (pp. 563–574). Humana-Springer.

Roberts, L. E. (2016). Mechanism and time course of tinnitus associated with hearing impairment. In D. Baguley and M. Fagelson (Eds.). *Tinnitus: Clinical and research perspectives* (pp. 13–33). Plymouth, U.K.: Plural Press.

Roberts, L. E., Bosnyak, D. J., Bruce, I. C., Gander, P. E., & Paul, B. T. (2015). Evidence for differential modulation of primary and non-primary auditory cortex by forward masking in tinnitus. *Hearing Research*, *327*, 9–27.

Roberts, L. E., Husain, F. T., & Eggermont, J. J. (2013). Role of attention in the generation and modulation of tinnitus. *Neuroscience and Biobehavioral Reviews*, *37*(8), 1754–1773. https://doi.org/10.1016/j.neubiorev.2013.07.007.

Roberts, L. E., Moffat, G., Baumann, M., Ward, L. M., & Bosnyak, D. J. (2008). Residual inhibition functions overlap tinnitus spectra and the region of auditory threshold shift. *JARO—Journal of the Association for Research in Otolaryngology*, *9*(4), 417–435. https://doi.org/10.1007/s10162-008-0136-9.

Roberts, M. T., & Trussell, L. O. (2010). Molecular layer inhibitory interneurons provide feedforward and lateral inhibition in the dorsal cochlear nucleus. *Journal of Neurophysiology*, *104*(5), 2462–2473. https://doi.org/10.1152/jn.00312.2010.

Roy, S., Ryals, M. M., Van Den Bruele, A. B., Fitzgerald, T. S., & Cunningham, L. L. (2013). Sound preconditioning therapy inhibits ototoxic hearing loss in mice. *Journal of Clinical Investigation*, *123*(11), 4945–4949. https://doi.org/10.1172/JCI71353.

Rüttiger, L., Singer, W., Panford-Walsh, R., Matsumoto, M., Lee, S. C., et al. (2013). The reduced cochlear output and the failure to adapt the central auditory response causes tinnitus in noise exposed rats. *PLoS ONE* *8*(3), e57247. https://doi.org/10.1371/journal.pone.0057247.

Salvi, R., Sun, W., Ding, D., Chen, G.-D., Lobarinas, E., Wang, J., . . . Auerbach, B. D. (2017). Inner hair cell loss disrupts hearing and cochlear function leading to sensory deprivation and enhanced central auditory gain. *Frontiers in Neuroscience*, *10*(January), 1–14. https://doi.org/10.3389/fnins.2016.00621.

Sametsky, E. A., Turner, J. G., Larsen, D., Ling, L., & Caspary, D. M. (2015). Enhanced GABA A-mediated tonic inhibition in auditory thalamus of rats with behavioral evidence of tinnitus. *Journal of Neuroscience*, *35*(25), 9369–9380. https://doi.org/10.1523/JNEUROSCI.5054-14.2015.

Sanchez, T. G., Moraes, F., Casseb, J., Cota, J., Freire, K., & Roberts, L. E. (2016). Tinnitus is associated with reduced sound level tolerance in adolescents with normal audiograms and otoacoustic emissions. *Scientific Reports, 6*(January), 27109. https://doi.org/10.1038/srep27109.

Sanchez, T. G., Yupanque Guerra, G. C., Lorenzi, M. C., Brandão, A. L., & Bento, R. F. (2002). The influence of voluntary muscle contractions upon the onset and modulation of tinnitus. *Audiology and Neuro-Otology, 7*(6), 370–375. https://doi.org/10.1159/000066155.

Schaette, R., & Kempter, R. (2006). Development of tinnitus-related neuronal hyperactivity through homeostatic plasticity after hearing loss: a computational model. *Eur. J. Neurosci., 23*, 3124–3138.

Schaette, R., & McAlpine, D. (2011). Tinnitus with a normal audiogram: Physiological evidence for hidden hearing loss and computational model, *31*(38), 13452–13457. https://doi.org/10.1523/JNEUROSCI.2156-11.2011.

Schaette, R., Turtle, C., & Munro, K. J. (2012). Reversible induction of phantom auditory sensations through simulated unilateral hearing loss. *PLoS ONE, 7*(6), 1–6. https://doi.org/10.1371/journal.pone.0035238.

Sedlacek, M., & Brenowitz, S. D. (2014). Cell-type specific short-term plasticity at auditory nerve synapses controls feed-forward inhibition in the dorsal cochlear nucleus, *8*(July), 1–12. https://doi.org/10.3389/fncir.2014.00078.

Sedley, W., Friston, K. J., Gander, P. E., Kumar, S., Griffiths, T. D., Shargorodsky, J., et al. (2016). An integrative tinnitus model based on sensory precision. *Trends in Neurosciences, 39*(12), 799–812. https://doi.org/10.1016/j.tins.2016.10.004.

Sedley, W., Parikh, J., Edden, R. A. E., Tait, V., Blamire, A., & Griffiths, T. D. (2015a). Human auditory cortex neurochemistry reflects the presence and severity of tinnitus. *Journal of Neuroscience: The Official Journal of the Society for Neuroscience, 35*(44), 14822–14828. https://doi.org/10.1523/JNEUROSCI.2695-15.2015.

Sedley, W., Gander, P. E., Kumar, S., Oya, H., Kovach, C. K., Nourski, K. V., . . . Griffiths, T. D. (2015b). Intracranial mapping of a cortical tinnitus system using residual inhibition. *Current Biology, 25*(9), 1208–1214. https://doi.org/10.1016/j.cub.2015.02.075.

Shaheen, L. A., Valero, M. D., & Liberman, M. C. (2015). Towards a diagnosis of cochlear neuropathy with envelope following responses. *JARO—Journal of the Association for Research in Otolaryngology, 16*(6), 727–745. https://doi.org/10.1007/s10162-015-0539-3.

Shargorodsky, J., Curhan, G. C., & Farwell, W. R. (2010). Prevalence and characteristics of tinnitus among U.S. adults. *American Journal of Medicine, 123*(8), 711–718. https://doi.org/10.1016/j.amjmed.2010.02.015.

Shargorodsky, J., Curhan, S. G., Curhan, G. C., & Eavey, R. (2010). Change in prevalence of hearing loss in U.S. adolescents. *JAMA: The Journal of the American Medical Association, 304*(7), 772–778. https://doi.org/10.1016/j.yped.2010.12.008.

Sheldrake, J., Diehl, P. U., & Schaette, R. (2015). Audiometric characteristics of hyperacusis patients. *Frontiers in Neurology, 6*(May), 1–7. https://doi.org/10.3389/fneur.2015.00105.

Sherlock, L. P., & Formby, C. (2005). Estimates of loudness, loudness discomfort, and the auditory dynamic range: Normative estimates, comparison of procedures, and test-retest reliability. *Journal of the American Academy of Audiology 16*, 85–100. doi:10.3766/jaaa.16.2.4.

Shi, L., Chang, Y., Li, X., Aiken, S. J., Liu, L., & Wang, J. (2016a). Coding deficits in noise-induced hidden hearing loss may stem from incomplete repair of ribbon synapses in the cochlea. *Frontiers in Neuroscience, 10*(May), 1–6. https://doi.org/10.3389/fnins.2016.00231.

Shi, L., Chang, Y., Li, X., Aiken, S., Liu, L., & Wang, J. (2016b). Cochlear synaptopathy and noise-induced hidden hearing loss. *Neural Plasticity*. https://doi.org/10.1155/2016/6143164.

Shi, L., Liu, L., He, T., Guo, X., Yu, Z., Yin, S., & Wang, J. (2013). Ribbon synapse plasticity in the cochleae of guinea pigs after noise-induced silent damage. *PLoS ONE, 8*(12). https://doi.org/10.1371/journal.pone.0081566.

Shore, S. E., Roberts, L. E., & Langguth, B. (2016). Maladaptive plasticity in tinnitus—triggers, mechanisms and treatment. *Nature Reviews Neurology, 12*(3), 150–160. https://doi.org/10.1038/nrneurol.2016.12.

Stefanescu, R. A., & Shore, S. E. (2017). Muscarinic acetylcholine receptors control baseline activity and Hebbian stimulus timing-dependent plasticity in fusiform cells of the dorsal cochlear nucleus. *Journal of Neurophysiology, 117*, 1229–1238.

Stellwagen, D., & Malenka, R. C. (2006). Synaptic scaling mediated by glial TNF-alpha. *Nature, 440*(7087), 1054–1059. https://doi.org/10.1038/nature04671.

Stracke, H., Okamoto, H., & Pantev, C. (2010). Customized notched music training reduces tinnitus loudness. *Communicative and Integrative Biology, 3*(3), 274–277.

Syka, J., Rybalko, N., & Popelář, J. (1994). Enhancement of the auditory cortex evoked responses in awake guinea pigs after noise exposure. *Hearing Research, 78*(2), 158–168. https://doi.org/10.1016/0378-5955(94)90021-3.

Tang, Z.-Q., & Trussell, L. (2017). 5-HT differentially modulates the output of auditory and multisensory inputs onto fusiform cells in the dorsal cochlear nucleus. Presented at the Annual Meeting of the Association for Research in Otolaryngology, Baltimore, MD (PS 270).

Tass, P. A., Adamchic, I., Freund, H. J., Von Stackelberg, T., & Hauptmann, C. (2012). Counteracting tinnitus by acoustic coordinated reset neuromodulation. *Restorative Neurology and Neuroscience, 30*(2), 137–159. https://doi.org/10.3233/RNN-2012-110218.

Terry, A. M. P., Jones, D. M., Davis, B. R., & Slater, R. (1983). Parametric studies of tinnitus masking and residual inhibition. *Br. J. Audiol., 17*, 245–256.

Turrigiano, G. G., & Nelson, S. B. (2008). Hebb and homeostasis in neuronal plasticity. *Current Opinion in Neurobiology, 10*, 358–364. http://dx.doi.org/10.1016/S0959-4388(00)00091-X.

Tzounopoulos, T., Rubio, M. E., Keen, J. E., & Trussell, L. O. (2007). Coactivation of pre- and postsynaptic signaling mechanisms determines cell-specific spike-timing-dependent plasticity. *Neuron, 54*(2), 291–301. https://doi.org/10.1016/j.neuron.2007.03.026.

Vogler, D. P., Robertson, D., & Mulders, W. H. A. M. (2011). Hyperactivity in the ventral cochlear nucleus after cochlear trauma. *Journal of Neuroscience: The Official Journal of the Society for Neuroscience, 31*(18), 6639–6645. https://doi.org/10.1523/JNEUROSCI.6538-10.2011.

Wang, H., Brozoski, T. J., Turner, J. G., Ling, L., Parrish, J. L., Hughes, L. F., & Caspary, D. M. (2009). Plasticity at glycinergic synapses in dorsal cochlear nucleus of rats with behavioral evidence of tinnitus. *Neuroscience, 164*(2), 747–759. https://doi.org/10.1016/j.neuroscience.2009.08.026.

Wehr, M., & Zador, A. M. (2005). Synaptic mechanisms of forward suppression in rat auditory cortex. *Neuron, 47*(3), 437–445. https://doi.org/10.1016/j.neuron.2005.06.009.

Weisz, N., Muller, S., Schlee, W., Dohrmann, K., Hartmann, T., & Elbert, T. (2007). The neural code of auditory phantom perception. *Journal of Neuroscience, 27*(6), 1479–1484. https://doi.org/10.1523/JNEUROSCI.3711-06.2007.

Whiting, B., Moiseff, A., & Rubio, M. E. (2009). Cochlear nucleus neurons redistribute synaptic AMPA and glycine receptors in response to monaural conductive hearing loss. *Neuroscience, 163*(4), 1264–1276. https://doi.org/10.1016/j.neuroscience.2009.07.049.

Wienbruch, C., Paul, I., Weisz, N., Elbert, T., & Roberts, L. E. (2006). Frequency organization of the 40-Hz auditory steady-state response in normal hearing and in tinnitus. *NeuroImage, 33*(1), 180–194. https://doi.org/10.1016/j.neuroimage.2006.06.023.

Winkler, I., Denham, S. L., & Nelken, I. (2009). Modeling the auditory scene: predictive regularity representations and perceptual objects. *Trends in Cognitive Sciences, 13*(12), 532–540. https://doi.org/10.1016/j.tics.2009.09.003.

Wu, C., Martel, D. T., & Shore, S. E. (2016). Increased synchrony and bursting of dorsal cochlear nucleus fusiform cells correlate with tinnitus. *Journal of Neuroscience, 36*(6), 2068–2073. https://doi.org/10.1523/JNEUROSCI.3960-15.2016.

Yang, S., Weiner, B. D., Zhang, L. S., Cho, S.-J., & Bao, S. (2011). Homeostatic plasticity drives tinnitus perception in an animal model. *Proceedings of the National Academy of Sciences of the United States of America, 108*(36), 14974–14979. https://doi.org/10.1073/pnas.1107998108.

Zeng, C., Nannapaneni, N., Zhou, J., Hughes, L. F., & Shore, S. (2009). Cochlear damage changes the distribution of vesicular glutamate transporters associated with auditory and nonauditory inputs to the cochlear nucleus. *The Journal of Neuroscience: The Official Journal of the Society for Neuroscience*, *29*(13), 4210–4217. https://doi.org/10.1523/JNEUROSCI.0208-09.2009.

Zeng, F. G. (2013). An active loudness model suggesting tinnitus as increased central noise and hyperacusis as increased nonlinear gain. *Hearing Research*, *295*(May), 172–179. https://doi.org/10.1016/j.heares.2012.05.009.

Zhao, Y., & Tzounopoulos, T. (2011). Physiological activation of cholinergic inputs controls associative synaptic plasticity via modulation of endocannabinoid signaling. *Journal of Neuroscience*, *31*(9), 3158–3168. https://doi.org/10.1523/JNEUROSCI.5303-10.2011.

Zheng, X., Giang, A., Vetsis, S., Bruce, I. C., & Voigt H. F. (2009). A computational modeling study of the effects of acoustic trauma on the dorsal cochlear nucleus. In: Vander Sloten, J., Verdonck, P., Nyssen, M., & Haueisen, J. (Eds.). 4th European Conference of the International Federation for Medical and Biological Engineering. IFMBE Proceedings, vol. 22. Berlin, Heidelberg: Springer.

7

Hyperacusis: Medical Diagnoses and Associated Syndromes

Don McFerran

Introduction

As our knowledge of disorders of sound tolerance increases it has become apparent that there is a family of conditions rather than a single entity: this chapter deliberates on conditions as disparate as the exaggerated startle reflex of a child with Cri du Chat syndrome, the heightened awareness of internal body sounds seen in Superior Semicircular Canal Dehiscence, supranormal hearing thresholds following spinal anesthesia, and the auditory pain reported in Acoustic Shock Syndrome or Meniere's disease. Yet all have been termed hyperacusis. There is no consensus on how to assess disorders of sound tolerance: hyperacusis tests used by studies in this chapter include testing the startle reflex, measuring loudness discomfort levels, measuring audiometric thresholds, patient report, parental report, structured interviews, and hyperacusis questionnaires. The pathophysiological mechanisms are still putative, and it is quite possible, indeed probable, that multiple mechanisms are at play.

The taxonomy of disorders of sound tolerance is still unsatisfactory with at least two competing classifications (see also Chapter 1). Jastreboff and Jastreboff (2002) divided disorders of sound tolerance into four subgroups: recruitment or abnormal loudness growth, attributed entirely to peripheral mechanisms secondary to outer hair cell loss in the cochlea; hyperacusis, defined as discomfort caused by exposure to a sound that would not evoke a similar reaction in an average listener; misophonia, defined as dislike or hatred of specific sounds due to enhanced reactivity of the limbic and autonomic systems; phonophobia, defined as a subsection of misophonia when fear is the dominant evoked emotion. Tyler et al. (2014) proposed a different classification comprised of loudness hyperacusis, annoyance hyperacusis, pain hyperacusis, and fear hyperacusis. Neither of these classifications seems fully fit for purpose and there are situations that do not seem to sit easily within either system. Formby, Sherlock, Hawley, and Gold (2017) have shown that sound tolerance can be improved in the case of recruitment which should not be possible if it was entirely due to outer hair cell damage. Misophonia has been redefined by some workers to describe a group of patients who experience anger, disgust, and anxiety in response to their trigger sounds which are typically sounds such as chewing, lip-smacking, or whistling. These patients display avoidant or aggressive behavior in response to the trigger sounds and there have been calls to redefine misophonia as a specific psychiatric condition (Schröder, Vulink, & Denys, 2013).

There would appear to be, potentially, considerable overlap between the categories proposed by Tyler et al. (2014): Is someone who has pain hyperacusis not also annoyed? In any case, the question of subtypes of hyperacusis is somewhat academic in the context of medical conditions associated with sound tolerance disorders—in most of the studies discussed in this chapter no attempt was made to subtype the associated sound tolerance disorder(s). Generally, in the following text, the word hyperacusis is used as an umbrella term to denote any impairment of sound tolerance. Some older works used the word to signify better than normal hearing thresholds.

Most review articles regarding hyperacusis and other disorders of sound tolerance include lists or tables of medical conditions associated with sound intolerance (Marriage & Barnes, 1995; Katzenell & Segal, 2001; Baguley, 2003; Tyler et al., 2014; Pienkowski et al., 2014). Many such publications are now easily available on the Internet, which means that it is a simple process to cut and paste lists of hyperacusis-associated medical conditions onto other information disseminating platforms. Therefore, the information is sometimes presented to the public in an uncritical fashion. For example, the table of potentially associated medical conditions described by Pienkowski et al. (2014) has been reproduced accurately by a patient information website, Hyperacusis Focus (2017). Unfortunately, the website includes no qualitative assessment of the copied information—it is presented as established fact. A search of the medical literature produced a long list of conditions with a possible link to disorders of sound tolerance (Table 7–1).

The evidence for a link between the conditions in Table 7–1 and disorders of sound tolerance is explored in more detail in the following text. For many of these conditions the evidence suggesting a link is based on case reports or small case series. To date there have been very few population-based studies on hyperacusis (Fabijanska, Rogowski, Bartnik, & Skarzynski, 1999; Andersson, Lindvall, Hursti, & Carlbring, 2002; Paulin, Andersson, & Nordin, 2016) and only one that has attempted to explore the potential comorbidities of impaired sound tolerance with any degree of scientific rigor. Paulin et al. (2016) used data supplied by participants in the Västerbotten Environmental Health Study. This is an ongoing series of different studies conducted on a sample of the population of Västerbotten, a county of northern Sweden with a population of approximately 260,000. A random sample of 8600 adults (age range 18 to 79) was invited to participate. Of these, 8520 could be contacted and 3406 ultimately agreed to participate. In this subsection of the study, participants were asked whether they had "been diagnosed with sound intolerance by a physician" and whether they had a "hard time tolerating everyday sounds that you believe most of the people can tolerate." There were 66 people who met the criterion for physician-diagnosed hyperacusis and 313 for self-reported hyperacusis. The responses from these groups were compared with those of a control group of 2995 people and data regarding a series of health conditions was collected for both the hyperacusis and control groups. Odds ratios for the presence of

Table 7–1. Conditions with a suggested association with hyperacusis. The best level of evidence supporting each potential association is denoted in the right-hand column. Source material regarding each condition is discussed in the text.

Disease Classification	Disease or Condition		Best Level of Evidence
Genetic	Williams syndrome		Controlled case series
	GM2 gangliosidoses	Tay-Sachs disease	Uncontrolled case series
		Sandhoff disease	Uncontrolled case series
	GM1 gangliosidosis, type 2		Case reports
	Cri du Chat syndrome		Uncontrolled case series
Otological	Hearing loss		Population study
	Tinnitus		Population study
	Associated with failure of the stapedial reflex due to facial nerve dysfunction	Bell's palsy	Uncontrolled case series
		Ramsay Hunt syndrome	Uncontrolled case series
	Associated with failure of the stapedial reflex due to direct dysfunction of the stapedius muscle	Post-stapedectomy	Uncontrolled case series
	Specific otological conditions	Superior canal dehiscence syndrome (SCDS)	Uncontrolled case series
		Lateral semicircular canal dysplasia	Uncontrolled case series
		Meniere's disease	Uncontrolled case series
		Acoustic shock syndrome	Uncontrolled case series
		Following surgical correction of conductive hearing loss: tympanoplasty, stapedectomy.	Uncontrolled case series
		Perilymph fistula	Uncontrolled case series

Table 7–1. (*continued*)

Disease Classification	Disease or Condition		Best Level of Evidence
Neurological	Migraine		Population study
	Other headaches		Uncontrolled case series
	Myasthenia gravis		Uncontrolled case series
	Multiple sclerosis		Case reports
	Spina bifida		Controlled case series
	Complex regional pain syndrome		Population study
	Chronic fatigue syndrome		Population study
	Cerebrovascular accidents		Case reports
Neuropsychological	Head injury		Controlled case series
	Posttraumatic stress disorder		Population study
Neurodevelopmental	Autism spectrum		Controlled experimental study
	Learning disability and stuttering		Controlled experimental study
	Attention deficit hyperactivity disorder		Population study
Psychological	Depression		Population study
	Anxiety		Population study
	Panic disorder		Population study
	Obsessive compulsive disorder		Uncontrolled case series
	Eating disorder		Uncontrolled case series
Endocrine	Adrenocortical insufficiency	Addison's disease	Controlled case series
		Pan-hypopituitarism	Controlled case series
	Hyperthyroidism		None
	Growth hormone deficiency		Controlled case series

Metabolic	Pyridoxine deficiency		None
	Magnesium deficiency		Animal research
Autoimmune	Cogan's syndrome		Case report
	Systemic lupus erythematosus		Controlled case series
Musculoskeletal	Back, joint, and muscle pain		Population study
	Temporomandibular disorder (TMD)		Controlled case series
	Fibromyalgia		Population study
Vascular	Carotid aneurysm		None
	Middle cerebral artery aneurysm		Case report
Gastrointestinal	Irritable bowel syndrome		Population study
Pharmacological	Drug withdrawal	Benzodiazepine	Randomized controlled trial
		Monoamine oxidase inhibitor (MOAI)	Uncontrolled experimental study
	Drug side effects		Case reports
Infective	Lyme disease		Case reports
	Creutzfeldt Jacob disease		Case reports
	Neurosyphilis		Case reports
	Typhoid fever		None
	Typhus		Case reports
Iatrogenic	Spinal anaesthesia		None
Environmental intolerance	Multiple chemical sensitivity		Population study
	Non-specific building-related symptoms		Population study
	Electromagnetic hypersensitivity		Population study

hyperacusis in association with any of the health conditions were calculated. This was the first large-scale population-based study to explore the medical conditions associated with hyperacusis and added considerably to our knowledge but as the authors freely admitted, the study did have potential weaknesses: only 40% of the initial random sample agreed to participate and nonparticipation was skewed toward those of younger age; this

Table 7–2. Prevalence and odds ratios (adjusted for age, sex, and level of education) for participants in the population-based study undertaken by Paulin et al. (2016). Confidence intervals (CI) in brackets.

	Self-Reported Hyperacusis n = 313		Physician-Diagnosed Hyperacusis n = 66	
Medical Condition	Prevalence (%)	Adjusted Odds Ratio (95% CI)	Prevalence (%)	Adjusted Odds Ratio (95% CI)
Post-traumatic stress disorder	4.8	12.80 (5.65–29.00)	12.1	44.68 (16.52–120.87)
Generalized anxiety disorder	5.1	11.50 (5.40–24.51)	10.6	31.69 (11.83–84.87)
Chronic fatigue syndrome	3.2	11.33 (4.48–28.00)	10.6	34.31 (12.40–94.96)
ADHD	2.6	10.19 (3.73–27.83)		
Tinnitus	24.0	8.63 (6.15–12.10)	43.9	16.55 (9.43–29.04)
Exhaustion syndrome	14.7	5.05 (3.44–7.43)	18.2	7.12 (3.61–14.03)
Depression	17.3	4.91 (3.44–7.01)	22.7	8.89 (4.72–16.72)
Hearing impairment	29.4	4.71 (3.47–6.40)	59.1	12.23 (6.89–21.70)
Panic disorder	3.5	2.57 (1.28–5.14)		
Back/joint/ muscle disorder	23.4	2.47 (1.83–3.34)	39.4	3.84 (2.26–6.52)
Fibromyalgia	4.2	2.19 (1.16–4.10)	10.6	5.08 (2.17–11.87)
Irritable bowel syndrome	4.8	2.10 (1.17–3.77)	9.1	4.34 (1.78–10.60)
Migraine	6.7	1.49 (0.92–2.42)	12.1	3.21 (1.48–6.98)

study relied on self-report of both hyperacusis and medical conditions; no audiological assessment was conducted and there were therefore no data on hearing threshold or loudness discomfort levels; the study made no attempt to distinguish between different subtypes of hyperacusis and made no attempt to determine the impact of any hyperacusis. Despite these limitations the study delivered some very useful information. Overall, hyperacusis was found to be more common in women, more common with advancing age, and possibly more common with higher levels of education. The overall point prevalence of hyperacusis in the study was approximately 1 in 10 which agrees with several previous prevalence studies (Fabijanska et al., 1999; Andersson et al., 2002). Co-morbidities included hearing impairment, tinnitus, back/joint/muscle disorders, and various psychiatric conditions and functional somatic syndromes (Table 7–2).

Individual Conditions Associated with Disorders of Sound Tolerance

Genetic Conditions

Williams Syndrome

Williams syndrome or Williams Beuren syndrome is a genetic condition caused by deletion of a portion of chromosome 7. Affected individuals have endocrine abnormalities, mild-to-moderate cognitive impairment, and increased risk of cardiovascular disease. Typically, they have characteristic facial features which are often described as elfin. Several studies have identified abnormal sound tolerance in individuals with Williams syndrome (Klein, Armstrong, Greer, & Brown, 1990; Nigam & Samuel, 1994; Gothelf, Farber, Raveh, Apter, & Attias, 2006). The prevalence of hyperacusis in children with Williams syndrome was reported to be as high as 95% (Klein et al., 1990). In a comprehensive review, Attias, Raveh, Ben-Naftali, Zarchi, and Gothelf (2008) identified various sound-related symptoms in Williams syndrome: auditory fascination defined as above normal attraction to certain sounds; phonophobia; hyperacusis; strong attraction to music. Attias (2013) also supplied a critique on the underlying pathophysiology of Williams syndrome: the genes coded by the missing portion of chromosome are known, leading to speculation that the sound tolerance issues may be linked to the elastin gene (ELN), general transcription factor Iii gene (GTF 21), or domain kinase one gene (LMK1). In addition, the majority of children with Williams syndrome have absent stapedial reflexes (Attias et al., 2008) and therefore could develop some of their sound tolerance issues in a similar way to other patients with abnormalities of the acoustic reflex.

GM2 Gangliosidoses: Tay-Sachs, Sandhoff, and GM2 Gangliosidosis AB Variant

Tay-Sachs disease is a rare autosomal recessive genetic disorder caused by mutations in the HEXA gene on chromosome 15. Sandhoff disease is a rare autosomal recessive genetic disorder caused by mutations in the HEXB gene on chromosome 5: it is clinically indistinguishable from Tay-Sachs disease. These inherited defects lead to an accumulation of a molecule called GM2 ganglioside in the brain. Affected babies appear to develop normally initially but as the ganglioside accumulates, a variety of neurological problems appear and most affected individuals die in early childhood. Milder juvenile and adult forms of the condition can occur. Developmental delay or regression is the usual mode of presentation. Hyperacusis has been described (Gordon et al., 1988; Arisoy, Ozden, Ciliv, & Ozalp 1995; Karimzadeh et al., 2014) with Karimzadeh et al. (2014) reporting it in 7 (39%) of a series of 18 patients, comprised of 9 who had Tay-Sachs disease and 9 who had Sandhoff disease. GM2 gangliosidosis AB variant disease is an extremely rare autosomal recessive genetic disorder that is clinically similar to Tay-Sachs and Sandhoff diseases, caused by a mutation of the GM2A gene on chromosome 5. Hyperacusis in association with AB variant disease has been reported in this condition (Sheth et al., 2016). The effect of Tay-Sachs on the auditory periphery remains unclear.

GM1 Gangliosidosis

GM1 gangliosidosis is a rare inherited lysosomal storage disorder that progressively destroys neurons in the central nervous system; however, its effect on the cochlea is undetermined. The disease is subdivided into three types based on the age of onset of the condition: early infantile (type 1); late infantile (type 2); and adult (type 3). Although the types differ in severity, their features overlap significantly. GM1 gangliosidosis is caused by mutations in the GLB1 gene on chromosome 3 and is inherited in an autosomal recessive manner. Two siblings presented with developmental arrest, gait disturbance, dementia, epilepsy, and hyperacusis in the second year of life and after investigation were diagnosed with GM1 gangliosidosis type 2 (Gascon, Ozand, & Erwin, 1992).

Cri du Chat Syndrome

Cri du Chat syndrome is a congenital condition characterized by learning disability, spasticity, abnormal facial features, and a cat-like cry in infancy. It is caused by partial deletion of the short arm of chromosome 5. Cornish and Pigram (1996) explored the developmental and behavioral characteristics of 27 children (13 boys and 14 girls, mean age 8.3 years) with Cri du Chat syndrome. During a structured interview with the families, the researchers completed a Society for the Study of Behavioural Phenotypes questionnaire for each child. In 81.4% of the study group hypersensitivity to sensory stimuli including sound was reported. The study was uncontrolled and no robust evidence regarding the state of the auditory periphery was presented.

Otological Conditions

Hearing Loss and Tinnitus

In the population-based study undertaken by Paulin et al. (2016) hearing loss and tinnitus were respectively the most common and second most common conditions co-morbid with hyperacusis. The association of tinnitus and hyperacusis tallies with previous work: among people presenting with a primary complaint of tinnitus, figures for the proportion with co-morbid hyperacusis vary from 40% (Fabijanska et al., 1999) to 63% (Andersson, Vretblad, Larsen, & Lyttkens, 2001). When people whose primary complaint is hyperacusis are considered, 86% have co-morbid tinnitus (Anari, Axelsson, Eliasson, & Magnusson, 1999). The position regarding an association of hearing loss and hyperacusis has been less clear. Nelson and Chen (2004) argued that tinnitus, hyperacusis, and hearing loss share a common pathophysiology but in a population-based study Hannula Bloigu, Majamaa, Sorri, and Mäki-Torkko (2011) reported no statistically significant relationship between hyperacusis and average hearing threshold loss. However, this study revealed that self-reported hearing impairment was far greater than hearing impairment defined by audiometric measurement in the range of 0.5 to 4 kHz. Self-reported hearing difficulties including tinnitus and hyperacusis seemed predictive of hearing impairment at high frequencies (4 to 8 kHz). The epidemiological study described by Paulin et al. (2016) has methodological weaknesses and its reliance on self-reported hearing loss was a shortcoming. The term "hearing loss" covers a wide range of different medical conditions. Nevertheless, this study did at least suggest that there is an association between hearing loss and hyperacusis.

Stapedial Reflex Dysfunction

The stapedius muscle contracts involuntarily in response to high-intensity sound, stiffening the ossicular chain and decreasing sound transmission to the cochlea. Failure of this stapedial, or acoustic reflex would therefore be expected to allow more sound energy through the conductive mechanism to the cochlea and thereby increase the range of sound levels that produce discomfort in affected individuals. The reflex involves the inner ear, auditory nerve, brainstem, facial nerve, stapedius muscle, and ossicular chain: pathology of any component of this arc can disrupt the reflex. Hyperacusis in association with stapedial reflex dysfunction has been reported with idiopathic or Bell's palsy (Adour & Wingerd, 1974; McCandless & Goering, 1974; McCandless & Schumacher, 1979), herpes zoster associated palsy or Ramsay Hunt syndrome (Wayman, Pham, Byl, & Adour, 1990), myasthenia gravis (considered separately: see below), and after surgical division of the tendon of the stapedius muscle during stapedectomy (Mathisen 1969; McCandless & Goering, 1974). However, Mathisen (1969) reported that stapedectomy-associated hyperacusis tends to improve with time suggesting that the hyperacusis might arise within the central auditory system rather than because of loss of the stapedial reflex. There are other suggestions that the role of the stapedial reflex in the generation of hyperacusis is not clear-cut: although it might appear obvious that impairment of the acoustic reflex could contribute to increased sound sensitivity there are several studies that contradict this supposition. Citron and Adour (1978) described 48 consecutive patients with Bell's palsy and reported that hyperacusis was unrelated to stapedial muscle paralysis. Liriano Magalhães, Barros, José, and Fukuda (2004) reported on 18 patients with Bell's palsy. All but one had impaired stapedial reflexes but only one complained of hyperacusis. Loudness discomfort levels were performed in this study and were slightly reduced on the affected side. The authors concluded that sound sensitivity was slightly increased but not enough to generate clinical symptoms in a majority of patients. A cohort study by de Seta et al. (2014) reported on 269 patients with Bell's palsy. Hyperacusis was an uncommon symptom in this cohort—the results were presented graphically, and an exact figure cannot be quoted but is approximately 5%, which is comparable to the prevalence of hyperacusis in the general population.

Superior Semicircular Canal Dehiscence

Superior semicircular canal dehiscence (SSCD) is a condition first described by Minor, Solomon, Zinreich, and Zee (1998) in which the bone overlying the superior semicircular canal, separating the canal from the middle cranial fossa, is deficient, creating a so-called third window into the labyrinth. Patients may report increased awareness or sensitivity to bone conduction sounds such as the sound of their own voice or internal body sounds including eye movements or heartbeat. This has been called conductive hyperacusis and needs to be carefully contrasted to the more typical hyperacusis triggered by external sound sources (see Chapter 1 for concerns regarding the terminology). Other common symptoms include dizziness and sound-induced vertigo, or Tullio phenomenon. In addition to hypersensitivity to internal sounds, a case series has been published describing increased sensitivity to external sounds (Saliba et al., 2014).

Lateral Semicircular Canal Dysplasia

Modugno and Brandolini (2014) reported three patients who presented with symptoms suggestive of superior semicircular canal dehiscence including hyperacusis to external sounds. CT scanning showed no evidence of bony dehiscence but revealed that all three had abnormal, dilated lateral semicircular canals.

Meniere's Disease

Meniere's disease is a condition characterized by episodic attacks of vertigo, hearing loss, tinnitus, and aural fullness. The exact pathophysiology remains unknown but both postmortem studies and high-resolution MRI scans have shown an association with endolymphatic hydrops—an expansion of the endolymphatic compartment of the inner ear. Several studies have reported hyperacusis in Meniere's. Hadj-Djilani and Gerster (1984) reported a retrospective study of 33 cases of Meniere's: three out of four patients who were tested had a pain threshold to sound of less than 100 dB HL. Herraiz, Tapia, and Plaza (2006) reported on 102 patients with Meniere's who had been referred to a tinnitus clinic. These patients met the diagnostic criteria for definite Meniere's as described in the American Academy of Otolaryngology Head and Neck Surgery guidelines (American Academy of Otolaryngology—Head and Neck Foundation, Inc., 1995). For 6 of their 102 patients hyperacusis was the most troublesome symptom of their Meniere's and presence of hyperacusis was associated with increased tinnitus severity. Although loudness recruitment commonly accompanies Meniere's, it is not clear from the currently available evidence whether hyperacusis is more common in Meniere's than other cases of sensorineural hearing loss and/or tinnitus.

Acoustic Shock

Toward the end of the twentieth century there was a series of occupational health reports from call centers describing a cluster of audiovestibular symptoms seen after employees had been subjected to unexpected sound through their telephone headsets. The causative sounds were not necessarily at a level that would be expected to harm the auditory system and the common factor of the sounds was their very short rise-time or suddenness. The condition became known as acoustic shock syndrome or simply acoustic shock (McFerran, 2016a). Pain, tinnitus, perturbation of balance and hyperacusis or auditory hypervigilance were the most commonly reported symptoms. Although the condition remains enigmatic, Westcott et al. (2013) has suggested that the condition might be caused by abnormal contraction of the tensor tympani muscle. Although tonic tensor tympani syndrome could explain some symptoms such as pain and aural fullness, it is less clear to see how such pathology could result in hyperacusis.

Surgical Correction of Conductive Hearing Loss

Although it is common to hear anecdotal reports of excessively sensitive hearing after ventilation tube or grommet insertion there is very little written in the medical literature regarding this. In a study of acoustic reflexes in relation to audio sensitivity, Gordon (1986) reported a 9-year-old boy who developed sound sensitivity after grommet insertion. Other surgical procedures that can improve hearing include tympanoplasty and stapedectomy. There is a single case report of hyperacusis arising after tympanoplasty, necessitating the use of a sound attenuating ear plug (Stange, Mir-Salim, & Berghaus, 2001). Hyperacusis following stapedectomy is discussed above.

Perilymph Fistula

Perilymph fistula refers to an abnormal connection between the inner ear and the middle ear. It has been reported following ear surgery, head injury, and barotrauma. More controversially, it has been suggested that the condition may arise spontaneously (Althaus, 1977). Symptoms are similar to other inner ear pathologies such as Meniere's disease. A series of 40 patients who had received a diagnosis of idiopathic perilymph fistula was reported by Fukaya and Nomura (1988) and in this series 62.5% of patients presented with hyperacusis. Given the skepticism regarding the concept of spontaneous perilymph fistula and the lack of other substantiating evidence, these reports must be interpreted with caution.

Neurological Conditions

Migraine

Migraine affects 14.70% of the global population (Vos et al., 2010). Classically, sufferers experience episodic headache affecting one half of the head that may be accompanied by nausea, vomiting, and increased sensitivity to light, odors, and sound. For those who experience impaired sound sensitivity this discomfort can occur during the prodrome or the pain phase. There is conflicting evidence as to whether migraineurs have increased sound sensitivity interictally. Woodhouse and Drummond (1993) suggested this is not the case and that patients experience excessive loudness only when experiencing a migraine. Vingen, Sand, and Stovner (1999), using different methodology, stated that migraineurs have increased sensitivity even when headache free. Sound hypersensitivity worsens during the headache period but is not related to the presence or absence of migrainous aura.

Paulin et al. (2016) demonstrated that migraine is a risk factor for hyperacusis though the odds ratio was relatively modest (1.49 for self-reported hyperacusis; 3.21 for physician-diagnosed hyperacusis). For a common component symptom of a common condition there has been remarkably little work done to characterize the nature of the altered sound sensitivity that people with migraine experience. The increased sound sensitivity is generally called phonophobia; using the alternative classification of hyperacusis proposed by Tyler et al. (2014) it has been labeled a form of fear hyperacusis. Vingen et al. (1999) defined migrainous phonophobia as "hypersensitivity to auditory stimuli, involving a feeling of discomfort or pain." There was no mention of fear or phobia in this description. Using audiological definitions of sound tolerance disorders (Jastreboff & Jastreboff, 2002), this definition of migrainous phonophobia would probably be best regarded as hyperacusis or, in the alternative classification of Tyler et al. (2104), pain hyperacusis. A non-scientific straw poll by the author of this chapter suggested that people with migraine find that sounds seem louder than normal and they become irritated or annoyed by sound during the headache period. None of the people questioned described a fear of sound. This is clearly an area that needs exploration.

Other Forms of Headache

Increased sensitivity to sound has been reported in association with other types of headache. Patients with cluster headache have been reported to have increased sound sensitivity during the active phase of their condition but not when the condition is inactive (Vingen, Pareja, & Stovner, 1998). Patients with tension-type and cervicogenic headache have also been observed with increased sensitivity to sound, though in these conditions the sensitivity is elevated even during the headache-free period (Vingen et al., 1999).

Myasthenia Gravis

Myasthenia gravis is a rare autoimmune disease affecting nerve synapses, leading to skeletal muscle weakness. The stapedius muscle is vulnerable to this pathology, and Laurian, Laurian, Sadov, Strauss, and Kalmanovitz (1983) showed abnormalities of the stapedial reflex in myasthenic patients with raised stapedial reflex thresholds and decreased amplitudes. No clinical correlation to loudness intolerance was made in this study. Morioka, Neff, Boisseranc, Hartman, and Cantrell (1976) reported a series of six patients who had myasthenia. Hyperacusis was noted together with raised stapedial reflex thresholds and both factors improved after treatment.

Multiple Sclerosis

Multiple sclerosis is a demyelinating condition of the central nervous system. The insulating myelin sheaths of nerve fibers are damaged, resulting in impaired conduction of neural signals. Plaques of demyelination can occur at multiple locations in the central nervous system and the potential for involvement of the auditory system has long been recognized (Von Leden & Horton, 1948). Cases of hyperacusis in association with multiple sclerosis have been reported (Weber, Pfadenhauer, Stöhr, & Rösler, 2002).

Spina Bifida

Spina bifida is a developmental defect in which babies are born with incomplete closure of the spinal column. Neural tissue may be exposed or may be covered by soft tissue. In the cases where neural tissue is exposed there is often associated hydrocephalus. Both genetic and nongenetic factors are thought to contribute to the etiology of the condition. Hyperacusis has been reported in children with spina bifida. In a controlled case series Oen, Begeer, Staal-Schreinemachers, and Tijmstra (1997) used oral interview of parents and a nondisclosed questionnaire to investigate 50 babies with spina bifida, reporting hyperreactivity to sound in 50%.

Complex Regional Pain Syndrome

Complex regional pain syndrome is a form of chronic pain that usually follows injury. Some affected patients develop movement disorders including tremor, myoclonus, or dystonia. De Klaver et al. (2007) evaluated the audiological function of 40 patients with complex regional pain syndrome related dystonia. Peripheral auditory function was normal, and 38% reported hyperacusis.

Chronic Fatigue Syndrome

Chronic fatigue syndrome or myalgic encephalomyelitis (ME) is a condition characterized by persistent severe fatigue and a variety of other symptoms including memory and concentration issues, joint and muscle pains, and headaches. Although various hypotheses exist, the exact pathophysiology remains unclear. There have been previous suggestions that hyperacusis is more common in this condition (Behan & Bakheit, 1991). The population-based study by Paulin et al. (2016) confirmed this association (Table 7–2).

Cerebrovascular Disease

Hyperacusis has been reported occurring rarely after both ischemic and hemorrhagic stroke (Fukutake & Hattori, 1998; Sand, Biller, Corbett, Adams, & Dunn, 1986).

Neuropsychological Conditions

Head Injury

Waddell and Gronwall (1984) studied 9 consecutive closed head injury patients, assessing their sensitivity to sound and light. Measures were compared to controls matched for age, sex, race, and socioeconomic status. Head injury patients were statistically more sensitive to light than the controls. Eight patients participated in the sound sensitivity tests: 4/8 reported that they were more sensitive to sound and 2/8 reported that they were much more sensitive. The sound intensity tolerated by the head injury patients was lower than in the control group (82 dB compared to 94 dB) but the difference did not reach statistical significance. Chapter 9 offers a detailed summary regarding the association between traumatic brain injury and sound tolerance issues.

Post-traumatic Stress Disorder

Post-traumatic stress disorder (PTSD) is a mental health condition that can develop after a person is exposed to a traumatic event. Criteria for making a diagnosis of PTSD are complex and include exposure to a traumatic event, intrusive thoughts, flashbacks, feeling of isolation, hypervigilance, heightened startle reaction, concentration problems, and insomnia. Fagelson (2007) reported PTSD in U.S. armed forces Veterans who were referred to a tinnitus clinic. Approximately 34% of 300 patients met the criteria for PTSD, were twice as likely as patients without PTSD to report sound tolerance problems, and three times as likely as patients without PTSD to report sound-evoked exacerbation of tinnitus. The large population-based study undertaken in Sweden, by Paulin et al. (2016), confirmed this co-morbidity (Table 7–2).

Neurodevelopmental Conditions

Autism Spectrum Disorders

Autism Spectrum Disorders (ASD) comprise a series of neurodevelopmental disorders in which affected individuals display persistent deficits in social communication and interaction and display restricted repetitive patterns of behavior, interests, or activities. Sensory hypersensitivity has long been recognized in ASD (Baron Cohen, Ashwin, Ashwin, Tavassoli, & Chakrabarti, 2009) and there are many anecdotal reports describing individual experiences of sound intolerance in autism (Tavassoli, 2013). The current *Diagnostic and Statistical Manual of Mental Disorders*, 5th ed. (DSM-5) (American Psychiatric Association, 2013) has added both hyperreactivity and hyporeactivity to sensory input to the diagnostic criteria for ASD. Although individuals with so-called high functioning ASD can describe their reactions to sensory stimuli, there are many autistic people who cannot interact with researchers in this fashion. This makes research in the field difficult and is reflected in the sometimes apparently contradictory nature of studies. Beers, McBoyle, Kakande, Dar Santos, and Kozak (2014) conducted a systematic review and concluded that there is no conclusive evidence that children with ASD are at increased risk of peripheral hearing loss. Matsuzaki et al. (2014) performed a magnetoencephalography (MEG) study on 21 boys with ASD, 12 of whom with auditory hypersensitivity and 9 without; 15 normally developing boys were used as a control group. Increased activity was seen in the group with autism and auditory hypersensitivity but in neither of the other groups. The authors speculated that auditory hypersensitivity in autism was caused by reduced inhibitory processing. Khalfa et al. (2004) performed a range of audiological tests on 11 children with autism and 11 without. The autistic children were found to have a smaller auditory dynamic range and increased perception of loudness. Rosenhall, Nordin, Sandström, Ahlsén, and Gillberg (1999) compared 199 children with autism (153 boys, 46 girls) against a control group finding hyperacusis in 18.0% of the autistic subjects versus 0% in the control group. Danesh et al. (2015) studied hyperacusis in individuals with Asperger's syndrome finding increased prevalence in the Asperger's group compared to both the general population and individuals with other forms of autism.

Learning Disability and Stuttering

Gordon (1986) described a study of 93 children with learning disability comprising 73 boys and 20 girls with a mean age of 9.4 years. Many, though the exact number was unspecified, had dyslexia. The children were allocated by parental report to one of three groups: audiosensitive defined as needing to turn the volume down on a TV, radio, or record player; noise intolerant defined as having any form of sound intolerance but not meeting the definition of audiosensitivity; tolerant to noise. Stapedial reflex abnormalities were reported more commonly in the audiosensitive group than the other two groups. MacCulloch and Eaton (1971) studied 44 children who had been referred because of stutter. There were 35 boys and 9 girls with a mean age of 12.5 years. An equal group of non-stuttering children was used as a control group. Loudness discomfort levels were tested and were found to be lower in the stuttering group than the non-stuttering controls. There was no report as to whether any of the test subjects were distressed by noise.

Attention Deficit Hyperactivity Disorder

Attention deficit hyperactivity disorder (ADHD) is a neurodevelopmental condition characterized by deficits in attention, organization, activity levels, and impulse control (Ramtekkar 2017). As part of a large population-based study of hyperacusis in Sweden, Paulin et al. (2013) asked participants about various health conditions including ADHD. Elevated odds ratios supported the hypothesis that ADHD is co-morbid with hyperacusis though the number of people self-reporting ADHD was very small (8 individuals) and this suggested association should be interpreted carefully.

Psychological Conditions

Hypersensitivity to sound has long been recognized as having co-morbidity with several mental health disorders including depression and anxiety (Stansfeld, 1992; Jüris, Andersson, Larsen, & Ekselius, 2013). Data from a large population-based study supports this assertion (Paulin, 2016) (Table 7–2). This study also demonstrated a co-morbidity between hyperacusis and panic disorder. Obsessive compulsive disorders and eating disorders have been described in case reports and case series of patients with misophonia (McFerran, 2016b).

Endocrine Conditions

Adrenocortical Insufficiency: Addison's Disease and Pan-Hypopituitarism

Adrenocortical insufficiency is a condition in which the adrenal glands fail to produce adequate quantities of steroids, particularly glucocorticoids. This can occur because of primary failure of the adrenal cortex due to autoimmune mechanisms in Addison's disease. Alternatively, it can arise because the pituitary gland is not producing the necessary hormones to control the adrenal gland. A study examined the auditory function of four patients with Addison's disease and four patients with adrenocortical insufficiency secondary to pan-hypopituitarism (Henkin, McGlone, Daly, & Bartter, 1968). Hearing thresholds of the study group were compared against 25 normal controls. The patients with adrenocortical insufficiency were found to have better hearing sensitivity across the audiometric range compared to the unaffected controls. The patients' hearing thresholds returned to normal after treatment with prednisolone. The paper did not mention whether any of the participants with adrenocortical insufficiency had clinical symptoms (i.e., loudness tolerance problems) related to their increased auditory sensitivity.

Hyperthyroidism

Hyperthyroidism, or overactivity of the thyroid gland, has been included in a table of clinical conditions associated with hyperacusis (Pienowski et al., 2014). Laurian et al. (1983) showed abnormalities of the stapedial reflex in patients with hyperthyroidism, with raised stapedial reflex thresholds and decreased amplitudes. No clinical correlation was made in this study and, in particular, there was no mention of hyperacusis.

Growth Hormone Deficiency

Growth hormone deficiency is a condition in which there is a complete or partial absence of growth hormone in the body. The condition most commonly presents in childhood, has a genetic basis, and results in the child failing to grow normally. It can also appear in adulthood most commonly secondary to tumors of the pituitary gland. Prado-Barreto et al. (2014) performed audiological evaluations on 26 individuals with isolated growth hormone deficiency and 25 normal controls. Misophonia and dizziness were significantly more common in the isolated growth hormone deficiency group and peripheral auditory function was also worse in this group.

Metabolic Conditions

Pyridoxine Deficiency

Pyridoxine, the most common form of vitamin B6, is a water-soluble vitamin that acts as a co-factor in a variety of the body's metabolic processes. Deficiency of this enzyme can result in anemia and peripheral neuropathy. Marriage and Barnes (1995) mention pyridoxine deficiency as a condition co-occurring with hyperacusis. This assertion was based on a personal communication (Oppe, 1992, personal communication, cited in Marriage & Barnes, 1995) and a thorough literature search has failed to reveal any more compelling evidence. Despite the weakness of the evidence, the putative link continues to be cited in print (Pienkowski et al., 2014) and online.

Magnesium Deficiency

Cevette, Vormann, and Franz (2003) in a review paper examined the evidence regarding magnesium in the auditory system, reporting auditory hyperexcitability in magnesium deficiency. These observations were based on animal research in rodents, specifically rats (Kruse, Orent, & McCollum, 1932), guinea pigs (Cevette, Franz, Brey, & Robinette, 1989), and mice (Bac et al., 1994). Magnesium is also being investigated as a potential otoprotectant (Le Prell, Hughes, & Miller, 2007). Despite these pieces of research highlighting magnesium's important role in the auditory system, there is no robust evidence that magnesium deficiency causes hyperacusis in humans.

Autoimmune Conditions

Cogan's Syndrome

Cogan's syndrome is an autoimmune condition characterized by interstitial keratitis of the eye together with vestibular and auditory dysfunction. A literature search revealed a single case report of hyperacusis in association with Cogan's syndrome (Schuknecht & Nadol, 1994).

Systemic Lupus Erythematosus

Systemic lupus erythematosus (SLE) is an autoimmune disease presenting predominantly in women that has a wide range of clinical presentations and can affect many body systems including the auditory system. Maciaszczyk, Durko, Waszczykowska, Erkiert-Polguj, and Pajor (2011) investigated the auditory manifestations of the condition in 35 consecutive patients with SLE, contrasted with 30 healthy age and sex matched patients. In the SLE group 9 patients (25.7%) reported hyperacusis. In the subgroup that had SLE and hearing loss, 4/10 reported hyperacusis. Unfortunately, the presence or absence of hyperacusis in the control group was not revealed. The authors discussed the use of ototoxic drugs in the management of SLE: 65.7% of the study group received chloroquine and all but two of the patients who had hearing loss had received this drug. All four patients who had both hearing loss and hyperacusis had received chloroquine. It therefore remains unclear whether SLE is a risk factor for developing hyperacusis or whether the symptom is a consequence of hearing loss caused by the medical treatment.

Musculoskeletal Conditions

Back, Joint, and Muscle Pain

As part of the large population-based study in Sweden, Paulin et al. (2013) asked participants about various health conditions including disorders of the back, joints, and muscles. The prevalence of joint and muscle disorders was 39.4% among participants with physician-diagnosed hyperacusis and 23.4% among those who self-reported hyperacusis. Elevated odds ratios supported the hypothesis that these forms of musculoskeletal pain are co-morbid with hyperacusis.

Temporomandibular Disorder

Temporomandibular disorder (TMD) is a common condition with a variety of symptoms related to the jaw joints and muscles of mastication and a huge number of synonyms including temporomandibular joint dysfunction, craniomandibular dysfunction, myofascial pain dysfunction syndrome, Costen syndrome, and many others. There have been suggestions that TMD is linked with various auditory system symptoms including tinnitus, hearing loss, and hyperacusis but there is still debate as to whether such coexistence of symptoms is coincidental or causal. Rubinstein and Erlandsson (1991) studied 42 patients who had tinnitus and craniomandibular dysfunction, comparing them to a control group that had tinnitus alone. A higher prevalence of hyperacusis was reported in the tinnitus and craniomandibular dysfunction group (71.4%) compared to the tinnitus alone group (58.3%). Hilgenberg, Saldanha, Cunha, Rubo, and Conti (2012) studied 100 people with tinnitus and a control group of 100 people without tinnitus. In the tinnitus group, 85% met the criteria for TMD, compared to 55% in the control group. Hyperacusis was also more common in the tinnitus group at 26%, compared to 12% in the controls. Schecklmann, Landgrebe, and Langguth (2014) analyzed data from the Tinnitus Research Initiative database which is a large multinational project that collects data on patients attending specialized tinnitus clinics using a standardized case report form. This data collection form includes questions such as, "Do sounds cause you pain or physical discomfort?" and "Do you suffer from temporomandibular disorder?" Information on TMD was available for 1674 patients and demonstrated a significantly increased prevalence of TMD in the tinnitus and hyperacusis group (26%) compared to the tinnitus alone group (16%).

Fibromyalgia

Fibromyalgia is a condition characterized by chronic pain throughout the body, tenderness to touch, and fatigue. The majority of affected individuals are female, and onset is generally in middle age. Sensitivity to other sensory stimuli has been reported and Geisser et al. (2008) conducted a study comparing 30 patients with fibromyalgia to 28 normal controls. Sensitivity to sound was statistically greater in the fibromyalgia group and this group also reported statistically significantly increased sensitivity to everyday sounds. Fibromyalgia was considered by Paulin et al. (2016): the prevalence was 10.6% among participants with physician-diagnosed hyperacusis and 4.2% among those who self-reported hyperacusis. Elevated odds ratios supported the hypothesis that fibromyalgia is co-morbid with hyperacusis.

Vascular Conditions

Carotid Aneurysm

An aneurysm is a pathological dilatation of the wall of a blood vessel and aneurysms can occur in both the intracranial and extracranial portions of the carotid arteries. Carotid aneurysms may be asymptomatic or may be associated with a variety of neurological symptoms and signs. Carotid aneurysm has been included in a table of clinical conditions associated with hyperacusis (Pienowski et al., 2014) but there is no source reference included in the paper to support this assertion.

Middle Cerebral Artery Aneurysm

Aneurysmal swelling of the middle cerebral artery is cited in many publications as a condition associated with hyperacusis. This is based on a solitary case report (Khalil, Ogunyemi, & Osborne, 2002): a 35-year-old patient presented with isolated episodic hyperacusis and investigation revealed a middle cerebral artery aneurysm. This was treated neuro-radiologically by Guglielmi detachable coil embolization, which resulted in complete resolution of the hyperacusis. The authors postulated that the aneurysm irritated the nearby auditory cortex thereby generating the hyperacusis.

Gastrointestinal Conditions

Irritable Bowel Syndrome

As part of the large population-based study in Sweden, Paulin et al. (2016) asked participants about various health conditions including irritable bowel syndrome. The prevalence of irritable bowel syndrome was 9.1% among participants with physician-diagnosed hyperacusis and 4.8% among those who self-reported hyperacusis. Elevated odds ratios (Table 7–2) supported the hypothesis that irritable bowel syndrome is co-morbid with hyperacusis.

Pharmacological Associations with Hyperacusis

Drug Withdrawal

Lader (1984) reported intolerance to noise in 6/10 patients who participated in a pilot, uncontrolled benzodiazepine withdrawal study. Following this pilot study, a double-blind placebo-controlled study was undertaken in which 18/24 patients reported hyperacusis. Benzodiazepine withdrawal was also mentioned as a potential cause of intolerance to noise in two other publications (Gordon 1981, 1986) but no data was available in these publications to support the assertions. Hyperacusis has also been reported as a component of monoamine oxidase inhibitor (MOAI) withdrawal, following research by Tyrer (1984). Patients withdrawing from either phenelzine (a monoamine oxidase inhibitor) or a tricyclic antidepressant drug were studied. Approximately 54 patients enrolled in the study with 51 completing, of which 34 were taking phenelzine and 17 taking a tricyclic antidepressant. Four of the phenelzine group developed hyperacusis during drug withdrawal compared to one of the tricyclic group.

Drug Side Effects

Sürer Adanir, Gizli Çoban, and Özatalay (2017) reported a case of an 11-year-old boy whose hyperacusis worsened when he was given risperidone for hyperactivity and behavioral problems. The hyperacusis improved when the drug was stopped but worsened again when it was restarted. Hyperacusis is mentioned as a potential side effect on the drug information leaflets of several different medications: Yang and Agarwal (2011) described hyperacusis as a possible side effect of the antiepileptic drug phenytoin.

Infective Conditions

Lyme Disease

Lyme disease is an infectious disease caused by spirochete bacteria of the borrelia genus, transmitted by ticks. Although deer ticks are the usual vector, the animal reservoir is in small mammals and birds rather than deer. When humans become infected, the first manifestation is usually an expanding painless circular rash called erythema migrans. Flu-like symptoms may also occur at this stage. The subsequent stages of the disease are divided into early and late disseminated stages, facial nerve palsy can occur during the early disseminated phase, potentially resulting in hyperacusis by affecting the stapedial reflex. A wide range of neurological, neuropsychiatric, and arthritic symptoms have been reported during the late disseminated phase. Hyperacusis in the absence of seventh nerve palsy has been described and this association is frequently cited in the hyperacusis literature. Case reports of hyperacusis in association with Lyme disease have been published (Fallon et al., 1992; Nields, Fallon, & Jastreboff, 1999) but the numbers are very small, and the suggested co-morbidity remains anecdotal rather than proven.

Creutzfeld Jacob Disease (CJD)

Merkler, Prasad, Lavi, and Safdieh (2014) reported a 52-year-old man who presented with a short history of impaired sound tolerance and difficulty discerning noises including speech and music. Initial otological and neurological examination was normal as was audiometry. He went on to develop myalgia, neck pain, dysarthria, and ataxia. He was comprehensively investigated and a diagnosis of CJD was ultimately confirmed on brain biopsy. He died 21 months after presentation. A few cases of hearing loss have been reported in CJD but no other cases of disordered sound tolerance. The patient's description of his sound intolerance was that he experienced sounds as jarring and unfamiliar rather than painful above certain intensities.

Syphilis/Neurosyphilis

There has long been a suggestion that syphilis is associated with hyperacusis: Perlman (1938), in a review article, discussed hyperacusis occurring in tabes dorsalis, one of the forms of neurosyphilis. Syphilis was mentioned as a possible cause of hyperacusis by Gordon (2000), but this suggestion was reached by a rather tortuous and nonscientific argument: the author noted that many classical music composers had audiosensitivity and had, or were thought to have had, otosyphilis. He therefore suggested that the two observations could be associated. Although an interesting hypothesis, this link remains unproven and possibly libelous! The only other published evidence is a case report of a 42-year-old man with multiorgan symptoms which included tinnitus and phonophobia (Abildgaard, Ottosen, Baggesen, & Vorum, 2014). He was found to have antibodies to *Treponema pallidum*. This is clearly an inadequate level of evidence to prove an association between the two conditions. There is no convincing evidence that syphilis is more likely to result in hyperacusis than other causes of hearing loss.

Typhoid Fever

Typhoid fever is a bacterial infection caused by *Salmonella typhi*. Symptoms include high fever, headache, general weakness, and skin rash. Late complications include delirium, encephalitis, intestinal hemorrhage, intestinal perforation, and septicemia. Typhoid has been included in a table of clinical conditions associated with hyperacusis (Pienowski et al., 2014) but there is no source reference included in the paper to support this assertion.

Typhus

Typhus is a group of infectious diseases caused by obligate intracellular bacteria of the Rickettsia or Orientia genera. Symptoms of infection include fever, headache, confusion, and a macular skin rash. Hyperacusis has been reported in both epidemic typhus caused by *Rickettsia prowazekii* (Cowan, 2000) and scrub typhus caused by *Orientia tsutsugumushi* (Kaki & Satyendra, 2016).

Iatrogenic Conditions

Hyperacusis has been cited as a complication of spinal anesthetic (Pienkowski et al.,

2014). There is certainly a publication titled "Hyperacusis after Spinal Anaesthetic" (Gordon, 1991). This is a letter to the editor of the journal, discussing a previous publication (Fog, Wang, Sundberg, & Mucchiano, 1990) in which hearing had been assessed before and after spinal anesthetic for prostatectomy. In this original study, hearing thresholds improved slightly in some patients following spinal anesthesia. Gordon is using the word "hyperacusis" to denote supra-normal hearing, not hyperacusis as we would currently understand. There was no evidence in the research undertaken by Fog et al. (1990) that the study patients had any negative experience associated with their improved pure tone audiometry.

Environmental Intolerance

Several conditions have been described in which people display intolerance to various facets of the environment. These include Multiple Chemical Sensitivity in which people react to very low levels of a variety of odorous chemicals, Non-Specific Building-Related Symptoms (Sick Building Syndrome), in which people complain of a variety of symptoms in particular buildings, and Electromagnetic Hypersensitivity in which individuals report symptoms when exposed to electromagnetic fields. Palmquist, Claeson, Neely, Stenberg, and Nordin (2014), using data from the Swedish Västerbotten Environmental Health Study, investigated the relation among these three environmental tolerances and sound intolerance. Among 3406 respondents, 21.6% reported sensitivity to at least one of the four triggers. This study showed that there was statistically significant overlap among all the environmental tolerances for both physician-diagnosed and self-reported cases except for physician-diagnosed sound intolerance and electromagnetic field intolerance.

Clinical Implications of Medical Conditions Associated with Hyperacusis

Hyperacusis is common, and there are many proven or suspected co-morbid conditions. Because of the wide range of these conditions it would be very difficult to devise a diagnostic algorithm and, given the associated effects on quality of life expressed across patients, it is doubtful if such a tool would be helpful in any case. In many instances, the co-morbid condition has been diagnosed long before the sound intolerance. In most co-morbidities there is no condition-specific treatment for any accompanying hyperacusis. The most commonly associated conditions are hearing loss and tinnitus, and a careful otological history, examination, and appropriate audiological testing should reveal these co-morbidities. The other common association is psychological disease, particularly depression and anxiety states. Being mindful of this possible connection and enquiring about the patient's mood during the process of taking the clinical history is recommended. Use of a mental health questionnaire such as the Hospital Anxiety Depression Scale (HADS) (Zigmond & Snaith, 1983) may be appropriate. One disorder that does have specific management strategies is superior semicircular canal dehiscence syndrome, but it is a moot point as to whether this can really be called a disorder of sound tolerance.

Management strategies for decreased sound tolerance are discussed later in this book. There is one interesting medical treatment that has recently been reported: Silverstein, Ojo, Daugherty, Nazarian, and Wazen (2016) described a novel surgical procedure to use fascia or perichondrium to reinforce the round and oval windows in the middle ear and reduce the amount of sound energy reaching the inner ear. The authors described the outcome for six patients who had undergone the procedure and reported improved sound tolerance and enhanced quality of life in this small cohort. Although the patients reported no significant change in hearing postoperatively, audiometry showed worse average pure tone thresholds in all but one operated ear. Clearly this treatment is at variance with most other hyperacusis management strategies which are designed at improving sound tolerance rather than blocking sound from the patient's auditory system.

Conclusions

Disorders of sound tolerance have been reported in numerous medical conditions and syndromes. In many cases the evidence for a link is poor, based on case reports or small uncontrolled case series. The best evidence for conditions associated with disorders of sound tolerance includes hearing loss, tinnitus, and neuroses, though even here the evidence is insufficient to show causality. Population-based surveys are emerging, but research is hampered by confusing and inconsistent terminology and a lack of both objective and subjective outcome measures for impaired sound tolerance. Because of the huge range of conditions that have already been reported in association with impaired sound tolerance, it is conceivable that it is a non-specific marker of illness, in which case this avenue of research may turn out to be pointless.

References

Abildgaard, S. K., Ottosen, S., Baggesen, K. L., & Vorum, H. (2014). [Visual symptoms by syphilis]. *Ugeskr Laeger*, *15*, 176(25A).

Adour, K. K., & Wingerd, J. (1974). Idiopathic facial paralysis (Bell's palsy): Factors affecting severity and outcome in 446 patients. *Neurology*, *24*, 1112–1116.

Althaus, S. R. (1977). Spontaneous and traumatic perilymph fistulas. *Laryngoscope*, *87*, 364–371.

American Academy of Otolaryngology—Head and Neck Foundation, Inc. (1995). Committee on Hearing and Equilibrium guidelines for the diagnosis and evaluation of therapy in Meniere's disease. *Otolaryngol. Head Neck Surg.*, *113*, 181–185.

American Psychiatric Association. (2013). *Diagnostic and statistical manual of mental disorders* (5th ed.). *DSM-5*. Arlington, VA: American Psychiatric Publishing.

Anari, M., Axelsson, A., Eliasson, A., & Magnusson, L. (1999). Hypersensitivity to sound–questionnaire data, audiometry and classification. *Scand. Audiol.*, *28*, 219–230.

Andersson, G., Lindvall, N., Hursti, T., & Carlbring, P. (2002). Hypersensitivity to sound (hyperacusis): A prevalence study conducted via the Internet and post. *Int. J. Audiol.*, *41*, 545–554.

Andersson, G., Vretblad, P., Larsen, H. C., & Lyttkens, L. (2001). Longitudinal follow-up of tinnitus complaints. *Arch. Otolaryngol. Head Neck Surg.*, *127*, 175–179.

Arisoy, A. E., Ozden, S., Ciliv, G., & Ozalp, I. (1995). Tay-Sachs disease: A case report. *Turk. J. Pediatr.*, *37*, 51–56.

Attias, J. (2013). New findings on hyperacusis in Williams syndrome. *ENT & Audiology News. 21*, 76–78.

Attias, J., Raveh, E., Ben-Naftali, N. F., Zarchi, O., & Gothelf, D. (2008). Hyperactive auditory efferent system and lack of acoustic reflexes in Williams syndrome. *J. Basic Clin. Physiol. Pharmacol.*, *19*, 193–207.

Bac, P., Pages, N., Herrenknecht, C., Dewulf, C., Binet, P., & Durlach, J. (1994). Effect of various serotoninergically induced manipulations on audiogenic seizures in magnesium-deficient mice. *Magnes. Res.*, *7*, 107–115.

Baguley, D. M. (2003). Hyperacusis. *J. R. Soc. Med.*, *96*, 582–585.

Baron-Cohen, S., Ashwin, E., Ashwin, C., Tavassoli, T., & Chakrabarti, B. (2009). Talent in autism: Hyper-systemizing, hyper-attention to detail and sensory hypersensitivity. *Philos. Trans. R. Soc. Lond. B. Biol. Sci.*, *364*, 1377–1383.

Beers, A. N., McBoyle, M., Kakande, E., Dar Santos, R. C., & Kozak, F. K. (2014). Autism and peripheral hearing loss: A systematic review. *Int. J. Pediatr. Otorhinolaryngol.*, *78*, 96–101.

Behan, P. O., & Bakheit, A. M. (1991). Clinical spectrum of postviral fatigue syndrome. *Br. Med. Bull.*, *47*, 793–808.

Cevette, M. J., Franz, K. B., Brey, R. H., & Robinette, M. S. (1989). Influence of dietary magnesium on the amplitude of wave V of the auditory brainstem response. *Otolaryngol. Head Neck Surg.*, *101*, 537–541.

Cevette, M. J., Vormann, J., & Franz, K. (2003). Magnesium and hearing. *J. Am. Acad. Audiol.*, *14*, 202–212.

Citron, D., 3rd, & Adour, K. K. (1978). Acoustic reflex and loudness discomfort in acute facial paralysis. *Arch. Otolaryngol.*, *104*, 303–306.

Cornish, K. M., & Pigram, J. (1996). Developmental and behavioural characteristics of cri du chat syndrome. *Arch. Dis. Child.*, *75*, 448–450.

Cowan, G. (2000). Rickettsial diseases: The typhus group of fevers—a review. *Postgrad. Med. J.*, *76*, 269–272.

Danesh, A. A., Lang, D., Kaf, W., Andreassen, W. D., Scott, J., & Eshraghi, A. A. (2015). Tinnitus and hyperacusis in autism spectrum disorders with emphasis on high functioning individuals diagnosed with Asperger's syndrome. *Int. J. Pediatr. Otorhinolaryngol.*, *79*, 1683–1688.

de Klaver, M. J., van Rijn, M. A., Marinus, J., Soede, W., de Laat, J. A., & van Hilten, J. J. (2007). Hyperacusis in patients with complex regional pain syndrome related dystonia. *J. Neurol. Neurosurg. Psychiatry*, *78*, 1310–1313.

De Seta, D., Mancini, P., Minni, A., Prosperini, L., De Seta, E., Attanasio, G., . . . Filipo, R. (2014). Bell's palsy: symptoms preceding and accompanying the facial paresis. *Scientific World Journal*, 801971.

Fabijanska, A., Rogowski, M., Bartnik, G., & Skarzynski, H. (1999). Epidemiology of tinnitus and hyperacusis in Poland. In: J. W. P. Hazell (Ed.), *Proceedings of the Sixth International Tinnitus Seminar* (pp. 569–571). London, U.K.: The Tinnitus and Hyperacusis Centre.

Fagelson, M. A. (2007). The association between tinnitus and posttraumatic stress disorder. *Am. J. Audiol.*, *16*, 107–117.

Fallon, B. A., Nields, J. A., Burrascano, J. J., Liegner, K., DelBene, D., & Liebowitz, M. R. (1992). The neuropsychiatric manifestations of Lyme borreliosis. *Psychiatr. Q.*, *63*, 95–117.

Fog, J., Wang, L. P., Sundberg, A., & Mucchiano, C. (1990). Hearing loss after spinal anesthesia is related to needle size. *Anesth. Analg.*, *70*, 517–522.

Formby, C., Sherlock, L. P., Hawley, M. L., & Gold, S. L. (2017). A sound therapy-based intervention to expand the auditory dynamic range for loudness among persons with sensorineural hearing losses: case evidence showcasing treatment efficacy. *Semin. Hear.*, *38*, 130–150.

Fukaya, T., & Nomura, Y. (1988). Audiological aspects of idiopathic perilymphatic fistula. *Acta Otolaryngol. Suppl.*, *456*, 68–73.

Fukutake, T., & Hattori, T. (1998). Auditory illusions caused by a small lesion in the right medial geniculate body. *Neurology*, *51*, 1469–1471.

Gascon, G. G., Ozand, P. T., & Erwin, R. E. (1992). GM1 gangliosidosis type 2 in two siblings. *J. Child. Neurol.*, *7*, Suppl, S41–50.

Geisser, M. E., Glass, J. M., Rajcevska, L. D., Clauw, D. J., Williams, D. A., Kileny, P. R., & Gracely, R. H. (2008). A psychophysical study of auditory and pressure sensitivity in patients with fibromyalgia and healthy controls. *J. Pain*, *9*, 417–422.

Gordon, A. G. (1981). Hyperactive acoustic reflexes and perilymphatic hypotension. *Arch. Otolaryngol.*, *107*, 774.

Gordon, A. G. (1986). Abnormal middle ear muscle reflexes and audiosensitivity. *Br. J. Audiol.*, *20*, 95–99.

Gordon, A. G. (1991). Hyperacusis after spinal anesthesia. *Anesth. Analg.*, *73*, 506–507.

Gordon, A. G. (2000). "Hyperacusis" and origins of lowered sound tolerance. *J. Neuropsychiatry Clin. Neurosci.*, *12*, 117–119.

Gordon, B. A., Gordon, K. E., Hinton, G. G., Cadera, W., Feleki, V., Bayleran, J., & Hechtman, P. (1988). Tay-Sachs disease: B1 variant. *Pediatr. Neurol.*, *4*, 54–57.

Gothelf, D., Farber, N., Raveh, E., Apter, A., & Attias, J. (2006). Hyperacusis in Williams syndrome: Characteristics and associated neuroaudiologic abnormalities. *Neurology, 66*, 390–395.

Hadj-Djilani, A., & Gerster, J. C. (1984). Meniere's disease and fibrositis syndrome (psychogenic rheumatism). Relationship in audiometric and nystagmographic results. *Acta Otolaryngol. Suppl., 406*, 67–71.

Hannula, S., Bloigu, R., Majamaa, K., Sorri, M., & Mäki-Torkko, E. (2011). Self-reported hearing problems among older adults: Prevalence and comparison to measured hearing impairment. *J. Am. Acad. Audiol., 22*, 550–559.

Henkin, R. I., McGlone, R. E., Daly, R., & Bartter, F. C. (1967). Studies on auditory thresholds in normal man and in patients with adrenal cortical insufficiency: The role of adrenal cortical steroids. *J. Clin. Invest., 46*, 429–435.

Herraiz, C., Tapia, M. C., & Plaza, G. (2006). Tinnitus and Meniere's disease: Characteristics and prognosis in a tinnitus clinic sample. *Eur. Arch. Otorhinolaryngol., 263*, 504–509.

Hilgenberg, P. B., Saldanha, A. D., Cunha, C. O., Rubo, J. H., & Conti, P. C. (2012). Temporomandibular disorders, otologic symptoms and depression levels in tinnitus patients. *J. Oral. Rehabil., 39*, 239–244.

Hyperacusis Focus. Retrieved from http://hyperacusisfocus.org/research/causes/.

Jastreboff, M. M., & Jastreboff, P. J. (2002). Decreased sound tolerance and tinnitus retraining therapy. *Aust. NZ J. Audiol., 24*, 74–84.

Jüris, L., Andersson, G., Larsen, H. C., & Ekselius, L. (2013). Psychiatric comorbidity and personality traits in patients with hyperacusis. *Int. J. Audiol., 52*, 230–235.

Kaki, A. R., & Satyendra, S. (2016). Scrub typhus with hyperacusis and tinnitus. *J. Assoc. Physicians India, 64*, 154.

Karimzadeh, P., Jafari, N., Nejad Biglari, H., Jabbeh Dari, S., Ahmad Abadi, F., Alaee M. R., . . . Ghofrani, M. (2014). GM2-gangliosidosis (Sandhoff and Tay Sachs disease): Diagnosis and neuroimaging findings (an Iranian pediatric case series). *Iran. J. Child. Neurol., 8*, 55–60.

Katzenell, U., & Segal, S. (2001). Hyperacusis: Review and clinical guidelines. *Otol. Neurotol., 22*, 321–326.

Khalfa, S., Bruneau, N., Rogé, B., Georgieff, N., Veuillet, E., Adrien, J. L., Barthélémy, C., & Collet, L. (2004). Increased perception of loudness in autism. *Hear. Res., 198*, 87–92.

Khalil, S., Ogunyemi, L., & Osborne, J. (2002). Middle cerebral artery aneurysm presenting as isolated hyperacusis. *J. Laryngol. Otol., 116*, 376–378.

Klein, A. J., Armstrong, B. L., Greer, M. K., & Brown, F. R., 3rd. (1990). Hyperacusis and otitis media in individuals with Williams syndrome. *J. Speech Hear. Disord., 55*, 339–344.

Kruse, H. D., Orent, E. R., & McCollum, E. V. (1932). Studies on magnesium deficiency in animals: I. Symptomatology resulting from magnesium deprivation. *J. Biol. Chem., 96*, 519–539.

Lader, M. (1984). Benzodiazepine dependence. *Prog. Neuropsychopharmacol. Biol. Psychiatry, 8*, 85–95.

Laurian, N., Laurian, L., Sadov, R., Strauss, M., & Kalmanovitz, M. (1983). New clinical applications of the stapedial reflex. *J. Laryngol. Otol., 97*, 1099–1103.

Le Prell, C. G., Hughes, L. F., & Miller, J. M. (2007). Free radical scavengers vitamins A, C, and E plus magnesium reduce noise trauma. *Free Radic. Biol. Med., 42*, 1454–1463.

Liriano, R. Y. G., Magalhães, S. L. B., Barros, F. T., José, R. G., & Fukuda, Y. (2004). Relation of hyperacusis and peripheral facial paralysis—Bell's palsy. *Revista Brasileira de Otorrinolaringologia, 70*, 776–779.

MacCulloch, M. J., & Eaton, R. (1971). A note on reduced auditory pain threshold in 44 stuttering children. *Br. J. Disord. Commun., 6*, 148–153.

Maciaszczyk, K., Durko, T., Waszczykowska, E., Erkiert-Polguj, A., & Pajor, A. (2011). Auditory function in patients with systemic lupus erythematosus. *Auris Nasus Larynx, 38*, 26–32.

Marriage, J., & Barnes, N. M. (1995). Is central hyperacusis a symptom of 5-hydroxytryptamine (5-HT) dysfunction? *J. Laryngol. Otol., 109*, 915–921.

Mathisen, H. (1969). Phonophobia after stapedectomy. *Acta Otolaryngol., 68*, 73–77.

Matsuzaki, J., Kagitani-Shimono, K., Sugata, H., Hirata, M., Hanaie, R., Nagatani, F., . . . Taniike, M.

(2014). Progressively increased M50 responses to repeated sounds in autism spectrum disorder with auditory hypersensitivity: A magnetoencephalographic study. *PLoS ONE, 9*, e102599.

McCandless, G. A., & Goering, D. M. (1974). Changes in loudness after stapedectomy. *Arch Otolaryngol.*, *100*, 344–350.

McCandless, G. A., & Schumacher, M. H. (1979). Auditory dysfunction with facial paralysis. *Arch Otolaryngol.*, *105*, 271–274.

McFerran, D. (2016a). Acoustic shock. In: D. M. Baguley & M. Fagelson (Eds.), *Tinnitus: Clinical and research perspectives* (pp. 181–196). San Diego, CA: Plural.

McFerran, D. (2016b). Misophonia and phonophobia. In: D. M. Baguley & M. Fagelson (Eds.), *Tinnitus: Clinical and research perspectives* (pp. 245–259). San Diego, CA: Plural.

Merkler, A.E., Prasad, M., Lavi, E., & Safdieh, J. (2014). Hyperacusis as the initial presentation of Creutzfeldt-Jakob disease. *Neurol. Neuroimmunol. Neuroinflamm.*, *1*, e32.

Minor, L. B., Solomon, D., Zinreich, J. S., & Zee, D. S. (1998). Sound- and/or pressure-induced vertigo due to bone dehiscence of the superior semicircular canal. *Arch Otolaryngol. Head Neck Surg.*, *124*, 249–258.

Modugno, G. C., & Brandolini, C. (2014). Can lateral semicircular canal dysplasia play a role in the genesis of hyperacusis. *Acta Otorhinolaryngol. Ital.*, *34*, 71–74.

Morioka, W. T., Neff, P. A., Boisseranc, T. E., Hartman, P. W., & Cantrell, R. W. (1976). Audiotympanometric findings in myasthenia gravis. *Arch Otolaryngol.*, *102*, 211–213.

Nelson, J. J., & Chen, K. (2004). The relationship of tinnitus, hyperacusis, and hearing loss. *Ear Nose Throat J.*, *83*, 472–476.

Nields, J. A., Fallon, B. A., & Jastreboff, P. J. (1999). Carbamazepine in the treatment of Lyme disease-induced hyperacusis. *J. Neuropsychiatry Clin. Neurosci.*, *11*, 97–99.

Nigam, A., & Samuel, P. R. (1994). Hyperacusis and Williams syndrome. *J. Laryngol. Otol.*, *108*, 494–496.

Oen, J. M., Begeer, J. H., Staal-Schreinemachers, A. I., & Tijmstra, T. (1997). Hyperacusis in children with spina bifida; a pilot-study. *Eur. J. Pediatr. Surg.*, *7* Suppl, 1, 46.

Palmquist, E., Claeson, A. S., Neely, G., Stenberg, B., & Nordin, S. (2014). Overlap in prevalence between various types of environmental intolerance. *Int. J. Hyg. Environ. Health*, *217*, 427–434.

Paulin, J., Andersson, L., & Nordin, S. (2016). Characteristics of hyperacusis in the general population. *Noise Health*, *18*, 178–184.

Perlman, H. B. (1938). Hyperacusis. *Annals Otol., Rhinol. Laryngol.*, *47*, 947–953.

Pienkowski, M., Tyler, R. S., Roncancio, E. R., Jun, H. J., Brozoski, T., Dauman, N., . . . Moore, B. C. (2014). A review of hyperacusis and future directions: Part II. Measurement, mechanisms, and treatment. *Am. J. Audiol.*, *23*, 420–436.

Prado-Barreto, V. M., Salvatori, R., Santos Júnior, R. C., Brandão-Martins, M. B., Correa, E. A., Garcez, F. B., . . . Aguiar-Oliveira, M. H. (2014). Hearing status in adult individuals with lifetime, untreated isolated growth hormone deficiency. *Otolaryngol. Head Neck Surg.*, *150*, 464–471.

Ramtekkar, U. P. (2017). DSM-5 changes in attention deficit hyperactivity disorder and autism spectrum disorder: Implications for comorbid sleep issues. *Children (Basel)*, *4*, E62.

Rosenhall, U., Nordin, V., Sandström, M., Ahlsén, G., & Gillberg, C. (1999). Autism and hearing loss. *J. Autism Dev. Disord.*, *29*, 349–357.

Rubinstein, B., & Erlandsson, S. I. (1991). A stomatognathic analysis of patients with disabling tinnitus and craniomandibular disorders (CMD). *Br. J. Audiol.*, *25*, 77–83.

Saliba, I., Maniakas, A., Benamira, L. Z., Nehme, J., Benoit, M., & Montreuil-Jacques, V. (2014). Superior canal dehiscence syndrome: clinical manifestations and radiologic correlations. *Eur. Arch Otorhinolaryngol.*, *271*, 2905–2914.

Sand, J. J., Biller, J., Corbett, J. J., Adams, H. P. Jr., & Dunn, V. (1986). Partial dorsal mesencephalic hemorrhages: Report of three cases. *Neurology*, *36*, 529–533.

Schecklmann, M., Landgrebe, M., Langguth, B., & TRI Database Study Group. (2014). Phenotypic characteristics of hyperacusis in tinnitus. *PLoS ONE*, *9*, e86944.

Schröder, A., Vulink, N., & Denys, D. (2013). Misophonia: Diagnostic criteria for a new psychiatric disorder. *PLoS ONE. 8*, e54706.

Schuknecht, H. F., & Nadol, J. B. Jr. (1994). Temporal bone pathology in a case of Cogan's syndrome. *Laryngoscope, 104*, 1135–1142.

Sheth, J., Datar, C., Mistri, M., Bhavsar, R., Sheth, F., & Shah, K. (2016). GM2 gangliosidosis AB variant: Novel mutation from India—a case report with a review. *BMC Pediatr., 16*, 88.

Silverstein, H., Ojo, R., Daugherty, J., Nazarian, R., & Wazen, J. (2016). Minimally invasive surgery for the treatment of hyperacusis. *Otol. Neurotol., 37*, 1482–1488.

Stange, T., Mir-Salim, P. A., & Berghaus, A. (2001). [Hyperacusis after tympanoplasty]. *HNO, 49*, 303–306.

Stansfeld, S. A. (1992). Noise, noise sensitivity and psychiatric disorder: Epidemiological and psychophysiological studies. *Psychol. Med. Monogr. Suppl., 22*, 1–44.

Sürer Adanir, A., Gizli Çoban, Ö., & Özatalay, E. (2017). Increased hyperacusis with risperidone in an autistic child. *Noro Psikiyatr Ars, 54*, 187–188.

Tavassoli, T. (2013). Sound tolerance in autism spectrum disorder. *ENT & Audiology News, 21*, 74–75.

Tyler, R. S., Pienkowski, M., Roncancio, E. R., Jun, H. J., Brozoski, T., Dauman, N., . . . Moore, B. C. (2014). A review of hyperacusis and future directions: Part I. Definitions and manifestations. *Am. J. Audiol., 23*, 402–419.

Tyrer, P. (1984). Clinical effects of abrupt withdrawal from tri-cyclic antidepressants and monoamine oxidase inhibitors after long-term treatment. *J. Affect. Disord., 6*, 1–7.

Vingen, J. V., Pareja, J. A., & Stovner, L. J. (1998). Quantitative evaluation of photophobia and phonophobia in cluster headache. *Cephalalgia, 18*, 250–256.

Vingen, J. V., Sand, T., & Stovner, L. J. (1999). Sensitivity to various stimuli in primary headaches: A questionnaire study. *Headache, 39*, 552–558.

Von Leden, H., & Horton, B. T. (1949). Auditory nerve in multiple sclerosis. *Arch Otolaryngol., 48*, 51–57.

Vos, T., Flaxman, A. D., Naghavi, M., Lozano, R., Michaud, C., Ezzati, M. . . . Memish, Z. A. (2012). Years lived with disability (YLDs) for 1160 sequelae of 289 diseases and injuries 1990–2010: A systematic analysis for the Global Burden of Disease Study 2010. *Lancet, 380*, 2163–2196.

Waddell, P. A., & Gronwall, D. M. (1984). Sensitivity to light and sound following minor head injury. *Acta Neurol. Scand., 69*, 270–276.

Wayman, D. M., Pham, H. N., Byl, F. M., & Adour, K. K. (1990). Audiological manifestations of Ramsay Hunt syndrome. *J. Laryngol. Otol., 104*, 104–108.

Weber, H., Pfadenhauer, K., Stöhr, M., & Rösler, A. (2002). Central hyperacusis with phonophobia in multiple sclerosis. *Mult. Scler., 8*, 505–509.

Westcott, M., Sanchez, T. G., Diges, I., Saba, C., Dineen, R., McNeill, C., . . . Sharples, T. (2013). Tonic tensor tympani syndrome in tinnitus and hyperacusis patients: a multi-clinic prevalence study. *Noise Health, 15*, 117–128.

Woodhouse, A., & Drummond, P. D. (1993). Mechanisms of increased sensitivity to noise and light in migraine headache. *Cephalalgia, 13*, 417–421.

Yang, L., & Agarwal, P. (2011). Systematic drug repositioning based on clinical side-effects. *PLoS ONE, 6*, e28025.

Zigmond, A. S., & Snaith, R. P. (1983). The hospital anxiety and depression scale. *Acta Psychiatr. Scand., 67*, 361–370.

8

Animal Models of Hyperacusis and Decreased Sound Tolerance

Jos J. Eggermont

Introduction

Hyperacusis describes an unusual hypersensitivity or discomfort induced by exposure to sound. It may be a composite of reduced sound level tolerance, which may start at low levels, and a reduced loudness discomfort level, which affects moderate to high sound levels. Many people with hyperacusis have "clinically normal" audiograms, thereby excluding as putative sources hypersensitive thresholds as well as hearing impairment (Anari et al., 1999). Hyperacusis is accompanied by increased amplitude of distortion product otoacoustic emissions (DPOAEs) in tinnitus patients without hearing loss (Sztuka et al., 2010), and may be caused by a reduced efferent system action. Jastreboff and Hazell (1993) described hyperacusis as a "manifestation of increased central gain" (Formby et al., 2003; Noreña & Chery-Croze, 2007), which may enhance the perception of loudness that accompanies stimulation from external signals.

What Are the Neural Correlates of Loudness and Hyperacusis in Humans?

Langers et al. (2007) found in people with normal hearing and those with symmetric high-frequency (4 and 8 kHz) hearing loss (40 to 70 dB HL) that it was the perceived loudness of stimuli and not the intensity level (dB SPL) that related strongly to cortical activation in these two groups of subjects. However, the activation measured in the participants with high-frequency hearing loss increased significantly more with stimulus intensity than in the normally hearing subjects. This reflects abnormal growth of loudness; a disproportionate increase in loudness with stimulus intensity. This demonstrates that fMRI activation at the level of the auditory cortex is more closely related to the percept of a stimulus (i.e., loudness) rather than to its physical characteristics (i.e., intensity), and suggests that fMRI activation may be interpreted as a correlate of the subjective strength of the stimulus percept.

Rohl and Uppenkamp (2012) used a psychophysical scaling procedure for quantifying the loudness percept in combination with fMRI. They, as well as Langers et al. (2007), observed an almost linear increase of perceived loudness and percent signal change (PSC) from baseline in all examined stages of the upper auditory pathway. Across individuals, the slope of the underlying growth function for perceived loudness was significantly correlated with the slope of the growth function for the PSC in the auditory cortex, but not in the inferior colliculus (IC) and thalamus.

These two studies suggest that loudness is reflected in the growth of the response-intensity function in auditory cortex but not in the IC.

Hyperacusis and the Startle Response

How can hyperacusis be studied in animal models? First, one needs a behavioral indicator for this hypersensitivity. The general approach taken is to use the magnitude of the startle reflex. Because the inducing sound of this reflex is very high (mostly 115 dB SPL; Turner & Larsen, 2016) one can likely only measure reduced loudness discomfort levels (Knudson & Melcher, 2016). Second, to locate the neural structures involved, the examiner often uses the amplitude-level functions of the local field potential (LFP), or the driven firing rate of single neurons.

Hyperacusis may be at the basis of observations (Ison et al., 2007) that mice with presbycusis also show exaggerated acoustic startle responses (see also Turner & Parrish, 2008; Sun et al., 2009). Sun et al. (2009) found that salicylate significantly increased the LFP in the auditory cortex but not in the IC. They also found that salicylate significantly increased the amplitude of the startle response. The increase in LFP amplitude and the increased startle reflex suggest that high doses of salicylate increase the gain in the central auditory system, presumably by down-regulating GABA-mediated inhibition. Such inhibition provides a complimentary mechanism for sustaining chronic, debilitating hyperacusis and underlies the importance of behavior modification, such as patients and physicians monitoring drug intake, in parallel to the specific desensitization techniques for management of hyperacusis (Noreña & Chery-Croze, 2007).

Recent work in mice has shown that noise exposure resulting in specific ribbon synapse damage can cause permanent degeneration of the auditory nerve despite complete recovery from temporary threshold shift (TTS; Kujawa & Liberman, 2009). This was suggested as a cause of hyperacusis as reflected in the enhanced acoustic startle reflex in these animals (Hickox & Liberman, 2014). However, Knudson and Melcher (2016) found that the human equivalent of the startle reflex (the eye-blink) is not related to hyperacusis but to a reduced loudness discomfort level. The authors distinguished hyperacusis from reduced loudness discomfort levels in functional terms as they asserted the former resulted in abnormal loudness sensation across a subject's dynamic range of audibility while the latter affected only the loudness experience at the upper limit of the dynamic range.

Central Gain Changes and Long-Term Non-Traumatic Noise Exposure

The original human study that drove animal research in directions addressing central gain changes in the auditory system was the finding by Formby et al. (2003) that 2-week exposure to a moderate wide band noise (~50 dB SPL) resulted in a 5 to 6 dB increase in loudness tolerance thresholds that were attributed to reductions in central gain. In contrast, blocking the ear canals for the same period of time resulted in decreased loudness tolerance that appeared related to an analogous increase in central gain.

We (Noreña et al., 2006) exposed normal hearing adult cats to a 4 to 20 kHz multifrequency sound (termed enhanced acoustic environment, EAE) for >4 months at 80 dB SPL, and found that this did not result in auditory brainstem response (ABR) threshold changes when results were compared to a large control group. Surprisingly, there was a strong reduction in the primary auditory cortex (A1) unit onset responses to tones with frequencies in the 4 to 20 kHz range, and a strong onset-response enhancement for frequencies <4 kHz and >20 kHz (Figure 8–1, A–C). In most of the enhanced response regions, the onset latencies were significantly lengthened compared to controls (Figure 8–1D).

These changes were also found for average (i.e., more than 100 ms post-stimulus) driven firing rates (Figure 8–2A) and LFP amplitudes (Figure 8–2B). Thus, whether loudness correlated with onset response or averaged driven firing rates, the findings suggested such changes occurred across a fairly large range of stimulus levels, that is, between 10 and 65 dB SPL.

Neural synchrony in auditory cortex may in principle also code for stimulus level. Eggermont (2000) found that, "For noise-burst stimulation, the onset correlation for between [cortical] area pairs was independent of stimulus intensity regardless [of] the difference in CF. In contrast, for tone-pip stimulation a significant dependence on intensity level of the peak correlation strength was found for pairs involving A1 and/or anterior auditory field (AAF) with CF difference less than one octave" (p. 2708). One octave corresponds in cat A1 with about 0.75 to 1 mm. After long-term exposure to non-traumatic sound (Noreña et al., 2006; Pienkowski & Eggermont, 2009) there was a significant change in the correlation distance, from <1 mm to ~3 mm, and doubling of the strength of the spontaneous peak correlation (neural synchrony), from ≤0.1 to 0.2 (Figure 8–3). These increases in correlation strength were for neurons with CFs outside the frequency range of the EAE.

Thus, increased onset- and average-firing rates, increased LFP amplitude, and increased neural synchrony may all be electrophysiological correlates of central gain changes provoked (somewhat unexpectedly) by stimuli presented at permissible SPLs. Because the short latency components of stimulus-driven LFPs reflect the output of thalamic neurons in the compound excitatory post-synaptic potential of cortical neurons, such gain changes are a thalamo-cortical phenomenon.

Similar data were obtained after a 6-week continuous exposure to steeply filtered 4 to 20 kHz noise, presented at a level of 68 dB SPL (Pienkowski et al., 2011). Figure 8–4 shows the frequency dependence of the multi-unit (MU) response (left) and LFP amplitude (right) for 65 dB SPL pure tone-pip stimulation. It is clear that compared to the average data in control cats (black) the responses of the EAE cats are greatly reduced from about 2.5 to 20 kHz, and greatly enhanced for frequencies below 2 kHz and above 20 kHz. This occurs both for MU firing rates and LFP amplitudes. Note that when the curves, which reflect the 95% confidence levels around the mean, do not overlap there is a significant difference at least at the $p < 0.05$ level. The difference between the control and EAE data show evidence for central gain changes, but without changes in distortion-product oto-acoustic

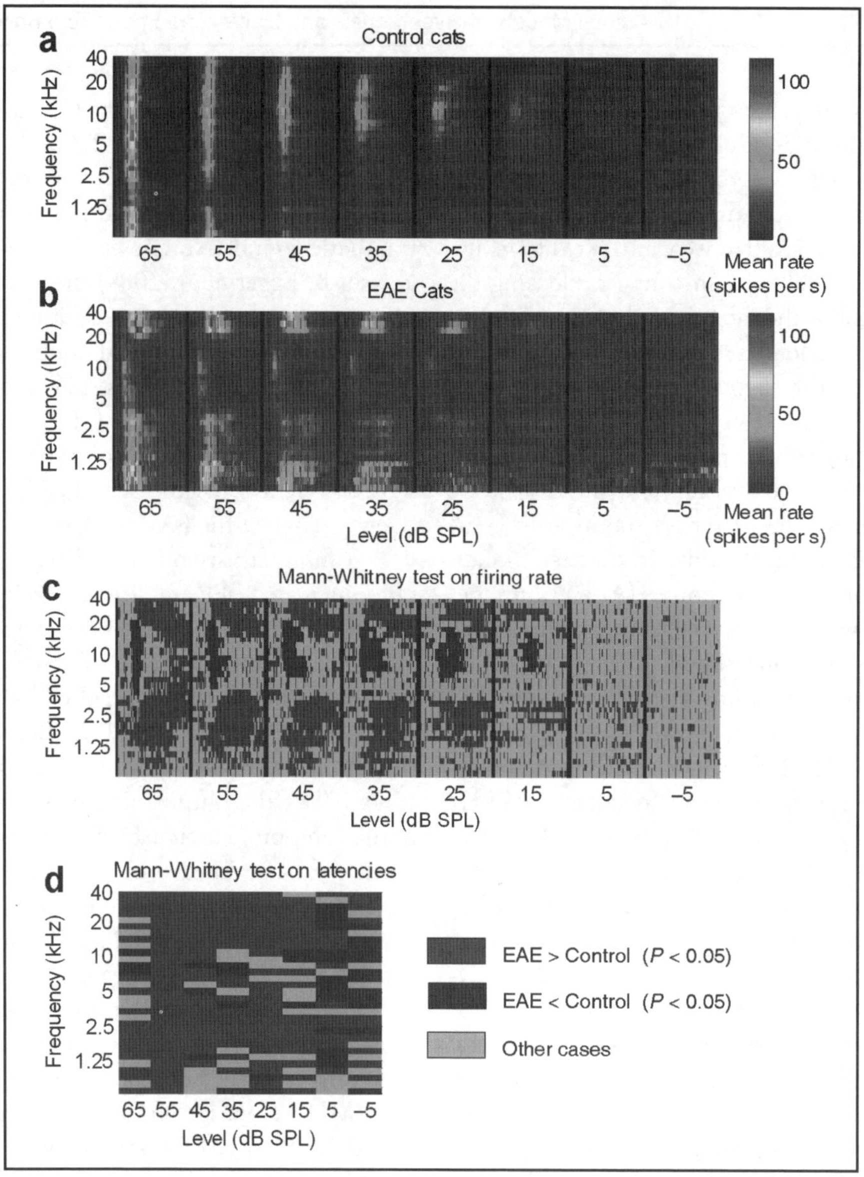

Figure 8–1. Averaged poststimulus time histograms across all control and EAE cats. (**a, b**) Averaged PSTHs (2-ms time bins) as a function of SPL, over a 100-ms time window, in control and EAE cats. Dashed lines, 10-ms intervals. Colored bars, mean firing rate. In control cats, the mean response suggested that the highest sensitivity (lowest thresholds) was to frequencies around 10 kHz and that the largest responses were to frequencies between 2.5 kHz and 10 kHz. In EAE cats, the most sensitive frequencies were those below 1.25 kHz and above 20 kHz. Note that neural responses in EAE cats were much more spread out over time compared to those in control cats. (**c, d**) Graphical representation of significant differences (Mann-Whitney test) between EAE and control groups in terms of (**c**) mean firing rate per frequency-latency bin and (**d**) mean latency per frequency-intensity bin. *Source*: From Noreña et al. (2006). To view this image in full color visit the Plural Publishing website for the book at http://pluralpublishing.com/publication_hdsi.htm.

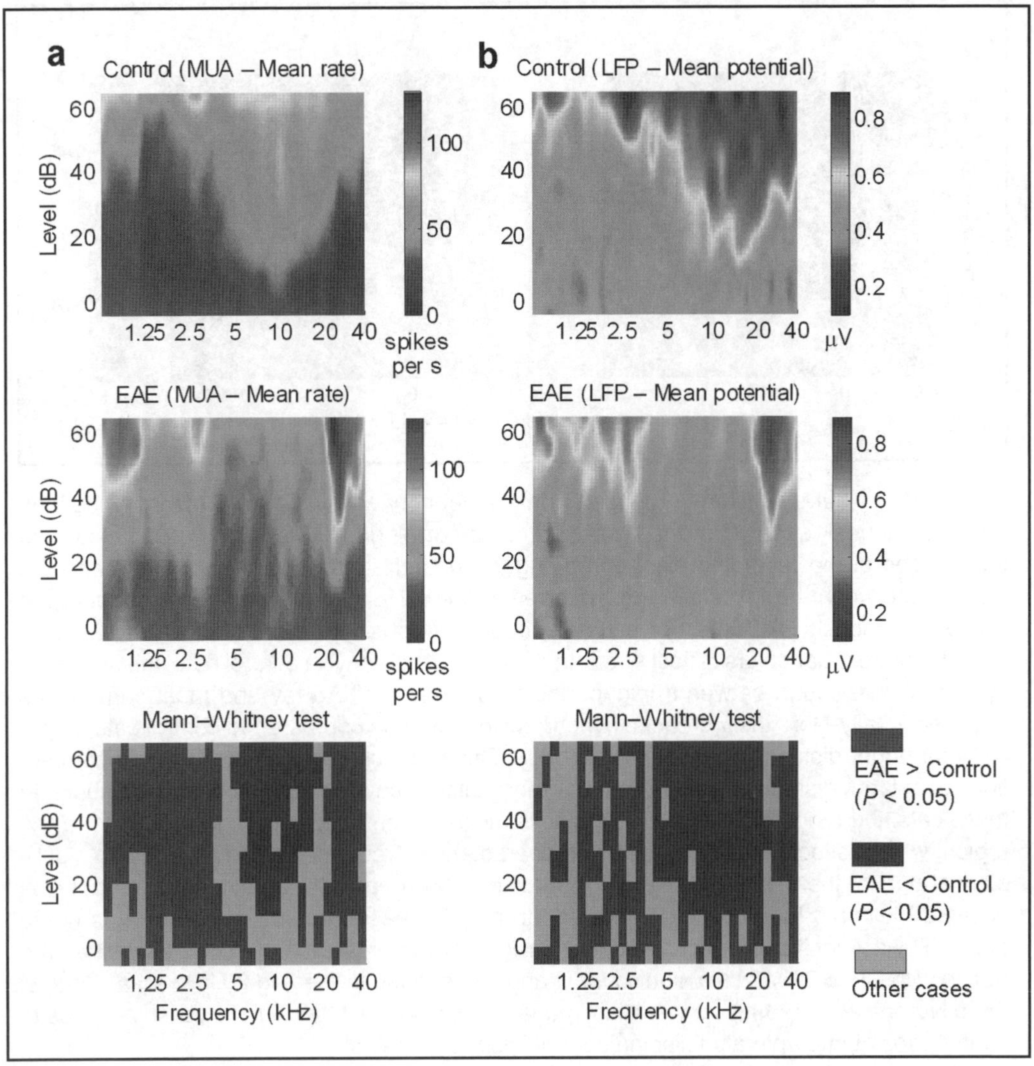

Figure 8–2. Averaged group multiunit firing rates and LFP amplitude as a function of frequency and intensity. First row, averaged multiunit firing rate; second row, averaged LFP amplitude; third row, results of statistical tests (Mann-Whitney) for comparisons between control and EAE cats. *Source*: From Noreña et al. (2006). To view this image in full color visit the Plural Publishing website for the book at http://pluralpublishing.com/publication_hdsi.htm.

emissions (DPOAEs) and ABRs (Pienkowski et al., 2011).

From the studies reviewed in this section, it is clear that central gain changes can be induced fairly quickly and that they are enabled via homeostatic plasticity mechanisms associated with either permanent or very long-lasting changes in the central auditory system. These changes could underlie hyperacusis in the absence of hearing loss.

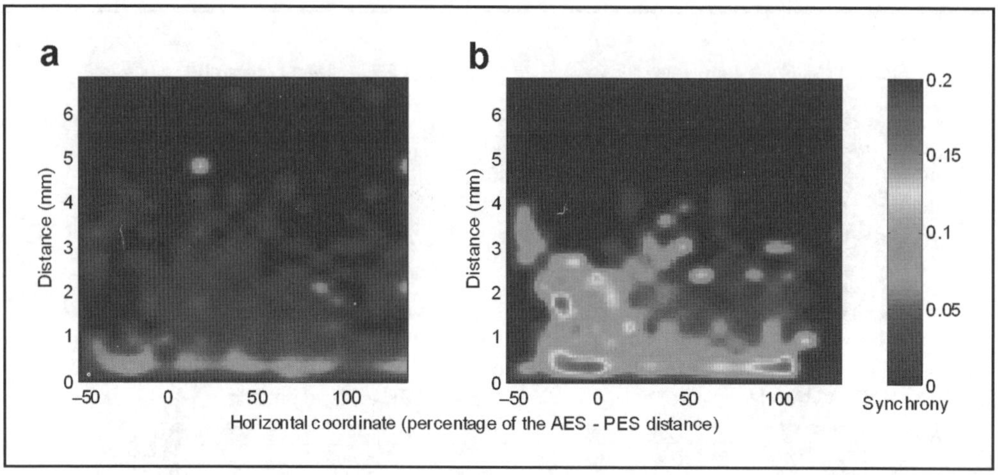

Figure 8–3. Neural synchrony maps in primary auditory cortex. (**a, b**) Synchrony, defined here as the peak strength of the corrected cross-correlogram (Methods), as a function of the position of the recording electrode along the postero-anterior axis (abscissa) and the distance between the two electrodes involved in the calculation of synchrony (ordinate), in (**a**) control and (**b**) EAE cats. For each electrode pair, positions along the postero-anterior axis are plotted. Bar colors reflect strength of neural synchrony. In control cats, the strongest synchrony was found between neighboring electrodes in the array and most correlations occurred locally. Note the increased synchrony in EAE cats compared to control cats, especially for larger distances between electrodes. This probably signifies the stronger connections over large distances (that is, into the reorganized region) made by horizontal fibers. In these cats, the range of strong correlations is much larger, especially in the –50% to +50% region, which reflects the entire area with characteristic frequencies <4 kHz but also a substantial part of the 5 to 20 kHz area. In addition, the area with characteristic frequencies above 20 kHz (70 to 125%) also showed strongly increased neural synchrony. It is noted that SFR was significantly increased in the region with putative CFs <4 kHz as well as the region with CFs >20 kHz. No significant change was found in the 5 to 20 kHz area. *Source*: From Noreña et al. (2006). To view this image in full color visit the Plural Publishing website for the book at http://pluralpublishing.com/publication_hdsi.htm.

Loudness Recruitment Is Central

Because hyperacusis often co-occurs with hearing loss, it is important to consider another well-studied consequence of sensorineural hearing loss (SNHL), namely loudness recruitment. This was previously thought to be a peripheral phenomenon (e.g., Eggermont, 1977; Phillips, 1987) but it may also, and more dominantly, involve the central auditory system.

Hyperactivity is seen in central auditory neurons after sensorineural hearing loss and is characterized by an abnormally rapid increase of response with stimulus intensity, by a heightened maximum response, or both (Salvi et al., 2000; Wang et al., 2002). This central hyperactivity is a potential contributor to amplitude growth of the LFPs, and must affect patterns of neural activity that code for per-

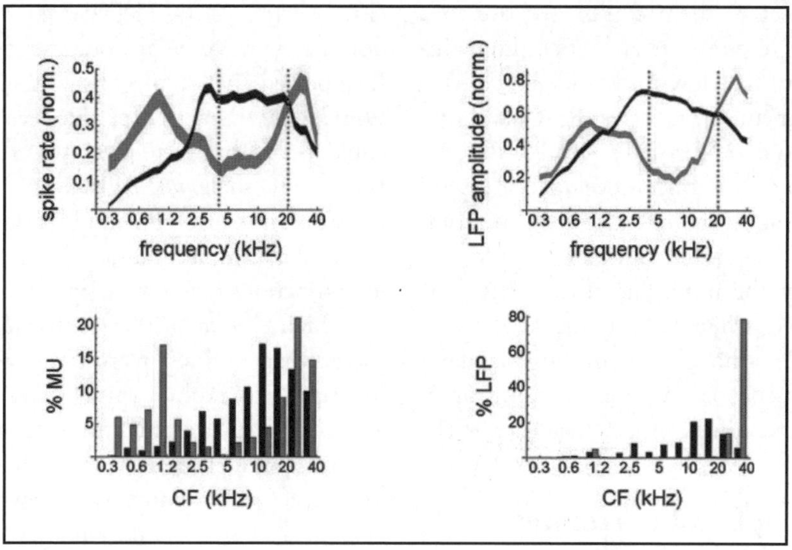

Figure 8–4. Population frequency tuning in A1, pooled across four individual noise-exposed (4 to 20 kHz steeply filtered noise, 68 dB SPL for 6 weeks) and control cats. Top row: averaged frequency marginals from control (black) and noise-exposed (red) cats. Curve thickness illustrates the Bonferroni-corrected 95% confidence interval for the mean, dotted lines mark the 4 to 20 kHz noise bandwidth. Left column based on MU activity, right column based on LFP amplitude. Bottom row: histogram distributions of response characteristic frequencies (CFs of frequency-tuning curves) or best frequencies (BFs of spectro-temporal receptive fields, STRFs) from control (black) and noise-exposed (red) cats (half-octave bin width). *Source*: Reprinted with permission from Pienkowski et al. (2011). To view this image in full color visit the Plural Publishing website for the book at http://pluralpublishing.com/publication_hdsi.htm.

ceived loudness. Coincidence-detecting cells in the ventral cochlear nucleus (VCN), which receive auditory nerve fiber (ANF) inputs with a narrow region of CFs, can potentially decode the spatiotemporal cue for sound level—the synchronous firing of a neural population. Such spatiotemporal processing could be performed at any level of the auditory brainstem wherein cells receive converging inputs from lower levels. For example, neurons recorded in VCN are typically classified based on temporal discharge patterns in response to tones. There is physiological evidence that cells in the anterior part of the VCN (AVCN) that receive convergent ANF inputs are sensitive to the temporal response pattern across the inputs (Carney, 1990). In particular, onset chopper response types (T-stellate cells) in the VCN, which are known to receive convergent inputs from ANFs with a wide range of CFs and to have wide dynamic ranges (Smith & Rhode, 1989), may act as coincidence—that is, synchrony—detectors coding for sound intensity. As synapses on inner hair cells (IHCs) and consequently ANFs span a range of different thresholds, synchronous activity detected from a subset of them could give rise to a population response related to sound intensity. Note that low-threshold ANFs have high spontaneous firing rates (SFR), and that high-threshold ANFs have low SFRs. After acquiring TTS, mice developed a loss of high-threshold ANFs, so that ABR thresholds and DPOAE characteristics were not affected. Additionally, the amplitude of the ABR wave I was reduced at high levels (Kujawa & Liberman, 2009), although this finding was later disputed based on compound action potential (CAP) recordings (Bourien et al., 2014).

Peripheral Correlates of Loudness Recruitment

Early findings suggested that in human ears with recruitment, the slopes of the CAP-level functions frequently were steeper than those obtained from control subjects (Eggermont, 1977), a result subsequently reported in animal studies of the ANF single-unit rate-level functions (reviewed in Phillips, 1987). More recent ANF single-unit studies, however, call these findings into question.

Liberman and Dodds (1984) reported that, following acoustic trauma, outer hair cell (OHC) loss is often accompanied by IHC damage, which compromises cochlear transduction and lowers the firing rates of ANFs (Liberman & Kiang, 1984). As a result, the slopes of their rate-level functions (RLFs) become shallower on average (Salvi et al., 1983; Heinz & Young, 2004). Additionally, in cats, the summed RLFs of ANFs following acoustic trauma, measured over either a narrow or wide range of CFs surrounding the stimulus frequency, did not show abnormally steep slopes (Heinz et al., 2005).

Although loudness recruitment could be the result of steeper rate-level functions in ANFs, increased total ANF firing rate due to spread of excitation, or increased neural synchrony across ANFs, Heinz et al. (2005) could not find evidence for any of these mechanisms. It appeared that if the loss was restricted to OHC only, then steeper rate-level functions could occur, but if the loss was restricted to IHCs only, shallower RLFs would be found. Because a mix of OHC and IHC loss typically is found after noise trauma, the effect on rate-level functions may not be significant.

Heinz et al. (2005) subsequently suggested that loudness recruitment was central in origin. To explore this, Cai et al. (2008) analyzed rate-level functions summed over various populations of VCN neurons following acoustic trauma and showed that the responses of non-primary-like types of neurons, especially chopper neurons, demonstrated changes in rate responses consistent with loudness recruitment (as suggested by Carney, 1990), whereas primary-like neurons did not, except in cases where spread of excitation in the population was included. Cai et al. (2008) suggested that the VCN was the most peripheral stage of the auditory pathway at which over-excitability of neurons appeared following acoustic trauma. Moreover, they again pointed to the synaptic processing in the non-primary-like, especially the stellate, cells as the initial locus of central compensation for reduced rate responses in the ANFs. An alternate view was offered by the LFP data from Wang et al. (2002), however, which put the most peripheral source of recruitment in the midbrain. Neural hyperexcitability at the LFP level is commonly reported in auditory cortex (AC) and IC (Qiu et al., 2000), but the results in cochlear nucleus have been mixed, with both positive (Saunders et al., 1972) and negative (Salvi et al., 1990) findings.

Summarizing, when considering loudness recruitment, one assumes that changes in the loudness function are mirrored by similar changes in neural response growth functions, that is, steeper neural growth functions correspond to steeper loudness growth starting likely at the IC. This behavior has been reported in the human auditory system through functional imaging at the level of the AC (Langers et al., 2007). These neural data match the expectation of loudness recruitment qualitatively in the sense that the neural responses of populations are stronger after cochlear damage; however, the changes may originate in a variety of areas in the auditory CNS.

Interaction between Loudness Recruitment and Hyperacusis

Interactions between mechanisms causing hyperacusis and loudness recruitment may be demonstrated through effects on firing rate, firing synchrony, and LFP amplitudes at elevated SPL. Following acoustic trauma, chopper neuron responses in the AVCN (Cai et al., 2008) showed sharply elevated amplitudes and discharge rates at high sound levels, consistent with findings related to loudness recruitment. Such changes may result in over-recruitment, in which intense sounds become too loud for comfortable listening (Sherlock & Formby, 2005; Nelson & Chen, 2004). In contrast, hyperacusis patients often cannot stand relatively soft sounds either and complain that they are too loud. We must look for a potential neural correlate that shows strongly increased neural responses starting just above threshold, and Noreña et al. (2006) already suggested that a central gain change may induce this.

Hyperacusis and Serotonin

Serotonin (5-hydroxytryptamine, 5-HT) has been suggested as a causal factor in hyperacusis (Marriage & Barnes, 1995; Simpson & Davies, 2000). Trauma to the cochlea or central affective dysfunction may alter the serotonergic regulation of the balance between excitation and inhibition. Serotonin-containing fibers innervate inhibitory gamma-aminobutyric acid (GABA) neurons, and in turn may produce symptoms such as phantom sounds and the excessive auditory gain potentially underlying hyperacusis (Hurley & Hall, 2011).

Sodium salicylate (SS), which is known to increase the central gain (Sun et al., 2009) increases 5-HT in IC and AC (Liu et al., 2003). Wang et al. (2006) subsequently demonstrated that SS attenuates inhibitory postsynaptic currents in the auditory cortex, suggesting a potential mechanism for tinnitus induced by SS in the central auditory system. This may occur because SS, through influencing serotonergic modulation of the GABAergic synaptic transmission, causes an imbalance between inhibition and excitation (Wang et al., 2008). This finding implies that at least a portion of the effects of SS and hyperacusis that may result are controlled via modulation of serotonin and its effects on GABAergic neurotransmission. Acoustic trauma is also capable of producing modest but significant decreases in the density of serotonergic fibers innervating the IC (Papesh & Hurley, 2012), which in turn could decrease inhibitory effects.

Audiogenic Seizures and Hyperacusis

A Rodent Model

Audiogenic seizures (AGS) are convulsions brought about by prolonged exposure to high frequency sound, particularly in rodents and rabbits and constitute a rodent model of generalized tonic-clonic epileptic seizures, induced in susceptible animals by high intensity (~110 dB SPL) acoustic stimulation (Garcia-Cairasco et al., 1993). Certain strains of mice are either genetically susceptible (e.g., DBA/2) or not susceptible (e.g., C57BL/6J) to AGS. However, seizure susceptibility can be induced in nonsusceptible strains by exposure to intense auditory stimulation during a neonatal sensitive period, a procedure known as "priming." As Saunders et al. (1972) showed that priming, usually done at high sound levels, caused cochlear damage, they proposed such exposures as an explanation for the fact that only mice with hearing loss exhibited AGS. Additionally, Garcia-Cairasco et al. (1993) reported that mice lacking serotonin 5-HT2c receptors were extremely susceptible to AGSs. The onset of susceptibility was between two and three months of age. AGS-induced immediate early gene expression indicated that AGSs were subcortical phenomena in auditory circuits.

Faingold et al. (1988) found that the IC was the most sensitive auditory center to the anticonvulsant drug AP7's action and that the imbalance between inhibitory and excitatory transmission within the IC might be crucial in the initiation of AGS in the genetically epilepsy-prone rat. In about 50% of IC neurons of normal rats, high-intensity acoustic stimulation produced neuronal firing reductions compared to lower level stimulation thereby resulting in a non-monotonic rate-level function.

However, a critical feature of all AGS models is the reduction of neural activity in the auditory pathways resulting from hearing loss during development. The initiation and propagation of AGS activity relies upon hyperexcitability in the auditory system, particularly the IC wherein bilateral lesions abolish AGS (Ross and Coleman, 2000). In AGS rats, the rate-level functions ceased to be non-monotonic and instead showed continuing increases with level, likely as a result of reduced GABA activity. A deficit in GABA-mediated inhibition in IC neurons was shown to be a critical mechanism in genetic and induced forms of AGS. In addition, excessive activation of the excitatory glutamate receptors in the IC is also strongly implicated as the other major mechanism in the pathophysiology of AGS. These neurotransmitter abnormalities result in excessive firing of IC neurons and act as the critical initiation mechanism for triggering seizures in response to intense acoustic stimuli (Faingold, 2002).

Repetition of audiogenic seizures (AGS kindling) increases the duration of convulsive behavior and the emergence of cortical epileptiform EEG activity (Feng & Faingold, 2002). The lateral amygdala (LAMG) is involved in this expanded network because after AGS kindling, LAMG neurons display a significantly increased incidence of onset-only patterns (93.3%, at 0.5 Hz), and mean acoustic responsiveness is also significantly increased (516.2% of control). LAMG neurons fire tonically during tonic convulsions and exhibit burst firing during post-tonic clonus. Greater acoustically-induced synchronization of LAMG firing, as indicated by elevated responsiveness and increased concentration of firing near the stimulus onset, may be critical for mediating the behavioral and EEG changes induced by AGS kindling. Faingold (2004) postulated that AGS qualify as an emergent property, since in AGS the acoustic stimulus evokes a non-linear output (motor convulsion), but the identical stimulus evokes minimal behavioral changes normally. The hierarchical neuronal network, underlying AGS in rodents, is initiated in IC and progresses to deep layers of superior colliculus, pontine reticular formation, and periaqueductal gray in genetic and ethanol withdrawal-induced AGS. External stimuli can induce emergent properties by producing oscillations that outlast the stimulus and induce synchronized burst firing in a neuronal population.

Faingold (2004) summarized these observations as follows: "In AGS, hyperresponsive pontine reticular formation (PRF) neurons receive an exaggerated output from IC and other sites in the AGS network, which results in a non-linear output of pontine reticular formation. The synchronized increase in reticular neuronal responses to sensory stimuli is a critical mechanism of sensory initiation of generalized seizures. Reticular neuronal responsiveness to sensory stimuli is highly constrained under normal conditions, resulting in minimal conduction of repetitive stimuli via reticular pathways. However, in seizure-susceptible states the extensive increases in neuronal responsiveness greatly enhance reticular output, synchronizing the firing of many neurons that receive reticular input, including the spinal cord, where the central pattern generators for the convulsive behaviors are localized. When the numbers and distribution of affected neurons reach a critical neural mass, the sensory stimulus initiates generalized seizures" (p. 77).

Seizures and Hyperacusis in Humans?

AGS also occur in humans and may be induced by early-onset hearing loss or music: "Musicogenic seizures usually occur in patients with focal symptomatic or cryptogenic epilepsies, but they have been reported in rare genetic epilepsies such as Dravet syndrome. A single LGI1 mutation has been described in a girl with seizures evoked by auditory stimuli. Interestingly, heterozygous knockout ($Lgi1^{+/-}$) mice show susceptibility to sound-triggered seizures. Moreover, in Frings and Black Swiss mice, the spontaneous mutations of MASS1 and JAMS1 genes, respectively, have been linked to audiogenic seizures" (p. 52) (Italiano et al., 2016). Recent clinical reports also suggest that early-age hearing loss may be related to hyperacusis. Coelho et al. (2007) found that hearing loss was often reported in children who experienced hyperacusis and tinnitus (~37%) and suggested that the mild hearing loss might be an associated risk factor for hyperacusis and tinnitus (Coelho et al., 2007). Related animal experiments suggest that early-age conductive hearing loss may provide an underlying cause.

Sun et al. (2011) demonstrated that early conductive hearing loss in rats may not only cause hyperacusis but also AGS. The authors tested the effects of tympanic membrane (TM) damage at an early age on sound perception development in rats. They found that two weeks after the TM perforation, more than 80% of the rats showed AGS when exposed to high sound levels (120 dB SPL white noise, <1 min). The susceptibility of AGS lasted at least 16 weeks after the TM damage, even after the hearing loss recovered. The TM-damaged rats also showed significantly enhanced acoustic startle responses compared to the rats without TM damage. Sun et al. (2011) also showed that the AGS can be suppressed by the administration of vigabatrin, an antiepileptic drug inhibiting catabolism of GABA. Vigabatrin also significantly reduced the loudness response (Sun et al., 2014). These results indicated that early-age conductive hearing loss could impair sound tolerance by reducing GABA inhibition in the IC, an effect possibly related to hyperacusis seen in children with otitis media.

Type II Auditory Nerve Fibers and "Pain" Hyperacusis

Recently, Flores et al. (2015) suggested that type II cochlear afferents might be involved in the detection of noise-induced tissue damage. They implied that such damage could contribute to a novel form of sensation, termed auditory nociception, potentially related to "pain hyperacusis" (Tyler et al., 2014). Using immunoreactivity to cFos, Flores et al. (2015) recorded neuronal activation in the brainstem of Vglut3$^{-/-}$ mice, in which the type-I afferents were silenced. In these deaf mice, the investigators found in cochlear nucleus neurons responses to hair-cell damaging noise, but not to non-traumatic noise. The responses were subsequently shown to originate in the cochlea. Flores et al. (2015) concluded that their findings "imply the existence of an alternative neuronal pathway from cochlea to brainstem that is activated by tissue-damaging noise and does not require glutamate release from IHCs" (p. 606) and does not necessarily encode acoustic-only stimulation. Corroboration of this idea that Type II afferents are nociceptors comes from Liu et al. (2015), who showed that type II afferents are activated when outer hair cells are damaged. This response depends on purinergic receptors, which are ubiquitous and mediate transport of neurotransmitters between cells. The purinergic receptors bind ATP released from nearby supporting cells in response to hair cell damage. Liu et al. reported that selective activation of the metabotropic purinergic receptors increased type II afferent excitability, a putative mechanism for pain hyperacusis. The effect of this activity as part of a nociceptive system could contribute to avoidance behaviors displayed by individuals with hyperacusis.

Summary

Hyperacusis in animals is indirectly inferred from the acoustic startle reflex and from the driven firing rate and/or LFP amplitude recorded along the auditory pathway. Steeper response-stimulus curves reflect increased central gain, which is present in all neural stations from the cochlear nucleus to the auditory cortex. The link between increased central gain and hyperacusis is only by inference, and often by the occurrence of "over recruitment," which is basically a combination of loudness recruitment augmented by the increased central gain; these factors cannot easily be disentangled. Evidence for decreased sound tolerance is only clear in animal strains that are prone to AGS. The relation to humans is putatively found in musicogenic seizures in patients with epilepsy. Pain hyperacusis was recently linked to a neural substrate in the type II auditory nerve fibers involving nociception and related avoidance behaviors.

References

Anari, M., Axelsson, A., Eliasson, A., & Magnusson, L. (1999). Hypersensitivity to sound–questionnaire data, audiometry and classification. *Scandinavian Audiology*, *28*, 219–230.

Bourien, J., Tang, Y., Batrel, C., Huet, A., Lenoir, M., Ladrech, S., . . . Wang, J. (2014). Contribution of auditory nerve fibers to compound action potential of the auditory nerve. *Journal of Neurophysiology*, *112*, 1025–1039.

Cai, S., Ma, W.-L. D., & Young, E. D. (2009). Encoding intensity in ventral cochlear nucleus following acoustic trauma: implications for loudness recruitment. *Journal of the Association for Research in Otolaryngology*, *10*, 5–22.

Carney, L. H. (1990). Sensitivities of cells in anteroventral cochlear nucleus of cat to spatiotemporal discharge patterns across primary afferents. *Journal of Neurophysiology*, *64*, 437–456.

Coelho, C. B., Sanchez, T. G., & Tyler, R. S. (2007). Hyperacusis, sound annoyance, and loudness hypersensitivity in children. *Progress in Brain Research*, *166*, 169–178.

Eggermont, J. J. (1977). Electrocochleography and recruitment. *Annals of Otology Rhinology and Laryngology*, *86*, 138–149.

Eggermont, J. J. (2000). Sound-induced synchronization of neural activity between and within three auditory cortical areas. *Journal of Neurophysiology*, *83*, 2708–2722.

Faingold, C. L. (2002). Role of GABA abnormalities in the inferior colliculus pathophysiology—

audiogenic seizures. *Hearing Research, 168*, 223–237.

Faingold, C. L. (2004). Emergent properties of CNS neuronal networks as targets for pharmacology: Application to anticonvulsant drug action. *Progress in Neurobiology, 72*, 55–85.

Faingold, C. L., Millan, M. H., Boersma, C. A., & Meldrum, B. S. (1988). Excitant amino acids and audiogenic seizures in the genetically epilepsy-prone rat. I. Afferent seizure initiation pathway. *Experimental Neurology 99*, 678–686.

Feng, H.-J., & Faingold, C. L. (2002). Repeated generalized audiogenic seizures induce plastic changes on acoustically evoked neuronal firing in the amygdala. *Brain Research, 932*, 61–69.

Flores, E. N., Duggan, A., Madathany, T., Hogan, A. K., Márquez, F. G., Kumar, G., . . . García-Añoveros, J. (2015). A non-canonical pathway from cochlea to brain signals tissue-damaging noise. *Current Biology, 25*, 1–7.

Formby, C., Sherlock, L. P., & Gold, S. L. (2003). Adaptive plasticity of loudness induced by chronic attenuation and enhancement of the acoustic background. *Journal of the Acoustical Society of America, 114*, 55–58.

Garcia-Cairasco, N., Terra, V. C., & Doretta, M. C. (1993). Midbrain substrates of audiogenic seizures in rats. *Behavioural Brain Research, 58*, 57–67.

Heinz, M. G., Issa, J. B., & Young, E. D. (2005). Auditory-nerve rate responses are inconsistent with common hypotheses for the neural correlates of loudness recruitment. *Journal of the Association for Research in Otolaryngology, 6*, 91–105.

Heinz, M. G., & Young, E. D. (2004). Response growth with sound level in auditory-nerve fibers after noise-induced hearing loss. *Journal of Neurophysiology, 91*, 784–795.

Hickox, A. E., & Liberman, M. C. (2014). Is noise-induced cochlear neuropathy key to the generation of hyperacusis or tinnitus? *Journal of Neurophysiology, 111*, 552–564.

Hurley, L. M., & Hall, I. C. (2011). Context-dependent modulation of auditory processing by serotonin. *Hearing Research, 279*, 74–84.

Ison, J. R., Allen, P. D., & O'Neill, W. E. (2007). Age-related hearing loss in C57BL/6J mice has both frequency-specific and non-frequency-specific components that produce a hyperacusis-like exaggeration of the acoustic startle reflex. *Journal of the Association for Research in Otolaryngology, 8*, 539–550.

Italiano, D., Striano, P., Russo, E., Leo, A., Spina, E., Zara, F., . . . Ferlazzo, E. (2016). Genetics of reflex seizures and epilepsies in humans and animals. *Epilepsy Research, 121*, 47–54.

Jastreboff, P. J., & Hazell, J. W. P. (1993). A neurophysiological approach to tinnitus: Clinical implications. *British Journal of Audiology, 27*, 7–17.

Knudson, I. M., & Melcher, J. R. (2016). Elevated acoustic startle responses in humans: relationship to reduced loudness discomfort level, but not self-report of hyperacusis. *Journal of the Association for Research in Otolaryngology, 17*, 223–235.

Kujawa, S. G., & Liberman, M. C. (2009). Adding insult to injury: Cochlear nerve degeneration after "temporary" noise-induced hearing loss. *Journal of Neuroscience, 29*, 14077–14085.

Langers, D. R. M., van Dijk, P., Schoenmaker, E. S., & Backes, W. H. (2007). fMRI activation in relation to sound intensity and loudness. *NeuroImage, 35*, 709–718.

Liberman, M. C., & Dodds, L. W. (1984). Single-neuron labeling and chronic cochlear pathology. II. Stereocilia damage and alterations of spontaneous discharge rates. *Hearing Research, 16*, 43–53.

Liberman, M. C., & Kiang, N. Y. (1984). Single-neuron labeling and chronic cochlear pathology. IV. Stereocilia damage and alterations in rate- and phase-level functions. *Hearing Research, 16*, 75–90.

Liu, J., Li, X., Wang, L., Dong, Y., Han, H., & Liu, G. (2003). Effects of salicylate on serotoninergic activities in rat inferior colliculus and auditory cortex. *Hearing Research, 175*, 45–53.

Liu, C., Glowatzki, E., & Fuchs, P. A. (2015). Unmyelinated type II afferent neurons report cochlear damage. *Proceedings of the National Academy of Sciences of the United States of America, 112*, 14723–14727.

Marriage, J., & Barnes, N. M. (1995). Is central hyperacusis a symptom of 5-hydroxytryptamine (5-HT) dysfunction? *Journal of Laryngology and Otology, 109*, 915–921.

Nelson, J. J., & Chen, K. (2004). The relationship of tinnitus, hyperacusis, and hearing loss. *Ear Nose and Throat Journal, 83*, 472–476.

Noreña, A. J., & Chery-Croze, S. (2007). Enriched acoustic environment rescales auditory sensitivity. *Neuroreport, 18*, 1251–1255.

Noreña, A. J., Gourévitch, B., Aizawa, N., & Eggermont, J. J. (2006). Spectrally enhanced acoustic environment disrupts frequency representation in cat auditory cortex. *Nature Neuroscience, 9*, 932–939.

Papesh, M. A., & Hurley, L. M. (2012). Plasticity of serotonergic innervation of the inferior colliculus in mice following acoustic trauma. *Hearing Research, 283*, 89–97.

Phillips, D. P. (1987). Stimulus intensity and loudness recruitment: Neural correlates. *Journal of the Acoustical Society of America. 82*, 1–12.

Pienkowski, M., & Eggermont, J. J. (2009). Recovery from reorganization induced in adult cat primary auditory cortex by a band-limited spectrally enhanced acoustic environment. *Hearing Research, 257*, 24–40.

Pienkowski, M., Munguia, R., & Eggermont, J. J. (2011). Passive exposure of adult cats to band-limited tone pip ensembles or noise rapidly leads to long-term response suppression in auditory cortex. *Hearing Research, 277*, 117–126.

Qiu, C. X., Salvi, R., Ding, D., & Burkard, R. (2000). Inner hair cell loss leads to enhanced response amplitudes in auditory cortex of unanesthetized chinchillas: Evidence for increased system gain. *Hearing Research, 139*, 153–171.

Röhl, M., & Uppenkamp, S. (2012). Neural coding of sound intensity and loudness in the human auditory system. *Journal of the Association for Research in Otolaryngology, 13*, 369–379.

Ross, K. C., & Coleman, J. R. (2000). Developmental and genetic audiogenic seizure models: Behavior and biological substrates. *Neuroscience and Biobehavioral Reviews, 24*, 639–653.

Salvi, R. J., Hamernik, R. P., Henderson, D., & Ahroon, W. A. (1983). Neural correlates of sensorineural hearing loss. *Ear & Hearing, 4*, 115–129.

Salvi, R. J., Saunders, S. S., Gratton, M. A., Arehole, S., & Powers, N. (1990). Enhanced evoked response amplitudes in the inferior colliculus of the chinchilla fallowing acoustic trauma. *Hearing Research, 50*, 245–258.

Salvi, R. J., Wang, J., & Ding, D. (2000). Auditory plasticity and hyperactivity following cochlear damage. *Hearing Research, 147*, 261–274.

Saunders, J. C., Bock, G. R., Chen, C.-S., & Gates, G. R. (1972). The effects of priming for audiogenic seizures on cochlear and behavioral responses in BALB/c mice. *Experimental Neurology, 36*, 426–436.

Sherlock, L. P., & Formby, C. (2005). Estimates of loudness, loudness discomfort, and the auditory dynamic range: normative estimates, comparison of procedures, and test-retest reliability. *Journal of the American Academy of Audiology, 16*, 85–100.

Simpson, J. J., & Davies, W. E. (2000). A review of evidence in support of a role for 5-HT in the perception of tinnitus. *Hearing Research, 145*, 1–7.

Smith, P. H., & Rhode, W. S. (1989). Structural and functional properties distinguish two types of multipolar cells in the ventral cochlear nucleus. *Journal of Comparative Neurology, 282*, 595–616.

Sun, W., Lu, J., Stolzberg, D., Gray, L., Deng, A., Lobarinas, E., & Salvi, R. J. (2009). Salicylate increases the gain of the central auditory system. *Neuroscience, 159*, 325–334.

Sun, W., Manohar, S., Jayaram, A., Kumaraguru, A., Fu, Q., Li, J., & Allman, B. (2011). Early age conductive hearing loss causes audiogenic seizure and hyperacusis behavior. *Hearing Research, 282*, 178–183.

Sun, W., Fu, Q., Zhang, C., Manohar, S., Kumaraguru, A., & Li, J. (2014). Loudness perception affected by early age hearing loss. *Hearing Research, 313*, 18–25.

Sztuka, A., Pospiech, L., Gawron, W., & Dudek, K. (2010). DPOAE in estimation of the function of the cochlea in tinnitus patients with normal hearing. *Auris Nasus Larynx, 37*, 55–60.

Turner, J. G., & Larsen, D. (2016). Effects of noise exposure on development of tinnitus and hyperacusis: Prevalence rates 12 months after exposure in middle-aged rats. *Hearing Research, 334*, 30–36.

Turner, J. G., & Parrish, J. (2008). Gap detection methods for assessing salicylate-induced tinnitus and hyperacusis in rats. *American Journal of Audiology, 17*, S185–192.

Tyler, R. S., Pienkowski, M., Roncancio, E. R., Jun, H. J., Brozoski, T., Dauman, N., . . . Moore, B. C. (2014). A review of hyperacusis and future directions: Part I. Definitions and manifestations. *American Journal of Audiology*, *23*, 402–419.

Wang, J., Ding, D., & Salvi, R. J. (2002). Functional reorganization in chinchilla inferior colliculus associated with chronic and acute cochlear damage. *Hearing Research*, *168*, 238–249.

Wang, H.-T., Luo, B., Zhou, K.-Q., Xu, T.-L., & Chen, L. (2006). Sodium salicylate reduces inhibitory postsynaptic currents in neurons of rat auditory cortex. *Hearing Research*, *215*, 77–83.

Wang, H.-T., Luo, B., Huang, Y.-N., Zhou, K.-Q., & Chen, L. (2008). Sodium salicylate suppresses serotonin-induced enhancement of GABAergic spontaneous inhibitory postsynaptic currents in rat inferior colliculus in vitro. *Hearing Research*, *236*, 42–51.

9

Traumatic Brain Injury and Auditory Processing

Melissa A. Papesh, Sarah M. Theodoroff, and Frederick J. Gallun

A Brief Background on Traumatic Brain Injury

Traumatic brain injury (TBI) is a form of acquired brain injury that occurs when a sudden external trauma damages the brain and disrupts neurological function. In 2010, approximately 2.5 million patients were seen in emergency departments across the United States for TBIs (CDC, 2015). Analysis of these visits reveals that falls account for the vast majority of TBIs in both young children (up to 4 years old) and in adults ages 45 and older. In other age groups, the causes of TBIs vary considerably and often involve falls, assaults, motor vehicle accidents, or striking the head against objects (Figure 9–1; CDC, 2015). Military personnel are also at risk of TBI from exposure to high-intensity blast discharges, such as those generated by improvised explosive devices (IEDs), in addition to the more typical causes of TBI that affect civilians. Since the start of U.S. military operations in Iraq and Afghanistan in 2000, more than 350,000 military service members have sustained TBIs, with blast-exposure being the leading cause of injury (DVBIC, 2016). In fact, blast exposure and resulting TBI are so common among military personnel that TBI is considered the "signature injury" of recent military conflicts (Hoge et al., 2008). For a review on the prevalence and risk factors of auditory-related problems in Veterans and military personnel of the recent conflicts in Iraq and Afghanistan, see Theodoroff et al. (2015).

Neurological damage from impact- and blast-related mechanisms results from the stretching or shearing of the elements comprising various neural pathways, contusions to the cortical surfaces that collide with the skull, injury to blood vessels, and the cascade of inflammatory responses to tissue injury that can both damage and heal the neural elements (Taber et al., 2006, 2015; Chafi et al., 2010; Tompkins et al., 2013). These effects can disrupt the functions of specific neural processing elements in the brainstem, thalamus, and cortex, as well as impair the functioning of synaptic structures and neural connections throughout the entire central nervous system (CNS). Additional structures affected include the corpus callosum and other long fiber tracts

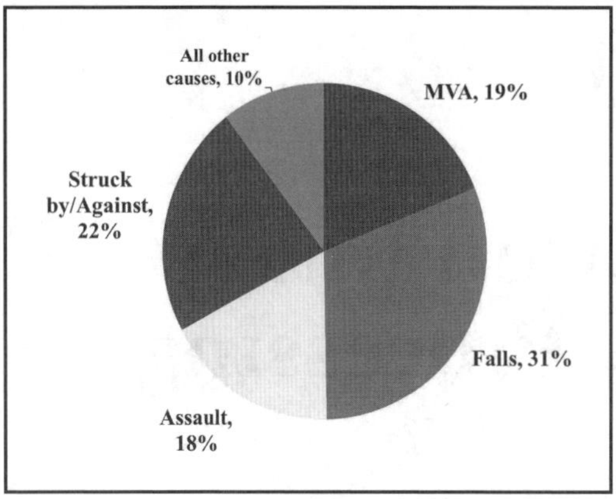

Figure 9–1. Primary causes of TBI-related emergency room visits for civilian patients between the ages of 5 and 64 years. Data were obtained from hospitals across the United States between 2001 and 2010. Overall, falls are the leading cause of injury for this age group (31% of TBIs), followed by the head being forcefully struck by or against a solid object (22%), motor vehicle accidents (MVA; 19%), and assaults (18%). *Source*: Data obtained from CDC (2015).

that are essential for coordination and distribution of information throughout the brain (Taber et al., 2006, 2015). Thus, TBI has the capacity to disrupt a wide array of neural functions including sensory, motor, cognitive, and emotional processes. Health effects most frequently associated with TBI include cognitive deficits in attention, memory, and executive function; behavioral and emotional disturbances spanning aggression, depression, and impulsivity; psychological injury such as post-traumatic stress disorder (PTSD); motor difficulties frequently affecting balance and muscle tone; changes in hearing and vision including increased sensitivity to light and noise; and somatic symptoms such as headaches, sleep disturbances, and chronic pain (Verfaellie et al., 2013; Godbolt et al., 2014; Fausti et al., 2009; Nampiaparampil, 2008; Bergemalm & Lyxell, 2005; Kapoor & Ciuffreda, 2002). The occurrence and persistence of these symptoms is heterogeneous across patients, even among those with the same etiology and similar severity of neural damage.

Of course, not all blows to the head result in TBI; diagnosis is based upon clinical symptoms of neural dysfunction observed during and shortly after the injury. Symptoms indicative of TBI include any period of loss of or decreased consciousness, retrograde or post-traumatic amnesia, neurological deficits such as muscle weakness, loss of balance and coordination, and sensory loss, as well as any alteration in mental state such as confusion and disorientation (CDC, 2015). The severity of these symptoms, in combination with structural imaging measures, is used to classify TBIs as mild, moderate, or severe (Table 9–1). The vast majority of TBIs incurred in both civilian and military populations fall within the mild classification (also known as a concussion) which is characterized by brief or no loss of consciousness, amnesia spanning no more than 24 hours, mild neurological symptoms, and lack of abnormal findings on standard clinical imaging tests immediately after injury. Most patients who sustain a mild TBI have a favorable outcome as symptoms resolve within a few weeks post-injury. However, estimates indicate that 10% to 15% of patients who incur a mild TBI will suffer from postconcussion syndrome (PCS) with symptoms lasting more than a year after injury (Alves, 1992; Gouvier et al., 1992; Binder et al., 1997). PCS specifically refers to the organic and psychogenic disturbances observed after closed head injuries including the subjective physical complaints (e.g., headache, dizziness), as well as cognitive, emotional, and behavioral changes (WHO, 1992). The likelihood of a patient displaying persistent PCS is influenced by many factors such as location and severity of injury, age at injury, and med-

Table 9–1. Symptoms used by medical professionals to classify the severity of TBI.

	TBI Classification		
	Mild/ Concussion	Moderate	Severe
Confusion/disorientation:	<24 hours	>24 hours	>24 hours
Loss of consciousness:	≤30 minutes	>30 minutes, <24 hours	>24 hours
Memory loss:	<24 hours	>24 hours, <7 days	>7 days
Brain imaging:	Normal	Abnormal	Abnormal
Glasgow coma scale:	13–15	9–12	3–8

ical history prior to injury including occurrence of previous head injuries (McAllister & Arciniegas, 2002; Munjal et al., 2010; Silver et al., 2011; Silverberg & Iverson, 2011).

Auditory Consequences of TBI

The entire CNS, including the peripheral and central auditory mechanism, is at risk of damage from TBI. The extreme mechanical forces that inflict TBI can produce damage to the auditory periphery in the form of tympanic membrane rupture, disarticulation of the ossicular chain, and/or inner ear damage caused by tearing of the oval or round window or fracture of the temporal bone (Darley & Kellman, 2010). Conductive and sensorineural hearing losses that result from these types of injuries may be remediated using traditional otological and audiological methods such as surgical repair of structural damage and/or provision of hearing assistive devices (Fausti et al., 2009; Darley & Kellman, 2010). However, between 50% and 75% of patients with previous TBI report auditory difficulties in spite of intact auditory periphery and normal pure tone hearing sensitivity (Oleksiak et al., 2012; Saunders et al., 2015; Gallun et al., 2012a,b, 2016). The difficulties reported by these patients are consistent with altered processing in the central auditory nervous system (CANS) and often include increased sensitivity to noise, poor speech understanding in competing background noise or reverberation, problems understanding on the telephone or when the talker's face is unseen, difficulty following conversations among groups of people, recalling auditory information, and auditory fatigue (Ryan & Warden, 2003; Fausti et al., 2009; Dikmen et al., 2010; Schultz et al., 2011; Papesh & Gallun, 2016; Saunders et al., 2015; Gallun et al., 2016). Current guidelines from the American Speech-Language-Hearing Association (ASHA; 2005) and the American Academy of Audiology (AAA, 2010) agree that even mild TBI commonly results in long-term CNS damage that may produce auditory dysfunction.

Auditory processing deficits can arise from damage specific to the auditory pathway as well as non-auditory-specific neural damage. Although a characteristic of mild TBI is lack of observable structural damage on standard clinical imaging scans, more advanced imaging techniques such as magnetic resonance spectroscopy (Jantzen, 2010), diffusion tensor imaging (Belanger et al., 2007), and resting state functional magnetic resonance imaging (Johnson et al., 2012) have recently been employed to examine neurological integrity in patients with mild TBI. Data from these studies combined with animal models of mild TBI have revealed the presence of chronic diffuse axonal injury (DAI) and neural restructuring in areas including the temporal and frontal cortices (Niogi & Mukherjee, 2010; Johnson et al., 2012), interhemispheric tracts including the corpus callosum (Koliatsos et al., 2011; Davenport et al., 2012; Petrie et al., 2014; Wright et al., 2016), cortical-subcortical tracts (Davenport et al., 2012; Petrie et al., 2014), fronto-parietal tracts (Davenport et al., 2012; Johnson et al., 2012), and the cerebellum (Koliatsos et al., 2011). Additional evidence of structural damage may include scarring of brain tissue at junctions between brain parenchyma and fluids, at junctions between gray and white matter (Shively et al., 2016), stunted dendritic outgrowths in GABAergic cortical neurons (Carron et al., 2016), mossy fiber sprouting in the hippocampus and increases in excitatory synapses (Hunt et al., 2011), and excitatory input to cortical pyramidal neurons (Jin et al., 2011). In the chronic phase of mild TBI, there is considerable evidence of hyperexcitability in sensory cortical areas (Alwis et al., 2012, 2013; Carron et al., 2016) largely due to decreased activity of inhibitory neurotransmitters and resulting imbalance of excitatory and inhibitory cortical networks (Yi et al., 2006; Buriticá et al., 2009; Pavlov et al., 2011). This pattern of cortical hyperexcitability is likely a consequence of maladaptive restructuring of cortical networks in response to widespread damage (Alwis et al., 2012, 2013; Greer et al., 2013). The resulting functional impairments in cognitive, motor, and sensory systems are frequently observed years after injury, even in cases of mild and moderate TBI (Draper & Ponsford, 2008; Little et al., 2010; Fischer et al., 2014; Song et al., 2016).

Many of the brain areas listed above are intimately involved in the processing of auditory information. The temporal lobe houses both the primary auditory cortex, which receives information from the medial geniculate body of the thalamus and lower auditory brainstem centers, and the auditory association cortex, which is involved in recognition and integration of auditory information with other neural processes. In cases of focal neural injury, damage to the auditory cortex is associated with a range of functional disabilities including impaired auditory pattern recognition (Musiek & Pinheiro, 1987; Musiek et al., 1990; von Steinbüchel et al., 1999), dichotic listening (Musiek, 1983; Mueller, 1987), and temporal discrimination (Mueller, 1987), as well as reduced performance on tests of speech perception in noise and rapidly spoken speech (Bergemalm & Borg, 2005). Damage to interhemispheric tracts including the corpus callosum produce deficits in dichotic listening performance (Musiek, 1983). Cortical and subcortical tracts carry auditory information between the cortex and brainstem and coordinate auditory processing with other neural regions. Damage to these pathways, as well as imbalance of excitatory and inhibitory neural responses in sensory cortices following brain injury, may reduce the ability to encode and discriminate basic characteristics of acoustic signals such as changes in the frequency, intensity, and timing of sounds (von Steinbüchel et al., 1999; Fausti et al., 2009). Such deficits may underlie more complex functional issues frequently reported by patients including increased sensitivity to noise and difficulty understanding degraded speech.

Mild TBI produces widespread and durable structural and functional changes that influence auditory function even when associated with damage to non-auditory-specific regions. Additional areas that frequently show chronic structural and physiological changes following mild TBI include regions involved in cognitive tasks such as the prefrontal cortex and hippocampus (McAllister et al., 1999; Palacios et al., 2013), the limbic system which regulates emotion (Capizzano et al., 2010; Zhu et al., 2014), and regions involved in multisensory integration such as the cerebellum (Spanos et al., 2007; Potts et al., 2009). Current theories of cognitive control indicate that brain centers associated with cognition modulate incoming sensory information, and provide top-down control which sculpts perception and behavioral responses (Mesulam, 2002; Wolf & Koch, 2016). Deficits in higher-order executive function including memory, attention, and cognitive capacity may impair auditory performance as such deficits reduce the availability of resources required to process auditory stimuli.

Mental health status is also known to affect auditory responses. PTSD and anxiety disorders amplify acoustic startle reflexes as indicated by larger amplitude and lower threshold reflexive myogenic responses to unexpected auditory stimuli (Morgan et al., 1996; Glover et al., 2011). Similarly, patients with depression are widely reported to have increased sensitivity to noise and abnormal electrophysiological findings that include significantly steeper cortical amplitude-intensity functions, increased P200 amplitudes, and prolonged P300 latencies compared to patients with no signs of depression (Vandoolaeghe et al., 1998; Gallinat et al., 2000; Gopal et al., 2004). Overall, these examples demonstrate that patients with previous TBI are at increased risk of poor neural regulation of both auditory stimuli and the responses they engender.

Sound Intolerance

It follows that poor pre- and post-attentive regulation of auditory information flow stemming from damage to auditory and non-auditory pathways likely contributes to sound intolerance in patients with previous TBI. The neuropsychological evaluation completed for all Veterans suspected of having sustained a TBI routinely has patients rate their sensitivity to noise on a scale from 1 (none/not a problem) to 5 (severe/cannot function without help) (DVA, 2007). Between 18 and 32% of these Veterans report being "bothered by noise" even after one year of recovery from TBI (Dikmen et al., 2010). Although sensitivity to noise is commonly reported in patients with previous TBI (Ryan & Warden, 2003; Cicerone & Kalmar, 1995; Jury & Flynn, 2001), the prevalence of this problem has not been well established (Halbauer et al., 2009; Reid et al., 2014). This gap in knowledge is due, in part, to the poorly defined nature of sensitivity to noise as well as lack of consistent terminology used to describe and report it (e.g., noise sensitivity, hyperacusis, phonophobia, misophonia, loudness intolerance). Often, these terms are used interchangeably by clinicians and researchers. Tyler et al. (2014) review the various definitions put forth in the literature and suggest a new nomenclature to describe various types of hyperacusis, although it is important to keep in mind that hyperacusis and noise sensitivity may be different types of sound intolerance disorders. Ideally, any classification system would be informed by objective measures sensitive to differentiating the various types of sound intolerance disorders rather than based solely on subjective report. It is likely that hyperacusis and noise sensitivity are distinct phenomena characterized by different patterns of physical and emotional responses to sound. For example, when a patient with previous TBI reports "noise sensitivity," their statement could indicate any of the following: (a) that high, moderate, or low noise levels induce physical sensations of pain; (b) that the patient has extreme difficulty listening to and understanding speech even in low levels of background noise; (c) that background noise induces emotional responses such as fear or agitation; or (d) some combination of these symptoms. Unfortunately, the majority of literature available on such sound intolerance disorders lacks well-defined self-report metrics and rarely includes rigorous psychophysical assessment of auditory function (for a rare exception, we refer readers to Ellermier et al., 2001). The validity of LDLs to assess sensitivity to noise has been questioned due to poor sensitivity for diagnosing hyperacusis (Sheldrake et al., 2015), the substantial influence of methodological differences across clinics and experimental protocols (Punch et al., 2004), and weak correlations between patients' LDLs and their self-reported intolerance of sound in everyday life (Zaugg et al., 2016).

Auditory Evaluation and Treatment of Patients with TBI

Because dysfunction stemming from TBI is often multifaceted in nature, a multidisciplinary team approach to assessment and treatment is warranted. A full assessment considering auditory as well as language, memory, and attention abilities is required as these higher-order functions are often affected in patients with TBI. Due to the interconnected nature of neural processing underlying sensory, cognitive, and emotional regulation, improvements in one of these areas often results in improvements in other areas. Thus, treatments for TBI-related cognitive or psychological disorders may in fact improve auditory function (Dundon et al., 2015). Unfortunately, there is often a tendency to attribute auditory dysfunction to co-morbidities rather than attempt to specifically treat the auditory concerns (Oleksiak et al., 2012). While patients are likely to benefit from treatment of co-morbid disorders, the need for auditory-specific rehabilitation should not be discounted; just as improvements in co-morbid conditions may result in improved auditory processing, improvements in auditory processing may reduce severity of co-morbid conditions as well.

Audiological evaluation of patients with previous TBI begins with a comprehensive examination including a thorough case history reviewing medical history, previous head injuries, and details of the specific difficulties the patient is having. As described above, patients who are found to have conductive or sensorineural hearing loss are routinely treated via traditional otological and audiological means, including surgical intervention for repairable structural damage and hearing aids for permanent hearing loss. Those who have auditory difficulties with normal audiometric thresholds should be further evaluated for central auditory processing disorders (APD). Even mild TBIs can produce chronic auditory processing deficits that are extremely varied across patients. Deficits may include poor auditory discrimination, decreased auditory temporal processing, sensitivity to noise, difficulty with auditory pattern processing, poor dichotic listening, and abnormally poor auditory performance in competing acoustic signals or when auditory signals are otherwise degraded (Bergemalm & Borg, 2005; Bressler et al., 2016; Downie et al., 2002; Dundon et al., 2015; Fausti et al., 2009; Gallun et al., 2012, 2016; Hoover et al., 2015; Mueller et al., 1987). Table 9–2 shows several common clinical tests of

Table 9–2. Rates of abnormal performance by patients with previous TBI on clinical tests of central auditory processing.

Central Auditory Processing Tests	% Abnormal Performance
Speech in Noise Comprehension	
Hearing in Noise Test (HINT); Words in Noise (WIN); Quick Speech-in-Noise (QuickSIN); Listening in Spatialized Noise; SCAN and SCAN-A	28–59.2%
Temporal Processing	
Gaps-in-Noise (GIN); Adaptive Tests of Temporal Resolution (ATTR)	31–60.7%
Auditory Pattern Recognition	
Frequency Patterns Test (FPT); Duration Pattern Test (DPT)	19–64%
Dichotic Listening Tests	
Dichotic Digits Test (DDT); Staggered Spondaic Words Test (SSW)	14–64%
Binaural Interaction	
Masking Level Difference Test (MLD)	10–20%

Note. Central auditory processing tests are grouped according to the specific auditory processes which they target. Abnormal percentages were derived from studies that included participants with at least one TBI or blast exposure incurred from 1 year to 10 years prior to testing. References for abnormal test performance values include Van Toor et al., 2006; Bergemalm & Lyxell, 2005; Turgeon et al., 2011; Gallun et al., 2012; Saunders et al., 2015; and Gallun et al., 2016.

central auditory processing grouped according to auditory tasks which are frequently found to be deficient in patients with previous TBI. The percentage of abnormal performance for each of these subgroups was derived from published studies of patients with normal pure tone audiograms who had sustained a mild TBI between 1 and 10 years prior to testing.

Electrophysiological assessments may also aid the evaluation and rehabilitation of auditory concerns following TBI (Fausti et al., 2009; Lew et al., 2007; Folmer et al., 2011). While responses generated by the auditory brainstem are generally found to be abnormal only in cases of moderate to severe brain damage (Jabbari et al., 1987; Folmer et al., 2011; Bressler et al., 2016), several studies indicate that changes in cortical and cognitive auditory evoked potentials (AEP) are often observable even in mild cases of TBI (Gallun et al., 2012; Duncan et al., 2011; Folmer et al., 2011; Lew et al., 2004). Cortical and cognitive AEPs used most often to probe auditory function in patients with TBI include the N100, P200, N200, mismatch negativity, and P300 responses. In comparison to healthy controls, patients who have suffered TBI most often demonstrate reduced response amplitudes, longer latencies, or both (Lew et al., 2004, 2007; Gallun et al., 2012; Bressler et al., 2016; Folmer et al., 2011; Elting et al., 2008; Rapp et al., 2015; Sun et al., 2015). AEP measures also reveal differences in brain activity when auditory tasks are compared between controls and TBI patients. Multiple studies have shown that although brain-injured patients are often able to perform simple auditory tasks with the same ability as healthy controls (albeit often with longer response times), the scalp topography of AEP responses clearly demonstrates differences in the recruitment of various brain regions to perform these tasks (Larson et al., 2007; Elting et al., 2008; Gallun et al., 2012; Kaipio et al., 2013).

Due to the heterogeneous nature of auditory deficits arising from head injury, a patient/deficit-specific approach to treatment is warranted (Bellis, 2002). Treatment strategies are often comprised of a combination of auditory training and general management interventions. With auditory training, the hope is to elicit experience-based neural plasticity within the auditory pathway designed to sharpen specific auditory functions (Ross-Swain et al., 2007; Chermak & Musiek, 2002). In patients with previous TBIs, such retraining targets encoding and regulation of auditory information (Murphy et al., 2011). Training is most effective during heightened states of neural plasticity, such as during youth and soon after the brain injury has been incurred (Chermak & Musiek, 2002). In order for training to produce optimal results, it must focus on a specific deficit and provide adequate challenge before progressing to more difficult tasks. The trainee must be motivated and actively participate to the best of their abilities; to do so, they must commit to the training exercises on a regular schedule (Chermak & Musiek, 2002). While some auditory training programs are available commercially, the majority of these are specifically designed for pediatric populations (Bamiou et al., 2006) and do not target specific TBI-related deficits.

Less-structured training programs, such as dichotic interaural intensity training for patients who have one ear that performs significantly better than the other, may also prove beneficial for TBI patients with APD (Musiek et al., 2004). This technique asks participants to select two different listening materials to be presented to each ear simultaneously. The intensity of the dichotic material is initially set so that the better-performing ear receives a signal at a lower sensation level compared to that presented to the poorer ear, thereby making it easier for the patient to hear the stimuli presented to the poorer ear. Over time, the level of the stimuli in the two ears is slowly adjusted with the goal of achieving similar levels of intensity and performance for both ears. A benefit to this type of intervention is that patients can choose their own training materials and times for training sessions.

Assistive devices for hearing have also proven helpful to many patients with normal hearing thresholds and APD (Johnston et al., 2009; Bamiou et al., 2006). Such devices prioritize improving the relative levels of speech and background noise, the so-called signal-to-noise ratio. A recent study examined the efficacy of administering a personal ear-level frequency modulation (FM) system to young and middle-aged patients with normal hearing thresholds who had suffered mild TBI within the past 10 years (Saunders et al., 2014). Study participants found numerous ways to use the FM systems to benefit them throughout the day, and usage remained high throughout the 8-week study duration. For example, several participants were students who reported difficulty hearing in classroom environments and expressed great benefit from being able to place the FM microphone near or on the instructor. This likely had the effect of both improving the signal-to-noise ratio of the instructor's voice as well as reducing the deleterious effects of reverberation in classrooms.

Individuals also reported benefit of the FM system in the workplace. One participant was required to attend weekly team meetings at which co-workers gathered around a large table to discuss relevant topics. He expressed difficulty following the conversation as it switched among talkers. However, by placing his FM microphone either in the center of the table or by passing it to various coworkers to speak into, he was able to keep up with the conversation and not miss out on important information. Another patient was employed at a canine kennel and had great difficulty hearing her co-workers in the reverberant kennel area, even when the dogs were being relatively quiet. By placing the FM microphone near the front desk, her co-workers were able to communicate with her effectively, thereby reducing stress and improving job satisfaction. Usage of the FM systems was so successful that many participants requested to keep their devices at the conclusion of the study.

Similar positive outcomes have been reported when assistive devices are provided for pediatric patients with APD (Johnston et al., 2009). Other interventions likely to improve auditory performance in normally hearing patients with APD concerns now include low-amplification hearing aids, as many employ algorithms designed to improve the signal-to-noise ratio in various listening environments and thus provide a less effortful listening experience for users (Stach et al., 1991; Pichora-Fuller, 2003). Although many audiology clinics provide FM systems or low-amplification hearing aids to normally hearing patients with APD concerns, the long-term benefits from such interventions are not yet known.

Lastly, all patients with previous TBI and auditory processing difficulties should receive communication counseling (Bellis, 2002; Bamiou et al., 2006). Validating auditory complaints in this population, and explaining that auditory issues can persist in spite of "normal" hearing thresholds, can substantially reduce the social and emotional burden of these problems on patients as such counseling helps convince both the patient and their support group of the need for rehabilitation and changes in communication strategies. Counseling should also include factors such as environmental modifications to improve listening, encouraging the patient to make active requests of communication partners to facilitate communication, and encouraging patients to use additional strategies such as communicating important messages in writing as opposed to verbally.

Research Priorities

Although significant advancements have been made regarding the long-term consequences of TBI on the auditory system, a considerable number of questions remain unanswered. For example, it is presently unclear whether the etiology of head injury is important when determining either the type or extent of auditory dysfunction that a patient may experience. It is currently unknown whether a TBI resulting from a fall is likely to cause the same types of auditory impairments as those resulting from vehicle accidents or exposure to high-intensity blast waves. A better understanding of how different traumatic insults to the brain could impair auditory function may improve our ability to detect and rehabilitate auditory conditions. This work will require increased application of advanced imaging techniques in patients with TBIs of varying etiologies, as well as long-term studies comparing the auditory behavioral and physiological outcomes of diverse types of TBI.

Another essential question that remains unanswered is why some individuals will sustain lasting auditory consequences from head injury while others will have full recovery of auditory function. Several factors are likely to contribute to such individual variability including the age at which the injury occurs, presence of preexisting behavioral, physical, or neurological conditions, genetic factors, socioeconomic factors, and life history. Additional large-scale studies are needed to tease out the impact of these various factors.

Case Study

A male Veteran (MV) recently presented to an audiology clinic in the US at the age of 52 stating that he had noticed a substantial decrease in his hearing ability following his military service as well as the onset of constant tinnitus. MV served in the Navy and Army National Guard between 1977 and 2009. He served many domestic and international service missions, including deployments to Egypt, Cuba, and Iraq. He was exposed to three bomb blasts during his time in Iraq, with the most severe resulting from an improvised explosive device in 2008, approximately 6 years prior to presenting in the VA audiology clinic. Bodily damage incurred from the blast included a TBI, ruptured discs and vertebrae throughout his spine, broken nose, permanent damage to his right arm and knee, and loss of teeth. In spite of his injuries, he managed to rescue three comrades from a burning vehicle, for which he was awarded a Purple Heart. At the time he was seen at the VA audiology clinic, he had previously undergone cognitive rehabilitation treatment through a polytrauma clinic, as well as treatment from speech language pathology services for concerns related to cognitive difficulties. His additional medical diagnoses included PTSD, anxiety, obstructive sleep apnea, chronic headaches, type 2 diabetes mellitus, sensitivity to light, colitis, chronic knee and back pain, hyperlipidemia, weakness and numbness of the right arm, and coronary heart disease. An intake interview revealed that his primary auditory complaints included difficulty hearing in noise and in the presence of multiple talkers, difficulty understanding on the telephone, problems paying attention to people speaking, and confusing similar-sounding words. Comprehensive audiological assessment revealed normal pure tone thresholds (Figure 9–2A), normal functioning on immittance measures, and present distortion product otoacoustic emissions from 750 to 8000 Hz in both the right and left ears. Word recognition scores were 100% in both ears when presented in quiet. MV was subsequently referred to the VA's auditory processing disorder clinic. Here, he was tested on the SCAN-A (including all subtests), Gaps-in-Noise test, the pitch pattern test, Words-in-Noise, QuickSIN, Dichotic Digits, and the Staggered Spondaic Words test. Results indicated performance within the normal range on all subtests of the SCAN-A, the Words-in-Noise test, the QuickSIN, Dichotic Digits, and the Staggered Spondaic Words test. However, his performance on the Gaps-in-Noise test revealed poor temporal acuity in both ears (thresholds of 8 and 10 ms in the right and left ears, respectively), as well as poor auditory pattern recognition on the Pitch Pattern Test (52% and 80% correct in the right and left ears, respectively). Additional testing indicated minimal benefit from spatial separation between sound sources, and electrophysiological measurement of the P300 in response to a tonal oddball paradigm revealed minimal response to a 1000 Hz rare tone embedded in a series of 500 Hz tones (Figure 9–2B).

MV was subsequently diagnosed with an auditory processing disorder stemming from poor temporal processing. His reduced temporal acuity likely accounted for poor recognition of auditory temporal patterns as well as lack of the benefit that most listeners receive from spatial separation between talkers of interest and competing background sounds. The temporal smearing of sounds resulting from poor temporal acuity was likely responsible for his reported difficulties hearing in complex listening environments and on the telephone as

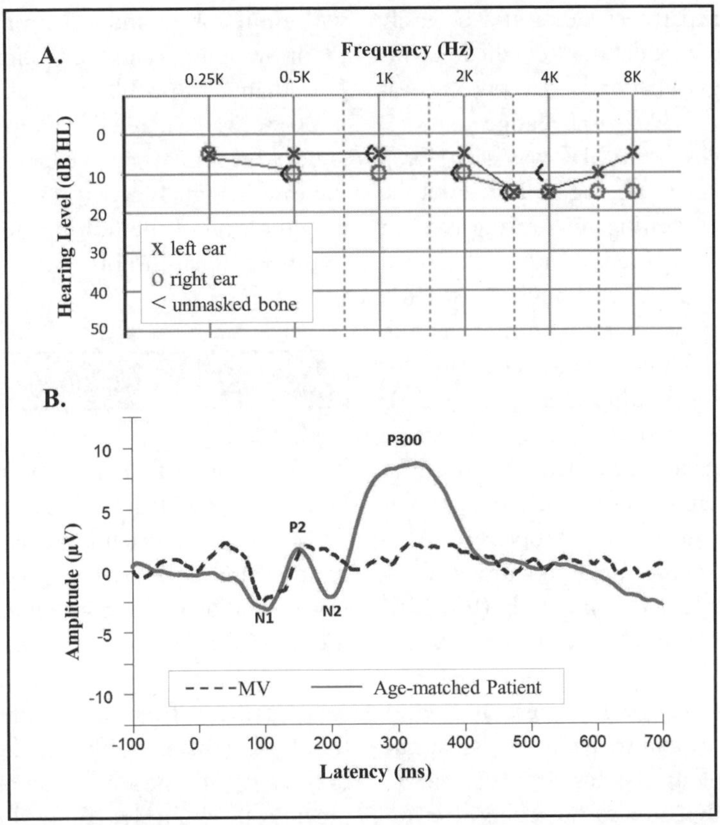

Figure 9–2. A. Pure tone thresholds obtained in the right and left ears of patient MV. **B.** Responses to the rare stimulus during a P300 oddball paradigm during which 80% of trials consisted of a 500-Hz tone (frequent stimulus) and 20% of trials consisted of a 1000-Hz tone (rare stimulus). The neural response of patient MV is shown in comparison to an age- and hearing-matched control participant.

well as his confusion of various word sounds. To remediate these issues, his audiologist prescribed a two-pronged approach including the use of low-amplification hearing aids with an FM streaming system, as well as counseling on environmental modifications and communication strategies to improve signal-to-noise ratios during listening. The low-amplification hearing aids, including directional microphones and the FM system would, in practice, increase the intensity of speech without commensurate increases in the intensity of competing sounds. This effect would putatively assist in difficult listening conditions. Communication strategies discussed included counseling on the types of environments that were most conducive to listening, making his communication partners aware of his hearing issues and asking them to get his attention before speaking to him, conversing in well-lit areas where his communication partner's face could be easily seen, and recommendations to schedule important meetings earlier in the day when he was well rested and less likely to be fatigued.

Eight weeks later, MV was seen for a follow-up visit. Data logging indicated that he was consistently wearing his hearing aids an average of 8 hours per day and he described them to be "perfect." Although it is often assumed that patients with normal hearing thresholds and PTSD are poor candidates for low-amplification hearing aids due to their increased startle response, MV stated that he felt his hearing aids provided him a better sense of his surroundings which reduced his overall level of anxiety and propensity to be startled. His responses on International Outcome Inventory for Hearing Aids (IOI-HA) and the Client Oriented Scale of Improvement (COSI) revealed significant improvements in his function in background noise and while on the telephone, and he reported less fatigue at the end of the day because it was "easier to hear." His family had also noted positive improvements, not only in his communication abilities but also regarding reduced frustration. Two years later, MV is still wearing his hearing aids regularly.

MV's perceived benefit from hearing aids likely stems from multiple factors. First, the noise reduction algorithms and directional microphones employed by the hearing as well as use of the FM system probably resulted in a more favorable signal-to-noise ratio, thus reducing MV's listening effort. Second, the nonlinear fast-acting compression characteristics of modern hearing aids, which favor amplification of low-level signals compared to higher level signals, have been shown to facilitate discrimination of speech signals from noise background and to improve listeners' ability to "listen in the dips" of fluctuating background noise (Gatehouse et al., 2003). Lastly, multiple lines of evidence suggest that higher signal levels and lower levels of background noise are associated with more robust and synchronous neural firing in response to auditory stimuli (Dallos & Cheatham, 1976; Billings et al., 2009). Thus, it is conceivable that MV's temporal processing issues were somewhat ameliorated by the slight increase in signal levels provided by the mild amplification of the hearing aid as well as the improved signal-to-noise ratio.

Summary

TBI, regardless of etiology, can result in a host of chronic neurological disorders affecting audition as well as cognition, emotion, motor control, and other sensory systems. For this reason, audiologists are important members of the multidisciplinary team needed for the appropriate assessment and rehabilitation of affected patients. Even when auditory pure tone thresholds remain within the clinically normal range, a significant proportion of patients with previous head injuries report chronic auditory problems. Common complaints include tinnitus, difficulty understanding speech in competing background noise and on the telephone, difficulty with rapid speech, problems attending to and recalling speech, and hypersensitivity to noise and other types of sound. The specific auditory processing deficits that underlie such concerns can vary considerably across patients even when the cause and severity of TBI is similar. For this reason, patients with auditory complaints should receive thorough examinations of auditory processing abilities in addition to careful probing of the specific situations and instances that are problematic. Rehabilitation efforts should focus on improving specific deficits and may include auditory training programs (when appropriate) and provision of assistive listening devices such as FM systems and/or low-amplification hearing aids. Communication counselling should be provided to all patients both to help them better understand the nature of their hearing deficits, and to empower them to actively participate in improving their communication abilities.

References

AAA. (2010). Taskforce to establish practice guidelines for the diagnosis, treatment and management of children and adults with central auditory processing disorder. Retrieved Aug, 2010, from http://www.audiology.org/resources/documentlibrary/Pages/CentralAuditoryProcessingDisorder.aspx.

Alves, W. M. (1992). Natural history of postconcussive signs and symptoms. *Physical Medicine and Rehabilitation, 6*, 21–32.

Alwis, D. S., Yan, E. B., Morganti-Kossmann, M. C., & Rajan, R. (2012). Sensory cortex underpinnings of traumatic brain injury deficits. *PLoS One, 7*(12), e52169.

Alwis, D. S., Johnstone, V., Yan, E., & Rajan, R. (2013). Diffuse traumatic brain injury and the sensory brain. *Clinical and Experimental Pharmacology and Physiology, 40*(7), 473–483.

American Speech-Language-Hearing Association. (2005). (Central) Auditory Processing Disorders [Technical Report]. Working Group on Auditory Processing Disorders. Rockville, MD: ASHA.

Bamiou, D. E., Campbell, N., & Sirimanna, T. (2006). Management of auditory processing disorders. *Audiological Medicine, 4*(1), 46–56.

Belanger, H. G., Vanderploeg, R. D., Curtiss, G., & Warden, D. L. (2007). Recent neuroimaging techniques in mild traumatic brain injury, *Journal of Neuropsychiatry and Clinical Neurosciences, 19*(1), 5–20.

Bellis, T. J. (2002). Developing deficit-specific intervention plans for individuals with auditory processing disorders. *Seminars in Hearing, 23*(4), 287–296.

Bergemalm, P. O., & Borg, E. (2005). Peripheral and central audiological sequelae of closed head injury: function, activity, participation and quality of life. *Audiological Medicine, 3*(3), 185–198.

Bergemalm, P. O., & Lyxell, B. (2005). Appearances are deceptive—long-term cognitive and central auditory sequelae from closed head injury. *International Journal of Audiology, 44*(1), 39–49.

Billings, C. J., Tremblay, K. L., Stecker, G. C., & Tolin, W. M. (2009). Human evoked cortical activity to signal-to-noise ratio and absolute signal level. *Hearing Research, 254*(1), 15–24.

Binder, L. M., Rohling, M. L., & Larrabee, G. J. (1997). A review of mild head trauma. Part I: Meta-analytic review of neuropsychological studies. *Journal of Clinical and Experimental Neuropsychology,19*, 421–431.

Bressler, S., Goldberg, H., & Shinn-Cunningham, B. (2016). Sensory coding and cognitive processing of sound in Veterans with blast exposure. *Hearing Research*. In press.

Buritica, E., Villamil, L., Guzman, F., et al. (2009). Changes in calcium-binding protein expression in human cortical contusion tissue. *Journal of Neurotrauma, 26*(12), 2145–2155.

Capizzano, A. A., Jorge, R. E., & Robinson, R. G. (2010). Limbic metabolic abnormalities in remote traumatic brain injury and correlation with psychiatric morbidity and social functioning. *The Journal of Neuropsychiatry and Clinical Neurosciences, 22*(4), 370–377.

Carron, S. F., Alwis, D. S., & Rajan, R. (2016). Traumatic brain injury and neuronal functionality changes in sensory cortex. *Frontiers in Systems Neuroscience, 10*, 47.

Centers for Disease Control and Prevention. (2015). *Report to Congress on Traumatic Brain Injury in the United States: Epidemiology and Rehabilitation*. National Center for Injury Prevention and Control; Division of Unintentional Injury Prevention. Atlanta, GA.

Chafi, M. S., Karami, G., & Ziejewski, M. (2010). Biomechanical assessment of brain dynamic responses due to blast pressure waves. *Annals of Biomedical Engineering, 38*(2), 490–504.

Chermak, G. D., & Musiek, F. E. (2002). Auditory training: principles and approaches for remediating and managing auditory processing disorders. *Seminars in Hearing, 23*(04), 297–308.

Cicerone, K. D., & Kalmar, K. (1995). Persistent postconcussion syndrome: The structure of subjective complaints after mTBI. *Journal of Head Trauma Rehabilitation, 10*, 1–17.

Dallos, P., & Cheatham, M. A. (1976). Compound action potential (AP) tuning curves. *The Journal of the Acoustical Society of America, 59*(3), 591–597.

Darley, D. S., & Kellman, R. M. (2010). Otologic considerations of blast injury. *Disaster medicine and public health preparedness, 4*(02), 145–152.

Davenport, N. D., Lim, K. O., Armstrong, M. T. et al. (2012). Diffuse and spatially variable white matter disruptions are associated with blast-related mild traumatic brain injury. *Neuroimage, 59*(3), 2017–2024.

Department of Veterans Affairs. (2007). *Screening and evaluation of possible traumatic brain injury in Operation Enduring Freedom (OEF) and Operation Iraqi Freedom (OIF) Veterans*. Washington (DC): Department of Veterans Affairs, Veterans Health Administration.

Dikmen, S., Machamer, J., Fann, J. R., & Temkin, N. R. (2010). Rates of symptom reporting following traumatic brain injury. *Journal of the International Neuropsychological Society, 16*(3), 401–411.

Defense and Veterans Brain Injury Center. (2016). *DoD TBI Worldwide Numbers since 2000*. Retrieved from http://dvbic.dcoe.mil/dod-worldwide-numbers-tbi.

Downie, A. L., Jakobson, L. S., Frisk, V., & Ushycky, I. (2002). Auditory temporal processing deficits in children with periventricular brain injury. *Brain and Language, 80*(2), 208–225.

Draper, K., & Ponsford, J. (2008). Cognitive functioning ten years following traumatic brain injury and rehabilitation. *Neuropsychology, 22*(5), 618.

Duncan, C. C., Summers, A. C., Perla, E. J., Coburn, K. L., & Mirsky, A. F. (2011). Evaluation of traumatic brain injury: Brain potentials in diagnosis, function, and prognosis. *International Journal of Psychophysiology, 82*(1), 24–40.

Dundon, N. M., Dockree, S. P., Buckley, V., Merriman, N., Carton, M., Clarke, S., . . . Dockree, P. M. (2015). Impaired auditory selective attention ameliorated by cognitive training with graded exposure to noise in patients with traumatic brain injury. *Neuropsychologia, 75*, 74–87.

Ellemeier, W., Eigenstetter, M., Zimmer, K. (2001). Psychoacoustic correlates of individual noise sensitivity, *Journal of the Acoustical Society of America, 109*(4), 1461–1473.

Elting, J. W., Maurits, N., van Weerden, T., Spikman, J., De Keyser, J., & van der Naalt, J. (2008). P300 analysis techniques in cognitive impairment after brain injury: Comparison with neuropsychological and imaging data. *Brain Injury, 22*(11), 870–881.

Fausti, S. A., Wilmington, D. J., Gallun, F. J., Myers, P. J., & Henry, J. A. (2009). Auditory and vestibular dysfunction associated with blast-related traumatic brain injury. *Journal of Rehabilitation Research and Development 46*(6), 797–810.

Fischer, B. L., Parsons, M., Durgerian, S. et al. (2014). Neural activation during response inhibition differentiates blast from mechanical causes of mild to moderate traumatic brain injury. *Journal of Neurotrauma, 31*(2), 169–179.

Folmer, R. L., Billings, C. J., Diedesch-Rouse, A. C. et al. (2011). Electrophysiological assessments of cognition and sensory processing in TBI: Applications for diagnosis, prognosis and rehabilitation. *International Journal of Psychophysics, 82*(1), 4–15.

Gallinat, J., Bottlender, R., Juckel, G., Munke-Puchner, A., Stotz, G., Kuss, H. J., . . . Hegerl, U. (2000). The loudness dependency of the auditory evoked N1/P2-component as a predictor of the acute SSRI response in depression. *Psychopharmacology, 148*(4), 404–411.

Gallun, F., Lewis, M., Folmer, R., Hutter, M., Papesh, M., Belding, H., and Leek, M. (2016). Chronic effects of exposure to high-intensity blasts: Results of tests of central auditory processing. *Journal of Rehabilitation Research and Development, 53*(6), 705–720.

Gallun, F. J., Diedesch, A. M., Kubli, L., Walden, T., Folmer, R. L., Lewis, M. S., . . . Leek, M. R. (2012a). Performance on tests of central auditory processing by individuals exposed to high-intensity blasts. *Journal of Rehabilitation Research and Development, 49*(7), 1005–1024.

Gallun, F. J., Lewis, M. S., Folmer, R. L., Diedesch, A. C., Kubli, L. R., McDermott, D. J., . . . Leek, M. R. (2012b). Implications of blast exposure for central auditory function: a review. *Journal of*

Rehabilitation Research and Development, 49(7), 1059–1074.

Glover, E. M., Phifer, J. E., Crain, D. F., Norrholm, S. D., Davis, M., Bradley, B., . . . & Jovanovic, T. (2011). Tools for translational neuroscience: PTSD is associated with heightened fear responses using acoustic startle but not skin conductance measures. *Depression and Anxiety, 28*(12), 1058–1066.

Godbolt, A. K., Cancelliere, C., Hincapié, C. A., Marras, C., Boyle, E., Kristman, V. L., . . . & Cassidy, J. D. (2014). Systematic review of the risk of dementia and chronic cognitive impairment after mild traumatic brain injury: Results of the International Collaboration on Mild Traumatic Brain Injury Prognosis. *Archives of Physical Medicine and Rehabilitation, 95*(3), S245–S256.

Gopal, K. V., Bishop, C. E., & Carney, L. (2004). Auditory measures in clinically depressed individuals. II. Auditory evoked potentials and behavioral speech tests. *International Journal of Audiology, 43*(9), 499–505.

Gouvier, W. D., Cubic, B., Jones, G., Brantley, P., & Cutlip, Q. (1992). Postconcussion symptoms and daily stress in normal and head-injured college populations. *Archives of Clinical Neuropsychology, 7*, 193–211.

Greer, J. E., Hånell, A., McGinn, M. J., & Povlishock, J. T. (2013). Mild traumatic brain injury in the mouse induces axotomy primarily within the axon initial segment. *Acta Neuropathologica, 126*(1), 59–74.

Halbauer, J. D., Ashford, J. W., Zeitzer, J. M., et al. (2009). Neuropsychiatric diagnosis and management of chronic sequelae of war-related mild to moderate traumatic brain injury. *Journal of Rehabilitation Research and Development, 46*(6), 757–796.

Hoge, C. W., McGurk, D., Thomas, J. L., et al. (2008). Mild traumatic brain injury in U.S. soldiers returning from Iraq. *New England Journal of Medicine, 358*(5), 453–463.

Hoover, E., Souza, P., & Gallun, F. (2015). Competing views on abnormal auditory results after mild traumatic brain injury. *SIG 6, Perspectives on Hearing and Hearing Disorders: Research and Diagnostics, 19*(1), 12–21.

Hunt, R. F., Scheff, S. W., & Smith, B. N. (2011). Synaptic reorganization of inhibitory hilar interneuron circuitry after traumatic brain injury in mice. *Journal of Neuroscience, 31*(18), 6880–6890.

Jabbari, B., Mueller, H. G., & Howard, D. K. (1987). Auditory brainstem response findings in the late phase of head injury. *Seminars in Hearing, 8*(3), 261–265.

Jantzen, K. J. (2010). Functional magnetic resonance imaging of mild traumatic brain injury. *Journal of Head Trauma Rehabilitation, 25*(4), 256–266.

Jin, X., Huguenard, J. R., & Prince, D. A. (2011). Reorganization of inhibitory synaptic circuits in rodent chronically injured epileptogenic neocortex. *Cerebral Cortex, 21*(5), 1094–1104.

Johnson, B., Zhang, K., Gay, M., Horovitz, S., Hallett, M., Sebastianelli, W., & Slobounov, S. (2012). Alteration of brain default network in subacute phase of injury in concussed individuals: Resting-state fMRI study. *Neuroimage, 59*(1), 511–518.

Johnston, K. N., John, A. B., Kreisman, N. V., Hall III, J. W., Crandell, C. C., Johnston, K. N., . . . & Crandell, C. C. (2009). Multiple benefits of personal FM system use by children with auditory processing disorder (APD). *International Journal of Audiology, 48*(6), 371–383.

Jury, M. A., & Flynn, M. C. (2001). Auditory and vestibular sequelae to traumatic brain injury: A pilot study. *New Zealand Medical Journal, 114*(1134), 286–288.

Kaipio, M. L., Cheour, M., Öhman, J., Salonen, O., & Näätänen, R. (2013). Mismatch negativity abnormality in traumatic brain injury without macroscopic lesions on conventional MRI. *Neuroreport, 24*(8), 440–444.

Kapoor, N., & Ciuffreda, K. J. (2002). Vision disturbances following traumatic brain injury. *Current Treatment Options in Neurology, 4*(4), 271–280.

Katz, J., & Smith, P. S. (1991). The staggered spondaic word test. *Annals of the New York Academy of Sciences, 620*(1), 233–251.

Keith, R. W. (1995). Development and standardization of SCAN-A: test of auditory processing disorders in adolescents and adults. *Journal of the American Academy of Audiology, 6*, 286–286.

Killion, M. C., Niquette, P. A., Gudmundsen, G. I., Revit, L. J., & Banerjee, S. (2004). Development of a quick speech-in-noise test for measuring signal-to-noise ratio loss in normal-hearing and hearing-impaired listeners. *The Journal of the Acoustical Society of America*, *116*(4), 2395–2405.

Koliatsos, V. E., Cernak, I., Xu, L. et al. (2011). A mouse model of blast injury to brain: initial pathological, neuropathological, and behavioral characterization. *Journal of Neuropathology and Experimental Neurology*, *70*(5), 399–416.

Larson, M. J., Kaufman, D. A., Schmalfuss, I. M., & Perlstein, W. M. (2007). Performance monitoring, error processing, and evaluative control following severe TBI. *Journal of the International Neuropsychological Society*, *13*(06), 961–971.

Lew, H. L., Lee, E. H., Pan, S. S., & Date, E. S. (2004). Electrophysiologic abnormalities of auditory and visual information processing in patients with traumatic brain injury. *American Journal of Physical Medicine & Rehabilitation*, *83*(6), 428–433.

Lew, H. L., Jerger, J. F., Guillory, S. B., & Henry, J. A. (2007) Auditory dysfunction in traumatic brain injury. *Journal of Rehabilitation Research and Development*, *44*(7), 921–928.

Little, D. M., Kraus, M. F., Joseph, J. et al. (2010). Thalamic integrity underlies executive dysfunction in traumatic brain injury. *Neurology*, *74*(7), 558–564.

McAllister, T. W., Saykin, A. J., Flashman, L. A. et al. (1999). Brain activation during working memory 1 month after mild traumatic brain injury: A functional MRI study. *Neurology*, *53*(6), 1300–1300.

McAllister, T. W., and Arciniegas, D. (2002). Evaluation and treatment of postconcussive symptoms. *NeuroRehabilitation*, *17*(4), 265–283.

Mesulam, M. M. (2002). The human frontal lobes: Transcending the default mode through contingent encoding. *Principles of Frontal Lobe Function*, 8–30.

Morgan, C. A., Grillon, C., Southwick, S. M., Davis, M., & Charney, D. S. (1996). Exaggerated acoustic startle reflex in Gulf War Veterans with posttraumatic stress disorder. *American Journal of Psychiatry*, *153*(1), 64–68.

Mueller, H. G. (1987). The staggered spondaic word test: Practical use. *Seminars in Hearing*, 8(3), 267–277.

Munjal, S. K., Panda, N. K., & Pathak, A. (2010). Relationship between severity of traumatic brain injury (TBI) and extent of auditory dysfunction. *Brain Injury*, *24*(3), 525–532.

Murphy, C. F. B., Fillippini, R., Palma, D., Zalcman, T. E., Lima, J. P., & Schochat, E. (2011). Auditory training and cognitive functioning in adult with traumatic brain injury. *Clinics*, *66*(4), 713–715.

Musiek, F. E. (1983). Assessment of central auditory dysfunction: The dichotic digit test revisited. *Ear and Hearing*, *4*(2), 79–83.

Musiek, F. E., & Pinheiro, M. L. (1987). Frequency patterns in cochlear, brainstem, and cerebral lesions. *Audiology*, *26*(2), 79–88.

Musiek, F. E., Baran, J. A., & Pinheiro, M. L. (1990). Duration pattern recognition in normal subjects and patients with cerebral and cochlear lesions. *Audiology*, *29*(6), 304–313.

Musiek, F. E. (1994). Frequency (pitch) and duration pattern tests. *Journal of the American Academy of Audiology*, *5*, 265–265.

Musiek, F. E., Baran, J. A., & Shinn, J. (2004). Assessment and remediation of an auditory processing disorder associated with head trauma. *Journal of the American Academy of Audiology*, *15*(2), 117–132.

Musiek, F. E., Shinn, J. B., Jirsa, R., et al. (2005). GIN (Gaps-In-Noise) test performance in subjects with confirmed central auditory nervous system involvement. *Ear and Hearing*, *26*(6), 608–618.

Nampiaparampil, D. E. (2008). Prevalence of chronic pain after traumatic brain injury: A systematic review. *Journal of the American Medical Association*, *300*(6), 711–719.

Niogi, S. N., & Mukherjee, P. (2010). Diffusion tensor imaging of mild traumatic brain injury. *Journal of Head Trauma Rehabilitation*, *25*(4), 241–255.

Nölle, C., Todt, I., Seidl, R., & Ernst, A. (2004). Pathophysiological changes of the central auditory pathway after blunt trauma of the head. *Journal of Neurotrauma*, *21*(3), 251–258.

Oleksiak, M., St Andre, J. R., Caughlan, C. M., & Steiner, M. (2012). Audiological issues and hearing loss among Veterans with mild traumatic brain injury. *Journal of Rehabilitation Research and Development, 49*(7), 995–1004.

Palacios, E. M., Sala-Llonch, R., Junque, C., et al. (2013). Long-term declarative memory deficits in diffuse TBI: correlations with cortical thickness, white matter integrity and hippocampal volume. *Cortex, 49*(3), 646–657.

Papesh, M., & Gallun, F. (2015). Auditory impacts of blast exposure. *Hearing Health & Technology Matters, Pathways.*

Pavlov, I., Huusko, N., Drexel, M. et al. (2011). Progressive loss of phasic, but not tonic, GABA A receptor-mediated inhibition in dentate granule cells in a model of post-traumatic epilepsy in rats. *Neuroscience, 194*, 208–219.

Petrie, E. C., Cross, D. J., Yarnykh, V. L. et al. (2014). Neuroimaging, behavioral, and psychological sequelae of repetitive combined blast/impact mild traumatic brain injury in Iraq and Afghanistan war Veterans. *Journal of Neurotrauma, 31*(5), 425–436.

Pichora-Fuller, M. K. (2003). Cognitive aging and auditory information processing. *International Journal of Audiology, 42*, 2S26–2S32.

Potts, M. B., Adwanikar, H., & Noble-Haeusslein, L. J. (2009). Models of traumatic cerebellar injury. *The Cerebellum, 8*(3), 211–221.

Punch, J., Joseph, A., & Rakerd, B. (2004). Most comfortable and uncomfortable loudness levels: six decades of research. *American Journal of Audiology*, 13, 144–157.

Rapp, P. E., Keyser, D. O., Albano, A., Hernandez, R., Gibson, D. B., Zambon, R. A., . . . & Nichols, A. S. (2015). Traumatic brain injury detection using electrophysiological methods. *Frontiers in Human Neuroscience, 9*, 11.

Reid, M. W., Miller, K. J., Lange, R. T. et al. (2014). A multisite study of the relationships between blast exposures and symptom reporting in a post-deployment active duty military population with mild traumatic brain injury. *Journal of Neurotrauma, 31*(23), 1899–1906.

Ross-Swain, D. (2007). The effects of auditory stimulation on auditory processing disorder: A summary of the findings. *The International Journal of Listening, 21*(2), 140–155.

Ryan, L. M., & Warden, D. L. (2003). Post concussion syndrome. *International Review of Psychiatry, 15*(4), 310–316.

Saunders, G. H., Frederick, M. T., Chisolm, T. H., Silverman, S., Arnold, M., & Myers, P. (2014). Use of a frequency-modulated system for Veterans with blast exposure, perceived hearing problems, and normal hearing sensitivity. *Seminars in Hearing, 35*(03), 227–238.

Saunders, G. H., Frederick, M. T., Arnold, M., et al. (2015). Auditory difficulties in blast-exposed Veterans with clinically normal hearing. *Journal of Rehabilitation Research and Development, 52*(3), 343.

Schultz, B. A., Cifu, D. X., McNamee, S., Nichols, M., & Carne, W. (2011). Assessment and treatment of common persistent sequelae following blast induced mild traumatic brain injury. *NeuroRehabilitation, 28*(4), 309–320.

Sheldrake, J., Diehl, P. U., & Schaette, R. (2015). Audiometric characteristics of hyperacusis patients. *Frontiers in Neurology*, May 15, *6* 105.

Shively, S. B., Horkayne-Szakaly, I., Jones, R. V. et al. (2016). Characterisation of interface astroglial scarring in the human brain after blast exposure: A post-mortem case series. *The Lancet Neurology.*

Silver, J. M., McAllister, T. W., and Yudofsky, S. C. (2011). *Textbook of Traumatic Brain Injury* (2nd ed.). Washington, D.C.: American Psychiatric Publishing Inc.

Silverberg, N. D., & Iverson, G. L. (2011). Etiology of the post-concussion syndrome: Physiogenesis and psychogenesis revisited. *NeuroRehabilitation, 29*(4), 317–329.

Song, H., Cui, J., Simonyi, A. et al. (2016). Linking blast physics to biological outcomes in mild traumatic brain injury: narrative review and preliminary report of an open-field blast model. *Behavioural Brain Research.*

Spanos, G. K., Wilde, E. A., Bigler, E. D., Cleavinger, H. B., Fearing, M. A., Levin, H. S., . . . Hunter, J. V. (2007). Cerebellar atrophy after moderate-to-severe pediatric traumatic brain injury. *American Journal of Neuroradiology, 28*(3), 537–542.

Stach, B. A., Loiselle, L. H., & Jerger, J. F. (1991). Special hearing aid considerations in elderly patients with auditory processing disorders. *Ear and Hearing, 12*(6), 131S–138S.

Sun, H. Y., Li, Q., Chen, X. P., & Tao, L. Y. (2015). Mismatch negativity, social cognition, and functional outcomes in patients after traumatic brain injury. *Neural Regeneration Research, 10*(4), 618.

Taber, K., Warden, D., & Hurley, R. (2006). Blast-related traumatic brain injury: what is known? *Journal of Neuropsychiatry and Clinical Neurosciences, 18*(2), 141–145.

Taber, K. H., Hurley, R. A., Haswell, C. C. et al. (2015). White matter compromise in Veterans exposed to primary blast forces. *Journal of Head Trauma Rehabilitation, 30*(1), E15.

Theodoroff, S. M., Lewis, M. S., Folmer, R. L., Henry, J. A., & Carlson, K. F. (2015). Hearing impairment and tinnitus: prevalence, risk factors, and outcomes in U.S. Service Members and Veterans deployed to the Iraq and Afghanistan wars. *Epidemiologic Reviews, 37*(1), 71–85.

Tompkins, P., Tesiram, Y., Lerner, M. et al. (2013). Brain injury: Neuro-inflammation, cognitive deficit, and magnetic resonance imaging in a model of blast induced traumatic brain injury. *Journal of Neurotrauma, 30*(22), 1888–1897.

Turgeon, C., Champoux, F., Lepore, F., Leclerc, S., & Ellemberg, D. (2011). Auditory processing after sport-related concussions. *Ear and Hearing, 32*(5), 667–670.

Tyler, R. S., Pienkowsi, M., Roncancio, E. R., Jun, H. J., Brozoski, T., Dauman, N., . . . Moore, B. C. J. (2014). A review of hyperacusis and future directions: Part I. Definitions and Manifestations. *American Journal of Audiology, 23*(4), 402–419.

Van Toor, T., Neijenhuis, K., Snik, A., & Blokhorst, M. (2006). Evaluation of auditory processing disorders after whiplash injury. *Audiological Medicine, 4*(4), 191–201.

Vandoolaeghe, E., van Hunsel, F., Nuyten, D., & Maes, M. (1998). Auditory event related potentials in major depression: Prolonged P300 latency and increased P200 amplitude. *Journal of Affective Disorders, 48*(2), 105–113.

Verfaellie, M., Lafleche, G., Spiro, A., Tun, C., & Bousquet, K. (2013). Chronic postconcussion symptoms and functional outcomes in OEF/OIF Veterans with self-report of blast exposure. *Journal of the International Neuropsychological Society, 19*(01), 1–10.

Verma, A., Anand, V., & Verma, N. P. (2007). Sleep disorders in chronic traumatic brain injury. *Journal of Clinical Sleep Medicine, 3*(4), 357–362.

von Steinbüchel, N., Wittmann, M., Strasburger, H., & Szelag, E. (1999). Auditory temporal-order judgement is impaired in patients with cortical lesions in posterior regions of the left hemisphere. *Neuroscience Letters, 264*(1), 168–171.

Wilson, R. H., & Weakley, D. G. (2005). The 500 Hz masking-level difference and word recognition in multitalker babble for 40- to 89-year-old listeners with symmetrical sensorineural hearing loss. *Journal of the American Academy of Audiology, 16*(6), 367–382.

Wilson, R. H., Carnell, C. S., & Cleghorn, A. L. (2007). The Words-in-Noise (WIN) test with multitalker babble and speech-spectrum noise maskers. *Journal of the American Academy of Audiology, 18*(6), 522–529.

Wolf, J. A., & Koch, P. F. (2016). Disruption of network synchrony and cognitive dysfunction after traumatic brain injury. *Frontiers in Systems Neuroscience, 10.*

World Health Organisation. (1992). *International Statistical Classification of Diseases and Related Health Problems*, 10th Revision (ICD-10). Geneva: WHO.

Wright, D. K., Trezise, J., Kamnaksh, A. et al. (2016). Behavioral, blood, and magnetic resonance imaging biomarkers of experimental mild traumatic brain injury. *Scientific Reports, 6.*

Yi, J. H., & Hazell, A. S. (2006). Excitotoxic mechanisms and the role of astrocytic glutamate transporters in traumatic brain injury. *Neurochemistry International, 48*(5), 394–403.

Zaugg, T. L., Thielman, E. J., Griest, S., & Henry, J. A. (2016). Subjective reports of trouble tolerating sound in daily life versus loudness discomfort levels. *American Journal of Audiology, 25*(4), 359–363.

Zhu, Y., Li, Z., Bai, L., Tao, Y., Sun, C., Li, M., . . . Zhang, M. (2014). Loss of microstructural integrity in the limbic-subcortical networks for acute symptomatic traumatic brain injury. *BioMedical Research International.*

10

Psychological Aspects and Management of Hyperacusis

Gerhard Andersson

Background

In spite of the prevalence of decreased sound tolerance in its more severe form—called hyperacusis—most research on the psychological mechanisms behind sound tolerance has been focused on noise sensitivity and the psychological consequences of noise in the general population (Baguley & Andersson, 2007; Stansfeld, 1992). It is an established fact that there is a substantial overlap between decreased sound tolerance and a range of medical and psychological conditions (Tyler et al., 2014), for example, migraine, post-traumatic stress disorder, and tinnitus, just to mention a few examples (Baguley & Andersson, 2007) (for further information see Chapters 1, 7, and 11 in this book). While audiologists and associated professionals are well acquainted with the phenomena of loudness recruitment and its role when fitting hearing aids, there is by no means a clear-cut difference between how patients with and without significant hearing loss experience sounds in terms of decreased sound tolerance. Symptoms of hyperacusis can be observed among persons across all ranges of hearing sensitivity and not only in the group with no marked hearing loss (a common definition in hyperacusis research). This chapter will focus on three aspects of decreased sound tolerance/hyperacusis. First, we will examine some of the associated non-auditory problems that might influence a patient's experience with sound. Second, we will propose potential psychological mechanisms that might be involved in disorders of sound tolerance, as would be consistent with a biopsychosocial understanding of the problem. Finally, a cognitive-behavioral treatment (CBT) approach will be described and in addition the initial evidence in favor of exposure-based CBT for hyperacusis. The chapter will conclude with a case and a discussion about future developments.

Associated Problems

There are a range of auditory conditions/disorders associated with decreased sound tolerance (see Chapters 2, 3, 7, and 9 in this book). It is important to note that patients may not easily distinguish between different categories of auditory problems that for them are perceived as a whole. Tinnitus is an example. Patients with decreased sound tolerance and tinnitus can experience a strong link between sound exposure and reactive tinnitus; this sensitivity can be linked to both annoyance and expectations of tinnitus becoming more disturbing during or following unwanted sounds. Additionally, hearing loss may cause a noisy social situation to be experienced as uncomfortable when it is hard to follow conversations or when loudness distresses the patient. In this example, there may be at least three reasons for a patient to avoid a situation, with only one being directly related to noise sensitivity: first, the sounds in the setting may be experienced as too loud, second, exposure to those sounds may be associated with tinnitus exacerbation (at least temporarily), and third, the situation is difficult from a listening and communicative perspective as the patient risks missing out on conversations, feeling embarrassed, or being overwhelmed by the ambient noise level. The point made here is that different problems are not easily distinguished, and patients can, for example, infer that "tinnitus is making it hard to hear" or that "sounds I cannot bear make it hard for me to communicate."

The second category of associated problems is in the psychiatric domain. Again, this is mentioned elsewhere (Tyler et al., 2014) and in this book (Chapters 9, 13, and 15), but different categories of psychiatric problems have been linked with decreased sound tolerance (e.g., mood and anxiety disorders). In two studies, Jüris and co-workers (2013 a,b) investigated links between hyperacusis and psychiatric problems. Psychiatric morbidity and personality traits were focused in one study, along with different sociodemographic and clinical characteristics (Jüris, Larsen, Andersson, & Ekselius, 2013). The study included 62 adult patients (mean age 40 years), who were interviewed using the mini-international neuropsychiatric interview (Sheehan et al., 1998), and the Swedish Universities Scales of Personality (Gustavsson et al., 2000). Results showed that as many as 56% of the patients had at least one psychiatric disorder, and 47% had an anxiety disorder. In addition, personality traits related to neuroticism were overrepresented relative to the general population. Using the same participants in another report, significant correlations between loudness discomfort levels (LDL) and symptoms of anxiety and depression were observed (Jüris, Ekselius, Andersson, & Larsen, 2013). In another study (Blaesing & Kroener-Herwig, 2012), 56 tinnitus patients with/without hyperacusis and 30 healthy controls were compared. Results showed that participants with hyperacusis tolerated significantly shorter exposure to a pure tone than non-hyperacusic subjects. Self-reported avoidance behaviors were significantly correlated with distress attributed to hyperacusis (r = 0.81), and with anxiety ratings. Other studies confirmed the role of personality in hyperacusis (Villaume & Hasson, 2017).

The biological underpinnings of the link between hyperacusis and anxiety/depression has been discussed for a long time (Marriage & Barnes, 1995), and it is a common finding that persons with hyperacusis also suffer from self-reported psychiatric problems such as post-traumatic stress disorder, chronic fatigue syndrome, generalized anxiety disorder, and depression (Paulin, Andersson, & Nordin, 2016).

We alluded to the social aspects of hyperacusis when referring to different reasons to avoid noisy situations. To the best of our knowledge, although many self-help networks and resources are available, there is a lack of literature addressing the shared aspects of hyperacusis, for example, occupationally, in educational settings, in family life, and not the least what many people regard as a favorite activity for relaxation—listening to music. Consequences of disordered sound tolerance at work are often reported by patients in the clinic and mentioned in the literature (Pienkowski et al., 2014), although this topic requires greater attention as well. A valuable early attempt was a qualitative study (Trulsson, Johansson, Jansson, Wiberg, & Hallberg, 2003), in which 21 patients with persisting hypersensitivity to sounds after an acute head trauma were interviewed. The authors reported that the patients became psychosocially vulnerable and suffered from a variety of symptoms including hypersensitivity to sounds, difficulties with concentrating and remembering, increased anxiety, and sensitivity to stress.

In sum, sound tolerance problems may include several associated issues with the clinical observation that hyperacusis, when severe, rarely appears as a single symptom/problem, and that it can have severe consequences in daily life.

Psychological Mechanisms

In this section psychological mechanisms will be proposed, bearing in mind that there are few studies on the psychology of hyperacusis. Avoidance is an inherent feature of hyperacusis and it is important to consider a patient's avoidance strategies to understand and manage their sound tolerance problem. Classical conditioning is likely to occur as certain sounds and situations become associated with, or "conditioned" to, negative reactions (both bodily and cognitively). Patients in clinic often report experiences of negative conditioning, for example, when they feel compelled to leave a situation because of sounds and subsequently report that they avoid that situation (for a similar discussion regarding tinnitus, see Andersson, Hesser, & McKenna, 2016). Briefly, in classical conditioning a neutral stimulus becomes paired with a negative reaction, for example, the sound of rain falling; an individual may not give the sound much thought until they survive a hurricane. The formerly neutral stimuli (rain falling) becomes paired with the reaction even in the absence of an actual hurricane (Schwartz, Wasserman, & Robbins, 2002). To be more specific, the person may start to fear and feel uncomfortable in a situation in which he or she has experienced loud or threatening storm-related sounds even when the situation poses no danger. This notion assumes that not all sounds lead to painful reactions and that in the life of a person with hyperacusis there are some sounds that are tolerated well and others that are experienced as pain or perhaps as a unique sensation of discomfort that, while not acute pain, would be extremely annoying and upsetting. A related condition is misophonia in which the reaction is mainly that of annoyance (often when confronted with everyday sounds such as other people eating) (Jastreboff & Jastreboff, 2006; Taylor, 2017). Interestingly, from first being observed and named in the field of audiology, misophonia is now being recognized in psychiatry (see Chapter 1). The different emotions involved in hyperacusis are not well investigated but in addition to irritation and being uncomfortable there is pain and even fear (Baguley & Andersson, 2007). The conditioned fear reaction can reach the level of a panic attack with strong anxiety, shortness of breath, sweating, and ultimately avoidance and reduced quality of life.

A second psychological perspective to consider concerns cognitions, including beliefs and information processing regarding the potential danger of sounds. Fears associated with anxiety and pain may involve catastrophic cognitions. In the pain field the "fear-avoidance" model has been very influential for the understanding and management of chronic pain (Vlaeyen & Linton, 2000). Briefly, the model proposes that individuals develop problems as a result of avoidant behavior based on fear.

In the case of hyperacusis, the avoidance of everyday sounds (and perhaps more importantly certain situations) is assumed to be influenced by inappropriate catastrophic beliefs. In addition to fear and to the patient considering avoiding a situation, it is also important to consider how actual exposure to sounds is experienced during the activity and reflected upon afterward. In my clinical work, hyperacusis patients report that they endure bothersome sounds (e.g., at a dinner party) but then subsequently regret that decision and tend to focus on negative aspects of the experience rather than the fact that they managed and might even (at least partly) have enjoyed the situation as it occurred. Selective attention to threat is common in anxiety disorders and the tendency to interpret situations in a negative manner typifies persons with mood disorders. It is important to note that selective attention to threatening sounds and negative interpretations should not be viewed as necessarily false (a common misunderstanding of cognitive therapy) and that the patient just needs to be informed that the situation is not dangerous and that it is better to think positively. Instead, the patient may benefit from learning more about the ways that thoughts can influence behavior (the classical cognitive model) and that avoidance can be negative in the long run. Other reactions sometimes seen in clinic include grief and feelings of bereavement. For example, a musician who has spent a large part of his life learning music and having it as a profession understandably suffers much loss and sadness with the prospect of not being able to enjoy music or continue in his profession. The negative emotional responses also exert an influence on quality of life as many social and occupational activities are loud and/or noisy. Patients sometimes report that hyperacusis has had a major impact on their social life and that they feel very sad about the perceived need to alter activities that were once routine.

A third psychological perspective concerns individual differences and the observation that some people report they are, and always have been, more sensitive to sounds than their friends and family members. This is well known in relation to neuropsychiatric conditions such as autism spectrum disorders (Khalfa et al., 2004), but also in the general population it is known that there are differences in sound sensitivity (Stansfeld, 1992). Thus, in clinic it is fairly common that patients tell us that they always have been sensitive to sounds but that it has worsened (sometimes in association with a noise trauma or negative life event). Stress vulnerability and stress reactions may also play a role, with patients reporting that they cannot handle stressful work conditions. Stress receives some attention in the clinical literature on hyperacusis and there is ongoing work linking stress responses to hyperacusis (Chen et al., 2017).

In sum, a psychological understanding of hyperacusis needs to consider a biopsychosocial approach stressing the importance of auditory dysfunction and its impact on social and psychological function. To date the psychological understanding has concerned behavioral mechanisms and the related role of cognitions. It can also be important to consider personality, individual differences, and finally the role of stress when a patient is confronted by or anticipating sounds that provoke pain or negative emotions. The next section will outline how hyperacusis can be managed using techniques derived from cognitive behavior therapy (CBT).

Treatment Based on Exposure and Cognitive Therapy

There is no published manual on how to conduct CBT for hyperacusis but there are descriptions in a book (Baguley & Andersson, 2007) and in a controlled trial (Jüris, Andersson, Larsen, & Ekselius, 2014), from which the current description is derived. In addition, I have worked with hyperacusis patients since the early 1990s and the current outline is informed by what I have learned from my patients.

The first step in the CBT management of hyperacusis consists of a clinical interview/case formulation and the use of screening measures for hyperacusis and anxiety/depression. The hyperacusis questionnaire (Khalfa et al., 2002) and the Hospital Anxiety and Depression Scale – HADS (Zigmond & Snaith, 1983) may be used in addition to a structured interview. It is important to cover history, associated medical problems, avoidance, use of hearing protection, and the influences of the condition on the patient's quality of life. Moreover, it is important to determine the ways in which the patient and his or her significant others view the problem. In association with formal assessments it is reasonable to adopt a motivational interviewing stance from the start (Miller & Rollnick, 2010). In practice, such an interviewing approach affirms that the patient needs to make a decision to confront the problems and be willing to spend time with the ensuing exercises and interventions. A motivational stance can include discussion about the pros and cons of avoidance and hearing protection. While important information should be conveyed, such as the experimental findings that protection can increase sensitivity in normal hearing individuals (Formby, Sherlock, & Gold, 2003), the therapist should show empathy and understanding when preparing the patient for treatment. I usually introduce home registrations, or maintaining a diary, at the first meeting in case the patient decides to continue clinic contact. Patients maintaining a diary aids the clinician's understanding of how problems affect the patient's daily life. While goals are briefly discussed at the first meeting, the more substantial work starts with the first treatment session (usually one week later). In the first treatment session a CBT-model for hyperacusis is outlined, informed by the initial assessments and the daily diary. A CBT session always starts with agenda setting and the first point is to discuss the homework (in this case, diary keeping). When developing a CBT model together with the patient, cognitions and consequences associated with the patient's negative reporting and experiences are covered. More specific goals, which need to be realistic and not overly optimistic, are set (McKenna, 1987). We then provide a rationale and descriptions for applied relaxation strategies. The approach is divided into four steps (sessions) starting with tense and relax (that's 1), relax without tensing first (2), controlled breathing (3), and then using a cue-word for rapid relaxation (with or without disturbing sounds) (4). Applied relaxation may support a variety of interventions but should not be used as a "safety behavior" or as a way to avoid a feared (imagined) catastrophe (McKenna, Handscomb, Hoare, & Hall, 2014). It can, however, be used as a coping technique that supports patients as they confront feared situations. Applied relaxation is a standard component in the Swedish approach to CBT for tinnitus (Andersson & Kaldo, 2006) that is presented in treatment sessions and then further practiced in the form of homework.

Regardless of the patient's use of applied relaxation, the main component of CBT for hyperacusis is exposure. The idea of working with exposure is not new (Scott, 1993), and indeed early work by Vernon (1987), tinnitus retraining (Jastreboff & Hazell, 2004) and Formby et al.'s (2003) investigation includes exposure to sounds. We present two ways to work with exposure. First, the patient begins by not avoiding sound in general, which can be described as "basic training." This can be accomplished with the help of soft music that should not be viewed as unbearable in any way. A metaphor of exercise in general can be useful in that listening practice may be considered a form of everyday physical exercise. The main challenge for the patient will remain exposure to feared or disliked sounds (intense exposure). Such exposures should be gradual and the patient well prepared. It may be that the patient cannot remain for long in the situation; we have found it can be more effective for the patient to stay longer in a less feared/annoying situation. I usually make two plans when giving exposure as homework.

One task should be less difficult, providing the patient a chance to excel before moving onto a second more difficult exposure. Sometimes patients come up with their own exercises and surprise the clinician. While exposure also can be completed in session, CBT requires that the patient practice in real life; most of the exposure is done as homework. It is crucial to discuss the exposure outcomes in subsequent sessions. Here, methods from cognitive therapy can be useful as the patient may hold negative beliefs even when exposure has worked. Therefore, it may not be wise to promise that the sensitivity/annoyance will reduce dramatically, but rather that the patient will be able to manage situations that do not pose a danger to hearing status. While the exposures should not be to sounds that can damage hearing, sometimes the patient is uncertain regarding risks and may need assurance and guidance; a form of risk assessment. The counseling can be supplemented with text descriptions/handouts for the patient to keep.

In terms of exposure and avoidance our clinic focuses on behavioral activation, which is an approach to the treatment of depression (Martell, Dimidjian, & Herman-Dunn, 2010). If the patient avoids situations and has become passive, then a focus on activation in general (not only in terms of exposure to sounds) can be useful. Behavioral activation involves values, or things that the patient believes are important that, in the end, influence quality of life. This approach is about more than being active in general (Kanter, Busch, & Rusch, 2009). Social interactions are inherently involved in

Table 10–1. Overview of CBT for hyperacusis.

First assessment	History, motivational interviewing, questionnaires
Session 1	CBT model for treatment, setting goals, applied relaxation 1, homework
Session 2	CBT model for treatment, applied relaxation 2, exposure, homework
Session 3	Risk assessment regarding sounds, applied relaxation 3, exposure, homework
Session 4	Applied relaxation 4, exposure, homework
Session 5	Behavioral activation applied relaxation 4, exposure, homework
Session 6	Behavioral activation relapse prevention, summary, and evaluation

Source: Based on Jüris et al. (2014).

the activation phase and in exposure; however, a challenge to the treatment may center on the patient's use of hearing protection in certain environments. The patient is encouraged to stop protecting the ears from everyday sounds and plan the exposure without the help of hearing protection. However, in our experience, there are situations in which use of hearing protection is the only way for the patient to be able to attend an event, such as a concert, hence it is also important to help the patient to be flexible and not adhere in all situations to fixed rules. One example could be going to the cinema; the endeavor has value but may be daunting for patients only recently introduced to the objectives of desensitization. The last session ends with a summary and evaluation of goals. A follow-up session is scheduled approximately two months later. A potential CBT program targeting hyperacusis appears in Table 10–1.

Research on Psychological Treatment

There are to date very few studies on the treatment of hyperacusis using CBT. One early case study showed promising outcomes (Scott, 1993), and in several texts on CBT for tinnitus, hyperacusis treatment has been included as part of a tailored approach to tinnitus management (Andersson, 2002). To my knowledge there is only one controlled trial on CBT for hyperacusis (Jüris et al., 2014). In that trial 60 patients with hyperacusis were randomized to CBT or to a waiting list control group. As outcome measures we used the Loudness Discomfort Level test, the Hyperacusis Questionnaire, the HADS, the Quality of Life Inventory (Frisch, Cornell, Villanueva, & Retzlaff, 1992), and the Tampa Scale of Kinesiophobia (Miller, Kori, & Todd, 1991), adapted for hyperacusis. We found significant between-group effects in favor of the CBT group on all measures except for the HADS anxiety scale. Effects were moderate to large (mean standardized differences approximately 0.65) on the primary outcomes and small to large on the other measures. Treatment results were largely maintained after 12 months. In comparison with tinnitus (Hesser, Weise, Zetterqvist Westin, & Andersson, 2011), there was far less evidence in favor of CBT (and indeed other treatment approaches as well), but the findings from this trial were promising.

Relatedly, a recent open trial on the use of CBT for misophonia was published (Schroder, Vulink, van Loon, & Denys, 2017), with a sample of 90 patients. Results showed that 48% of the patients demonstrated a significant reduction of misophonia symptoms following the CBT protocol. Another important outcome was that the authors found that severity of misophonia and the presence of disgust were positive predictors of treatment response.

In sum, there is a need for more research on hyperacusis and related conditions, but if taken together with the fact that CBT is an evidence-based approach for anxiety and mood disorders (Hofmann, Asnaani, Vonk, Sawyer, & Fang, 2012), referral to a qualified CBT therapist should be considered for patients with hyperacusis, in particular when avoidance and anxiety play a major role.

Case Example

Ingrid worked as preschool teacher, but had a history of burnout syndrome (depression mixed with strong anxiety) and had been on sick-leave for three months when returning to work. Previously she had enjoyed her work with small children but increasingly (she was now 53 years old) experienced that she reacted strongly to loud sounds and this was even worse now that she had returned to work. She wore hearing protection on the bus to work and also with the children. This was, however, problematic as she needed to hear what the children said. She also experienced tinnitus but did not consider that as a major problem. She was referred to a psychologist via the ENT audiological physician for a first assessment session. During the interview it became clear that she had experienced some sensitivity to sounds all her life, but also that she had enjoyed singing in the church choir, which she unfortunately discontinued after her sick-leave period. The more severe symptoms of hyperacusis began before the sick-leave and she believed they could be related to a specific event that included loud sounds at work when a child accidently turned on a radio with the volume at a high level. She was not fully convinced that this episode caused the sound tolerance problem, but she was now skeptical about her work and doubted if she would be able to continue. At home all was very calm as she had a husband and two grown-up children who did not live at home. She usually rested in silence after work and the weekends tended to be very calm as well. In fact, she avoided noisy situations including parties and cinemas, and increasingly used hearing protection. The case formulation clearly showed that things were going in the wrong direction; she understood that the avoidance of sounds was not a reasonable response, but she still doubted her ability to handle her work. She and her therapist decided to try the CBT approach and the treatment started as described above. She responded positively to the relaxation and had no immediate problems introducing soft sounds in her life at home, as she liked music. The gradual exposure was more difficult at work as she could not easily control the kids at all times. In response, the therapist and she came up with alternative solutions to gradually increase the work-related exposures. As she hoped to continue her work a decision was made to only gradually remove hearing protection in that setting. When planning for sound exposures it became clear that she most of all wanted to return to the choir again. She did so gradually and brought the hearing protection with her. To her great surprise she managed to return to the choir and found that she benefitted from the predictable nature of the sounds she experienced in that setting. During therapy there was one setback when she had to leave a family gathering at which there was a band playing live music. When discussing this event, it became clear that she had not been alone doing this and that other people as well had thought it was too loud for them. When finishing the therapy, she felt she had made great progress but was also aware that she needed more time and practice to maintain the achievement and that some sensitivity would likely remain. At work she managed to get some alternative tasks and she also benefited from a change in policy when the preschool devoted work more with outdoor activities (which for her was much easier to handle).

Discussion

Hyperacusis can be a severely debilitating condition to handle for patients and hard to treat for clinicians. In addition, patients may differ in their response to sounds and environments substantially. For example, treating a child who refuses to go to school because of noise sensitivity is very different from treating a musician who wants to work but just cannot continue. Despite differences in management, relaxation and gradual exposure are important to consider for most cases, and as with other medical problems a biopsychosocial understanding facilitates and should inform assessment, treatment, and research. Our experience affirms that hyperacusis patients should be seen in the audiology clinic and preferably within the setting of multidisciplinary teams. A common objection against CBT is that there are few trained CBT clinicians with an interest in audiology. One potential complement could be to develop Internet interventions for hyperacusis, as was done for tinnitus and which can be supported by audiologists with basic knowledge about CBT (Beukes, Baguley, Allen, Manchaiah, & Andersson, in press). On the other hand, there will most likely always be patients in need of specialized face-to-face CBT for their hyperacusis, and there remains a need for more treatment research on this often neglected condition.

References

Andersson, G. (2002). Psychological aspects of tinnitus and the application of cognitive-behavioral therapy. *Clinical Psychology Review, 22*, 977–990. doi:10.1016/S0272-7358(01)00124-6.

Andersson, G., Hesser, H., & McKenna, L. (2016). Psychological mechanisms and tinnitus. In D. M. Baguley & M. Fagelson (Eds.), *Tinnitus. Clinical and research perspectives* (pp. 63–73). San Diego, CA: Plural.

Andersson, G., & Kaldo, V. (2006). Cognitive-behavioral therapy with applied relaxation. In R. S. Tyler (Ed.), *Tinnitus treatment. Clinical protocols* (pp. 96–115). New York, NY: Thieme.

Baguley, D. M., & Andersson, G. (2007). *Hyperacusis: Mechanisms, diagnosis, and therapies*. San Diego, CA: Plural.

Beukes, E. W., Baguley, D. M., Allen, P. M., Manchaiah, V., & Andersson, G. (In press). Audiologist guided Internet-based cognitive behaviour therapy for adults with tinnitus in the United Kingdom: A randomised controlled trial. *Ear and Hearing*.

Blaesing, L., & Kroener-Herwig, B. (2012). Self-reported and behavioral sound avoidance in tinnitus and hyperacusis subjects, and association with anxiety ratings. *International Journal of Audiology, 51*, 611–617. doi:10.3109/14992027.2012.664290.

Chen, Y. C., Chen, G. D., Auerbach, B. D., Manohar, S., Radziwon, K., & Salvi, R. (2017). Tinnitus and hyperacusis: Contributions of paraflocculus, reticular formation and stress. *Hearing Research, 349*, 208–222. doi:10.1016/j.heares.2017.03.005.

Formby, C., Sherlock, L. P., & Gold, S. L. (2003). Adaptive plasticity of loudness induced by chronic attenuation and enhancement of the acoustic background. *Journal of the Acoustical Society of America, 114*, 55–58.

Frisch, M. B., Cornell, J., Villanueva, M., & Retzlaff, P. J. (1992). Clinical validation of the Quality Of Life Inventory: A measure of life satisfaction for use in treatment planning and outcome assessment. *Psychological Assessment, 4*, 92–101. doi:10.1037/1040-3590.4.1.92.

Gustavsson, J. P., Bergman, H., Edman, G., Ekselius, L., von Knorring, L., & Linder, J. (2000). Swedish universities Scales of Personality (SSP): Construction, internal consistency and normative data. *Acta Psychiatrica Scandinavica, 102*, 217–225.

Hesser, H., Weise, C., Zetterqvist Westin, V., & Andersson, G. (2011). A systematic review and meta-analysis of randomized controlled trials of cognitive-behavioral therapy for tinnitus distress. *Clinical Psychology Review, 31*, 545–553. doi:10.1016/j.cpr.2010.12.006.

Hofmann, S. G., Asnaani, A., Vonk, I. J., Sawyer, A. T., & Fang, A. (2012). The efficacy of cognitive behavioral therapy: A review of meta-analyses. *Cognitive Therapy and Research, 36*, 427–440. doi:10.1007/s10608-012-9476-1.

Jastreboff, P. J., & Hazell, J. (2004). *Tinnitus retraining therapy: Implementing the neurophysiological model.* Cambridge: Cambridge University Press.

Jastreboff, P. J., & Jastreboff, M. M. (2006). Tinnitus retraining therapy: A different view on tinnitus. *ORL; Journal for Oto-Rhino-Laryngology and Its Related Specialties, 68*, 23–29.

Jüris, L., Andersson, G., Larsen, H.-C., & Ekselius, L. (2014). Cognitive behavioural therapy for hyperacusis: A randomized controlled trial. *Behaviour Research and Therapy, 54*, 30–37. doi: 10.1016/j.brat.2014.01.001.

Jüris, L., Ekselius, L., Andersson, G., & Larsen, H.-C. (2013). The hyperacusis questionnaire, loudness discomfort levels, and the hospital anxiety and depression scale. A cross-sectional study. *Hearing, Balance and Communication, 11*, 72–79.

Jüris, L., Larsen, H.-C., Andersson, G., & Ekselius, L. (2013). Psychiatric comorbidity and personality factors in patients with hyperacusis. *International Journal of Audiology, 52*, 230–235. doi:10.3109/14992027.2012.743043.

Kanter, J. W., Busch, A. M., & Rusch, L. C. (2009). *Behavioral activation*. London, U.K.: Routledge.

Khalfa, S., Bruneau, N., Roge, B., Georgieff, N., Veuillet, E., Adrien, J. L., Barthelemy, C., & Collet, L. (2004). Increased perception of loudness in autism. *Hear. Res., 198*, 87–92.

Khalfa, S., Dubal, S., Veuillet, E., Perez-Sdiaz, F., Jouvent, R., & Collet, L. (2002). Psychometric normalisation of a Hyperacusis Questionnaire. *ORL, 64*, 436–442.

Marriage, J., & Barnes, N. M. (1995). Is central hyperacusis a symptom of 5-hydroxytryptamine (5-HT) dysfunction? *The Journal of Laryngology and Otology, 109*, 915–921.

Martell, C. R., Dimidjian, S., & Herman-Dunn, R. (2010). *Behavioral activation for depression. A clinician's guide*. New York, NY: Guilford Press.

McKenna, L. (1987). Goal planning in audiological rehabilitation. *British Journal of Audiology, 21*, 5–11.

McKenna, L., Handscomb, L., Hoare, D. J., & Hall, D. A. (2014). A scientific cognitive-behavioral model of tinnitus: novel conceptualizations of tinnitus distress. *Front. Neurol., 5*, 196. doi:10.3389/fneur.2014.00196.

Miller, R. P., Kori, S. H., & Todd, D. D. (1991). The Tampa Scale: A measure of kinisophobia. *The Clinical Journal of Pain, 7*, 51–52.

Miller, W. R., & Rollnick, S. (2010). *Motivational interviewing* (3rd ed.). New York, NY: Guilford Press.

Paulin, J., Andersson, L., & Nordin, S. (2016). Characteristics of hyperacusis in the general population. *Noise & Health, 18*, 178–184. doi:10.4103/1463-1741.189244.

Pienkowski, M., Tyler, R. S., Roncancio, E. R., Jun, H. J., Brozoski, T., Dauman, N., . . . Moore, B. C. (2014). A review of hyperacusis and future directions: Part II. Measurement, mechanisms, and treatment. *Am J Audiol, 23*, 420–436. doi:10.1044/2014_aja-13-0037.

Schroder, A. E., Vulink, N. C., van Loon, A. J., & Denys, D. A. (2017). Cognitive behavioral therapy is effective in misophonia: An open trial. *Journal of Affective Disorders, 217*, 289–294. doi:10.1016/j.jad.2017.04.017.

Schwartz, B., Wasserman, E. A., & Robbins, S. J. (2002). *Psychology of learning and behavior* (5th ed.). New York, NY: Norton.

Scott, B. (1993). *A graded exposure treatment for patients with hyperacusis*, Paper presented at the 19th Annual Convention of the Association for Behavior Analysis, Chicago, May.

Sheehan, D. V., Lecrubier, Y., Sheehan, K. H., Amorim, P., Janavs, J., Weiller, E., . . . Dunbar, G. C. (1998). The Mini-International Neuropsychiatric Interview (M.I.N.I.): The development and validation of a structured diagnostic psychiatric interview for DSM-IV and ICD-10. *The Journal of Clinical Psychiatry, 59 Suppl 20*, 22–33.

Stansfeld, S. A. (1992). Noise, noise sensitivity and psychiatric disorder: Epidemiological and psychophysiological studies. *Psychological Medicine, Monograph Supplement 22*, 1–44.

Taylor, S. (2017). Misophonia: A new mental disorder? *Medical Hypotheses, 103*, 109–117. doi:10.1016/j.mehy.2017.05.003.

Trulsson, U., Johansson, M., Jansson, G., Wiberg, A., & Hallberg, L. R. (2003). Struggling for a new self: In-depth interviews with 21 patients with hyperacusis after an acute head trauma. *J Health Psychol, 8*(4), 403–412. doi:10.1177/13591053030084001.

Tyler, R. S., Pienkowski, M., Roncancio, E. R., Jun, H. J., Brozoski, T., Dauman, N., . . . Moore, B. C. (2014). A review of hyperacusis and future directions: Part I. Definitions and manifestations. *American Journal of Audiology, 23*, 402–419. doi:10.1044/2014_aja-14-0010.

Vernon, J. A. (1987). Pathophysiology of tinnitus: A special case—Hyperacusis and a proposed treatment. *American Journal of Otology*, *8*, 201–202.

Villaume, K., & Hasson, D. (2017). Health-relevant personality is associated with sensitivity to sound (hyperacusis). *Scandinavian Journal of Psychology*, *58*, 158–169. doi:10.1111/sjop.12350.

Vlaeyen, J. W., & Linton, S. J. (2000). Fear-avoidance and its consequences in chronic musculoskeletal pain: A state of the art. *Pain*, *85*, 317–332.

Zigmond, A. S., & Snaith, R. P. (1983). The hospital anxiety and depression scale. *Acta Psychiatrica Scandinavia*, *67*, 361–370.

SECTION III

Auditory Disorders: Manifestations

11

Reflections on the Association between Hyperacusis and Tinnitus

David M. Baguley

Introduction

In the minds of many clinicians and researchers, hyperacusis and tinnitus are inextricably linked (Hazell & Sheldrake, 1992). As I will discuss, patients with these symptoms often follow similar referral pathways, and there is an undoubted and well-documented coincidence of these experiences. This may not indicate direct association, nor common mechanisms, however, and it may be that the elements of divergence between tinnitus and hyperacusis are sufficient for them to be considered as separate entities, although with some neurobiological overlap. These and other issues will be considered below; the present state of knowledge likely ensures that there are at least as many questions as answers.

Epidemiology

One aspect that hyperacusis and tinnitus do share is that estimates of the prevalence and recognized severity of each symptom are very strongly influenced by the question asked (Nemholt-Rosing, 2016a). This adversely affects the interpretation of research findings for each symptom alone, and when they are considered together, the problem is compounded. However, there is a consensus that many patients presenting with a primary complaint of tinnitus have experienced decreased sound tolerance (DST), and vice versa. What is largely missing from the literature, however, are data indicating how many patients with a primary complaint of one of these symptoms have *bothersome* experiences of the other. Also lacking are indications that these symptoms are somehow coupled in time of onset, or whether and to what degree they fluctuate over time (either in synchrony or reciprocally). These unanswered questions present a problem when it comes to determination of the association or mutually reinforcing elements between the symptoms.

As the literature on tinnitus is more extensive than that on hyperacusis, an initial review could consider the experiences of hyperacusis in patients with a primary complaint of tinnitus. Jack Vernon (1987) reported on a large series of patients undergoing clinical care for troublesome tinnitus, and while his study was ground-breaking in that it considered decreased sound tolerance at all, he noted:

> In our Tinnitus Clinic, where more than 4,000 patients have been seen, hyperacusis has been seen only four times.

Vernon defined hyperacusis as "unusual tolerance to ordinary environmental sounds," and one reflection might be that incorporation of the word *unusual* into a definition was an indication of an assumption that the symptom, or its trigger, was rare. As more attention was given to symptoms of reduced sound tolerance, it became clear that such symptoms were more common in people with tinnitus than Vernon had indicated. Initial reports of the prevalence of hyperacusis in patients presenting with troublesome tinnitus included figures of 40% (Jastreboff, Gray & Gold, 1996; Bartnik, Fabijanska, & Rogowski, 1999) and 60% (Andersson et al., 2001). In a study aiming to validate the Multiple-activity Scale for Hyperacusis, Dauman and Boscau-Faure (2005) recruited a series of 249 adult patients with tinnitus, reporting that 79% also had hyperacusis. It was noted that with treatment the hyperacusis impact decreased more frequently than that of tinnitus, although it was unclear to what extent this was due to time, treatment effects, or the way in which hyperacusis was defined to participants.

In a substantial series of 4993 adult patients with tinnitus, Hiller and Goebel (2005) reported that hyperacusis (definition not given) was present in 7.3%, a significant proportion of whom reported high levels of tinnitus loudness and annoyance. This finding was echoed by Fagelson (2007), who reported that patients with trauma histories who rated their tinnitus as severe were more likely than patients who did not suffer trauma to report severe co-occurring sound tolerance issues.

More recent research has provided data that is more nuanced. Scheckelman et al. (2014) reported a series of 2333 adult patients, 1713 of whom presented with a primary complaint of tinnitus. Asking the question, "Do sounds cause you pain or physical discomfort?" produced positive answers in 935 patients (55%), although 620 patients either did not answer the question or replied, "I don't know," and therefore the rate could conceivably be higher. Those patients deemed to have hyperacusis had better hearing thresholds than those without, and were younger. The two groups did not differ in gender nor in any of the tinnitus characteristics analyzed. Patients reporting both tinnitus and sound induced discomfort/pain were more likely to be undergoing psychiatric treatment, and had higher scores on the Tinnitus Handicap Inventory, the Beck Depression Inventory, and lower self-reported quality of life. The authors reflected that patients with both tinnitus and sound induced discomfort/pain were experiencing a form of hypervigilance to their symptoms, and that these co-incident auditory symptoms represented a specific subtype of tinnitus.

Yang et al. (2015) reported a consecutive series of 207 adult patients seen for troublesome tinnitus in whom the tinnitus was unilateral in 105 (50.7%) and bilateral in

102 (49.3%). The authors did not report the question used to differentiate the groups, nor did they discuss the experiences of patients in whom the experience of tinnitus was either central (filling the head) or the source appeared to be located externally. It was reported that of the patients with unilateral tinnitus, 5 (4.8%) experienced hyperacusis, as did 13 of those with bilateral tinnitus (12.7%): this difference was not statistically significant. The question used to identify hyperacusis was not given. While this work raised an interesting question regarding the perceived tinnitus "location" and DST, limited information could be gleaned about the physiological association between hyperacusis and tinnitus.

A further series of 81 adult tinnitus patients was described by Degeest et al. (2016). The data collected included Loudness Discomfort Levels (LDLs), and validated Dutch versions of the Tinnitus Handicap Inventory (THI) and the Hyperacusis Questionnaire (HQ). Statistically significant correlations were found between THI scores and LDL measures (albeit weak, $r = 0.265$), and HQ scores ($r = 0.729$). The mean HQ score in the group was 18.5 (s.d. 10.1) but the authors did not report how many patients met the HQ criteria for clinical significance. The association between the HQ and THI scores is of interest; causality aside, it may be a result of general distress driving both tinnitus and hyperacusis measures rather than a specific physiological association between the symptoms.

Less attention has been paid to patients with a primary complaint of hyperacusis, and whether they experience tinnitus. Anari et al. (1999) reported data from a series of 100 adult patients with a primary compliant of "hypersensitivity to sounds." noting that 86% of them "suffer from tinnitus," although formal evaluation of severity or impact was not reported. Fagelson (2007) reported that patients with trauma histories who experienced both tinnitus and hyperacusis were more likely to indicate that the sound tolerance issues outweighed the problems associated with tinnitus. In that chart review, 62% of the patients with both tinnitus and hyperacusis reported the sound tolerance as a more severe impairment.

Some other data is available regarding experiences of tinnitus and hyperacusis in the general population. In a conference proceedings, Fabijanska et al. (1999) reported findings from a postal questionnaire study in Poland with 10,349 respondents, of whom 20.1% reported tinnitus, and 15.2% hyperacusis. The questions used were not reported. Of those with tinnitus, the proportion also reporting hyperacusis approximated 40%. The proportion with hyperacusis indicating that they had tinnitus was not reported. In a more comprehensive study, originating from Sweden, Paulin et al. (2016) contacted 8520 adult individuals, of whom 3406 (40.0%) agreed to participate. Of those, 66 answered affirmatively when asked, "Have you been diagnosed with sound intolerance by a physician?"

A further 313 (9.2%) answered affirmatively to the question, "Do you have a hard time tolerating everyday sounds that you believe most other people can tolerate?" and were regarded as self-diagnosing with hyperacusis. Of those with a physician diagnosis, 29 (43.9%) reported tinnitus (tinnitus question not given), while of the self-diagnosed, 75 (24.0%) reported tinnitus. If it were the case that a person seeking advice from a physician about DST had more severe problems than a person who self-diagnosed, then this could be an indication that tinnitus is more prevalent when hyperacusis is more severe, but other factors could well be at work here, such as listening demands, and history of noise exposure.

Thus, there are fundamental problems in the interpretation of the published data regarding the co-incidence of hyperacusis and tinnitus in adults. These challenges are even more evident when one considers children and adolescents. A systematic review (Nemholt-Rosing et al., 2016a) of tinnitus and hyperacusis in these populations identified 25 papers examining tinnitus and/or hyperacusis in childhood (see also Chapter 13), but concluded that the variability in definitions and criteria for both hyperacusis and tinnitus were so great that meaningful meta-analysis was not possible. Nevertheless, the co-incidence of hyperacusis and tinnitus in childhood was addressed by Baguley et al. (2012) who considered the pediatric referrals of 4 well-established tinnitus clinics in Europe in the year 2009. During that time 88 children and adolescents were treated for a primary complaint of tinnitus, and in 34 (38%) hyperacusis (not defined) was also reported.

A series (Nemholt-Rosing, 2016b) of 81 young children and adolescents was referred to secondary care for tinnitus and/or hyperacusis in Southern Denmark in the period June 2014–February 2015. Of these, 9 cases (12.8%) had a primary complaint of hyperacusis, and both tinnitus and hyperacusis were the cause of complaint in 11 cases (15.7%).

An epidemiological study (Hall et al., 2016) considered the prevalence of hyperacusis and its relationship with tinnitus in a cohort of 11-year-old children in the United Kingdom who had enrolled in a longitudinal study entitled Avon Longitudinal Study of Parents and Children (ALSPAC). Of the participating children, 261/7092 (3.7%) reported hyperacusis, defined by the question, "Do you ever experience over-sensitivity or distress to particular sounds?"

Tinnitus of any severity or type was reported by 109 (41.7%) of these children. As discussed in Chapter 13, risk factors for hyperacusis included higher maternal education, male gender, and a readmission to the hospital in the first 4 weeks of life. Regarding tinnitus experiences (Humphriss et al., 2016), 218/7092 (3.1%) children reported clinically-significant tinnitus, defined by persistence and being described as bothersome. Of these, 21/218 (9.6%) reported hyperacusis. As with adults, the experience of tinnitus in persons with hyperacusis is more common than that of hyperacusis in persons with tinnitus.

In summary, the literature concerning the co-incidence of hyperacusis and tinnitus is complex and problematic. Variability in definitions and criteria is marked, and little attention has been paid to severity or impact of either tinnitus or hyperacusis as a secondary condition to the other. While it is possible to note that these symptoms commonly occur together, it is not possible to make other inferences about the possible causality or associations that exist between the two symptoms, or their relation over time. It can be noted, however, that it is entirely possible to have hyperacusis or tinnitus without the other symptom, and by no means is it an obligatory experience to have both. Having reflected on the epidemiology of hyperacusis and tinnitus, attention can now be directed toward when and how these symptoms converge, and then how they diverge.

Convergence

It has been mentioned above that even when the symptoms do not co-occur, in most health systems patients will be seen in the same clinics, and by the same professional groups, although this will vary country by country. Another area of convergence is the relation of hyperacusis, and of tinnitus, to psychological issues such as anxiety, fear, distress, and depression. Chapter 10 contains some discussion of the mutual reinforcement between hyperacusis and anxiety, as well as tinnitus experiences that can also be strongly influenced by psychological state. It would make sense, therefore, that when hyperacusis and tinnitus occur together, they too would be influenced in some form of coupling with a psychological state, although empirical evidence of this is sparse to date. The clinical implication is that just as tinnitus therapy consisting of audiology-based counseling and sound therapy can have increased efficacy if augmented with elements of psychological therapy (Cima et al., 2012), such combined interventions are likely to be of great value in cases of co-occurring hyperacusis and tinnitus.

Divergence

There are several ways in which the experience of hyperacusis, and of tinnitus, diverge from each other. The first is that while unilateral or strongly lateralized tinnitus is common, comprising 47% of the patient population, lateralized or unilateral hyperacusis is not common (Axelsson, 1995), although robust empirical data in that regard is not yet available. When DST is unilateral, the finding is most usually associated with a unilateral injury, such as an acoustic shock (McFerran & Baguley, 2007) or a specific lesion. Boucher and colleagues (2013) described a three-patient series each with a lesion of the insular cortex in whom a presenting symptom was unilateral hyperacusis.

Second, while the somatic modulation of tinnitus is common, this is not the case for hyperacusis. In the author's clinical experience this is very rarely volunteered by patients, and on questioning, is not commonly reported either. It has been proposed (Sanchez, 2016) that the somatic modulation of tinnitus involves interaction between the somatosensory systems and the auditory system within the dorsal cochlear nucleus, and if further investigation of the somatic modulation of hyperacusis confirms its low prevalence rate, then the implication might be that hyperacusis involves pathways extrinsic to those involved in the modulation of tinnitus. Further work is needed in this area.

Tinnitus can be an intermittent or transient experience, although it can also be unremittingly consistent, and this can vary both between individuals, and in a single individual's day to day experience. The severity of tinnitus can also vary, and emotional/psychological state is one factor that influences this. Hyperacusis, however, appears to be a more consistent phenomenon, in that once it begins it is persistent and consistent, and in general, while it may influence emotions, it does not vary with emotional state. One reported exception to this is the psychological stress associated with the anticipation of pain or distress associated with an impending sound event (Lupien et al., 2009). Imagine an adult waiting for a telephone call, sitting with their cell phone on the table in front of them: the call to come will bring some important news, perhaps of examination results, or the findings of an important medical investigation. As the person waits, their anticipation increases their auditory gain, so that when the phone rings, they startle, even though that was the very sound that they were expecting. Other examples include an anxious mother listening for her sick child to cough during the night, or a householder waiting for their noisy neighbor to return home and begin playing their intense and intrusive music.

Finally, hyperacusis seems to be related to some conditions that have little or nothing to do with tinnitus, such as misophonia, Williams syndrome, and autistic spectrum disorders. Misophonia, which may correspond to annoyance hyperacusis in Tyler et al.'s (2014) categorization scheme, is a condition where specific sounds evoke disgust or rage (McFerran, 2016). Common triggers include eating sounds, throat clearing, or audible breathing. The behavioral consequence is avoidance, and as the most common age of onset coincides with adolescence, the family/social consequences can be catastrophic. Functional imaging studies of misophonia (Kumar et al., 2017) have indicated abnormal functional connectivity between the anterior insular cortex and emotion processing centers such as the amygdala, and that this may be a disorder in the patient's evaluation of the salience or meaning of the trigger sounds. As such, misophonia differs substantially from hyperacusis, which is a general decreased tolerance to sound likely related to a disorder of auditory gain; however, the emotional aspects of hyperacusis would indicate that abnormal functional connectivity between sound perception and emotion may be an element of its neurobiological substrate. While this could also be proposed as being the case in some cases of tinnitus, hyperacusis and misophonia appear related in some ways that do not map onto tinnitus.

Williams syndrome (WS) is a neurodevelopmental disorder, associated with abnormalities on chromosome 7 (see Chapter 7). People with WS have distinctive elfin-like facial features, developmental delay, cardiac problems, with a behavioral phenotype of and inappropriate, or readily-displayed trust of strangers, perhaps viewed as excessive friendliness. Sound tolerance issues can be the first feature of WS noticed by the person's family, and have been said to involve over 90% of people with a diagnosis of WS (Klein et al., 1990; Van Borsel et al., 1997; Levitin et al., 2005). Investigation of such patients using the HQ did not indicate a severe hyperacusis (Blomberg et al., 2006), however, the extent to which the HQ derives meaningful data in the WS population is unknown. A model of hyperactivity in the auditory system of persons with WS was proposed (Zarchi et al., 2010) and some auditory evoked potential data supported this model (Zarchi et al., 2015). To the author's knowledge, there is no published data regarding tinnitus in persons with WS, and it may well be that WS is a condition characterized by reduced sound tolerance but without any associated tinnitus.

Abnormal tolerance of sound is a notable feature of autistic spectrum disorders (ASD; Rosenhall et al., 1999). Professor Temple Grandin has written about her auditory experiences in the context of her ASD:

> My hearing is like having a hearing aid with the volume control stuck on "super loud." It is like an open microphone that picks up everything. I have two choices: turn the mike on and get deluged with sound, or shut it off. . . . . . . I can't modulate incoming auditory stimulation. (Grandin, 1992)

While it is widely known that people with ASD have unusual auditory experiences, surprisingly little data regarding severity or patient profiles is available. Potentially this could be ascribed to the challenges of researching purely subjective phenomena in people with reduced abilities to communicate emotional or qualitative experiences. In a study investigating tinnitus and hyperacusis in persons with ASD, Danesh et al. (2015) reported data from 55 individuals with a diagnosis of Asperger's syndrome. Hyperacusis was reported by 69% of the series, although the mean score of the Hyperacusis Questionnaire (HQ) was 21 (of a potential maximum of 42), which did not indicate a severe problem; perhaps the result was indicative of a mismatch between the subjective experiences and those aspects of hyperacusis that the HQ aimed to measure (see Chapter 2). The prevalence of tinnitus was 35%, with a mean THI score of 23 (of a potential maximum of 100); while this score would exceed that of the general population, it was not indicative of severe tinnitus. The prevalence of both tinnitus and hyperacusis was 31%. Some caution must be advised when interpreting these results: the age range of the participants was 4 to 42 years (i.e., perhaps too wide to be meaningful), the response rate was only 16%, and the extent to which the THI and HQ provided meaningful data in this population, given both the diagnosis and the young age of some participants, was uncertain.

These reflections on areas of divergence between hyperacusis and tinnitus may have some implications. There are some conditions in which sound tolerance issues are pathognomonic, but that do not seem to involve tinnitus. There are some aspects of hyperacusis that have markedly different characteristics to tinnitus, including the characteristic lack of lateralization and of somatic modulation, and the relentless consistency of hyperacusis rather than the labile nature often ascribed to tinnitus. Does this mean that hyperacusis and tinnitus are essentially separate phenomena? Given the present sparse data we have, a definitive answer is not yet possible. However, while there is some neurobiological overlap, it does seem that there is sufficient divergence that the traditional grouping of hyperacusis with tinnitus can be called into question. An analogy to use with patients might be to describe hyperacusis and tinnitus as cousins rather than siblings: related, yet with substantial, distinctive, and important differences.

Unanswered Questions

As with several other chapters in this book, the number of unanswered questions identified is considerable. Some of these are offered below:

- What is the prevalence of hyperacusis and tinnitus as a secondary symptom to the other in adults and children?
- What is the severity of hyperacusis and tinnitus as a secondary symptom to the other in adults and children?
- When hyperacusis and tinnitus are co-incident, which is precursive of the other, and what is the natural history?
- When hyperacusis and tinnitus are co-incident, which responds more quickly and effectively to treatment?

It is our hope that colleagues in the auditory community, researchers, clinicians, and patients, might identify areas of interest, and undertake controlled trials to further our knowledge. There is much to do in that regard!

References

Anari, M., Axelsson, A., Eliasson, A., & Magnusson, L. (1999). Hypersensitivity to sound: Questionnaire data, audiometry, and classification. *Scandinavian Audiology*, *28*, 219–230.

Baguley, D. M., Bartnik, G., Kleinjung, T., Savastano, M., & Hough, E. A. (2013). Troublesome tinnitus in childhood and adolescence: Data from expert centres. *Int. J. Ped. Otorhinolaryngol.*, *77*(2), 246–251.

Blomberg, S., Rosander, M., and Andersson, G. (2006). Fears, hyperacusis and musicality in Williams syndrome. *Res. Dev. Disabil.*, Nov-Dec, *27*(6), 668–680.

Boucher, O., Turgeon, C., Champoux, S., Ménard, L., Rouleau, I., Lassonde, M., . . . Nguyen, D. K. (2015). Hyperacusis following unilateral damage to the insular cortex: A three-case report. *Brain Res. 5*, 1606, 102–12

Cima, R. F., Maes, I. H., Joore, M. A., Scheyen, D. J., El Refaie, A., Baguley, D. M., . . . Vlaeyen, J. W. (2012). Specialised treatment based on cognitive behaviour therapy versus usual care for tinnitus: A randomised controlled trial. *Lancet*, *379*(9830), 1951–1959.

Danesh, A. A., Lang, D., Kaf, W., Andreassen, W. D., Scott, J., & Eshraghi, A. A. (2015). Tinnitus and hyperacusis in autism spectrum disorders with emphasis on high functioning individuals diagnosed with Asperger's Syndrome. *Int. J. Pediatr. Otorhinolaryngol.*, Oct, *79*(10), 1683–1688.

Dauman, R., & Bouscau-Faure, F. (2005). Assessment and amelioration of hyperacusis in tinnitus patients. *Acta Otolaryngologica, 125*(5), 503–509.

Degeest, S., Corthals, P., Dhooge, I., & Keppler, H. (2016). The impact of tinnitus characteristics and associated variables on tinnitus-related handicap. *J. Laryngol. Otol., 130*(1), 25–31.

Fabijanska, A., Rogowski, M., Bartnik, G., & Skarzynski, H. (1999). Epidemiology of tinnitus and hyperacusis in Oland. In Hazell, J. W. P. (Ed.). *Proceedings of Sixth International Tinnitus Seminar* (pp. 569–571). London: The Tinnitus and Hyperacusis Centre.

Fagelson, M. A. (2007). The association between tinnitus and posttraumatic stress disorder. *Am. J. Aud.*, (16), 107–117.

Grandin, T. (1992). An inside view of autism. In Scopler, E. & Meribov, G. B. (Eds.). *High functioning individuals with autism* (pp. 105–126). New York, NY: Springer.

Hall, A. J., Humphriss, R., Baguley, D. M., Parker, M., & Steer, C. D. (2016). Prevalence and risk factors for reduced sound tolerance (hyperacusis) in children. *International Journal of Audiology, 55*(3), 135–141.

Hiller, W., & Goebel, G. (2006). Factors influencing tinnitus loudness and annoyance. *Arch Otolaryngol. Haed Neck Surg., 132*(12), 1323–1330.

Humphriss, R., Hall, A. J., & Baguley, D. M. (2016). Prevalence and characteristics of tinnitus in 11-year-old children. *Int. J. Audiol., 55*(3), 142–148.

Jang, C., Jung, J., Kim, S. H., Byun, J. Y., Park, M. S., & Yeo, S. G. (2015). Comparison of clinical characteristics in patients with bilateral and unilateral tinnitus. *Acta Oto-Laryngologica 135*(11), 1128–1131.

Jastreboff, P. J., Gray, W. C., & Gold, S. L. (1996) Neurophysiological approach to tinnitus patients. *Am. J. Otol., 17*(2), 236–240.

Klein, A. J., Armstrong, B. L., Greer, M. K., & Brown, F. R. 3rd. (1990). Hyperacusis and otitis media in individuals with Williams syndrome. *J. Speech Hear. Disord.*, May, *55*(2), 339–344.

Kumar, S., Tansley-Hancock, O., Sedley, W., Winston, J. S., Callaghan, M. F., Allen, M., . . . Griffiths, T. D. (2017). The brain basis for misophonia. *Curr. Biol., 27*(4), 527–533.

Levitin, D. J., Cole, K., Lincoln, A., & Bellugi, U. (2005). Aversion, awareness, and attraction: Investigating claims of hyperacusis in the Williams syndrome phenotype. *J. Child Psychol. Psychiatry*, May, *46*(5), 514–523.

Lupien, S. J., McEwen, B. S., Gunnar, M. R., & Heim, C. (2009). Effects of stress throughout the lifespan on the brain, behaviour and cognition. *Nature Reviews Neuroscience, 10*(6), 434–445.

McFerran, D. J. (2016). Misophonia and phonophobia. In Baguley, D. M., & Fagelson, M. (Eds.). *Tinnitus: Clinical and research perspectives* (pp. 254–260). San Diego, CA: Plural.

McFerran, D. J., & Baguley, D. M. (2007). Acoustic shock. *J. Laryngol. Otol., 121*(4), 301–305.

Nemholt-Rosing, S., Hvass Schmidt, J., Wedderkopp, N., & Baguley, D. M. (2016a). Prevalence of tinnitus and hyperacusis in children and adolescents: A systematic review. *BMJ Open 6*, 1–20.

Nemholt-Rosing, S., Kapandais, A., Schmidt, J. H., & Baguley, D. M. (2016b). Demographic data, referral patterns and interventions used for children and adolescents with tinnitus and hyperacusis in Southern Denmark. *Int. J. Ped. Otorhinolaryngol., 89*, 112–120.

Paulin, J., Andersson, L., & Nordin, S. (2016). Characteristics of hyperacusis in the general population. *Noise & Health, 18*(3), 178–184.

Rosenhall, U., Nordin, V., Sandstrom, M., Ahlsen, G., & Gillberg, C. (1999). Autism and hearing loss. *J. Autism Devel. Dis., 29*(5), 349–357.

Sanchez, T. G. (2016). Clinical aspects of somatic modulation of tinnitus. In Baguley, D. M., Fagelson, M. (Eds.). *Tinnitus: Clinical and research perspectives* (pp. 111–127). San Diego, CA: Plural.

Scheckleman, M., Landgrebe, M., Langguth, B., & TRI Database Study Group. (2015). Phenotypic characteristics of hyperacusis in tinnitus. *PLOS One, 9*(1): e86944.

Tyler, R. S., Pienkowski, M., Roncancio, E. R., Jun, H. J., Brozoski, T., Dauman, N., . . . Moore, B. C. (2014). A review of hyperacusis and future directions: Part I. Definitions and manifestations. *American Journal of Audiology, 23*(4), 402–419.

Van Borsel, J., Curfs, L. M., Fryns, J. P. (1997). Hyperacusis in Williams syndrome: A sample survey study. *Genet. Couns.*, *8*(2), 121–126.

Vernon, J. A. (1987). Pathophysiology of tinnitus: A special case—hyperacusis and a proposed treatment. *Am. J. Otol.*, *8*(3), 201–202.

Zarchi, O., Attias, J., & Gothelf, D. (2010). Auditory and visual processing in Williams syndrome. *Isr. J. Psychiatry Relat. Sci.*, *47*(2), 125–131.

Zarchi, O., Avni, C., Attias, J., Frisch, A., Carmel, M., Michaelovsky, E., . . . Gothelf, D. (2015). Hyperactive auditory processing in Williams syndrome: Evidence from auditory evoked potentials. *Psychophysiology*, *52*(6), 782–789.

12

Diplacusis

Marc Fagelson

Introduction

Diplacusis occurs when a listener perceives at least two distinctly different pitches as a pure tone signal or musical note or chord is presented simultaneously to both ears. Musicians appear more sensitive to the effects of diplacusis, likely because they can recognize when notes in a song are not in tune (i.e., dissonance or roughness is present when it should not be) with a greater degree of resolution and accuracy than other listeners. The term "diplacusis binauralis" is attributed to Shambaugh Sr. (1907; cited by Albers & Wilson, 1968) and several case studies over the years describe challenges to musicians' performances and listening experiences. It is implicated in the effectiveness of cochlear implant fittings and mapping (Reiss et al., 2007, 2011), although diplacusis is diagnosed and reported far less often than other manifestations of disordered sound tolerance (Jastreboff & Jastreboff, 2015). The needs of these diverse patient groups dictate that diplacusis merits consideration from clinicians and researchers working with patients who require audiologic rehabilitation.

At least three forms of diplacusis receive attention in the literature. Diplacusis monauralis refers to the observation that a single tone may be perceived as multiple tones or as a noise, in the stimulated ear. Such observations may be made by patients with profound unilateral hearing loss; the "better" ear produces the aberrant perception without contribution from the "poorer" ear. Diplacusis binauralis is the most common form of the disorder in which a single tone audible to both ears is perceived as two distinct tones or as a noisy signal. The two ears may appear to hear the tone(s) with a slightly different timing as well. Diplacusis dysharmonia (occasionally diplacusis harmonica) is a rarely used term, and, similar to diplacusis binauralis, relates to distinct tones or musical notes being perceived when only one note is presented.

Prevalence of diplacusis remains unknown and is difficult to determine definitively. Colin et al. (2016) indicate that prevalence among patients with hearing loss exceeds that of normal-hearing individuals, and that asymmetric hearing losses most often accompany the unusual pitch event. Small study samples, few patient reports, and difficulty measuring the pitch disparities are among the reasons prevalence data remain lacking. A search for primary care data indicates that 83 cases with diplacusis as the primary diagnosis are on record for 2009 in the United States (2013; ProQuest Document #1267703683).

In an analysis of musicians with histories of noise exposure, Jansen et al. (2009) compared prevalence of various auditory impairments including hearing loss, hyperacusis, diplacusis, and others. Of 241 musicians sampled, 190 (79%) reported hyperacusis, or issues with loudness tolerance, 121 (51%) reported tinnitus, 57 (24%) reported "distortion" of musical tones, and 17 (7%) experienced diplacusis. The experience of distortion may be a result of processing impairment related to diplacusis (i.e., the roughness produced by two different and unresolved notes), but in any case, the musician reports suggested that diplacusis was far less common than hyperacusis and tinnitus. In this study, prevalence of diplacusis was about 10% that of hyperacusis.

Most of us understand pitch to be the psychological correlate of a sound's frequency. In some cases, the terms are inaccurately used interchangeably; this mistake is understandable as, in general, the frequency of a sound is proportional to the pitch perception it creates. However, the situation is not so simple. For example, tangible pitch perceptions can arise through manipulations of complex sounds' spectra that eliminate energy in the cochlear frequency region from which the pitch perception would appear to arise, forming the so-called "residue" or "virtual" pitch (e.g., Terhardt, 1974; Pantev et al., 1996). In other cases, the sensation of pitch may be altered following onset of hearing loss, particularly single-sided loss, to the point that a pure tone signal can produce a pitch that differs across a listener's ears. Musicians experiencing this unusual event can on occasion map the pitch anomalies, and state with confidence the notes or range of notes that contribute to the disordered pitch sensation. The realization that perceived pitch may not be accurate can drive a musician away from playing, and can limit the enjoyment one experiences listening to music. Analogous pitch-related disorders can influence the effectiveness of cochlear implants as well. The diplacusis phenomenon remains incompletely understood, however, a few recent cases highlight the challenges associated with clinical management of such patients. In this chapter we will review causes and manifestations of disordered pitch perception, as well as review two cases of patients with varying degrees of hearing loss and diplacusis.

Review of Pitch Perception Mechanisms

The sensation of pitch is derived from two complimentary but distinct processing events. First, an environmental sound produces displacement of the eardrum, middle ear bones, and ultimately the sensory surface of the inner ear, the basilar membrane. Because the basilar membrane displays different resonance frequencies at specific locations along its length, the perception of pitch is related to, and generated by, the displacement pattern on the basilar membrane. The place theory of hearing emerges from our understanding of cochlear traveling waves and displacement patterns, and the place theory may be pictured as analogous to the relation between pitch and place along the length of a piano keyboard. Consider that displacement of the keyboard surface on the instrument's left side produces low-frequency notes that are progressively higher in pitch and frequency as one moves from the left side of the keyboard to the right side. The basilar membrane is similarly organized or mapped with respect to frequency of vibration such that the left side of the piano corresponds to the apical region of the cochlea while the right-hand side of the piano corresponds to the basal region. Therefore, an environmental sound generates inner ear activity at the location along the membrane that resonates when exposed to the spectral content of the sound; the cochlea converts frequency to place, and initiates the process by which the central mechanism propagates a neurally encoded version of the sound. The neural representation of the sound, under normal conditions, emphasizes the energy associated with the most substantial physical displacements of the membrane, thereby resulting in a salient pitch perception.

The place theory provided a clear and easily understood explanation for pitch perception during many routine listening tasks; however, some interesting contradictions to its basic assumptions were identified. For example, Plomp (1967), Schouten et al. (1962), and Terhardt (1974) identified spectral components of complex stimuli that produced the sensation of pitch even when the stimulus presented to listeners lacked energy at the frequency corresponding to the pitch. A harmonic complex of 800, 1000, and 1200 Hz would produce a pitch sensation corresponding to a 200-Hz sinusoid despite the absence of 200 Hz in the presented signal. This pitch experience arose from a stimulus that lacked energy at the cochlear place associated with the pitch frequency, and the pitch was termed a "residue" of the harmonic complex. Because no displacement occurred at the 200-Hz place, the listener extracted pitch by using a mechanism other than the place information described above. A pitch perception that was assumed to rely upon displacement along the basilar membrane at a specific location arose without such activation; a "virtual pitch." Plomp, Terhardt, and others ultimately reported that the highest common factor in the harmonic train would correspond in most cases to the perceived pitch. Indeed, Pantev et al. (1996) demonstrated that the virtual pitch event produced activation in the same cortical area that would have been stimulated by a sound with the matching spectral content. That is, a sequence of 8 tones at integer multiples of 250 Hz (but that did not include 250 Hz) not only produced the pitch sensation of 250 Hz, it produced brain activity in the 250 Hz region of the auditory cortex despite the omission of energy at that frequency from the sound's spectrum.

Although frequency and intensity were long considered independent physical attributes of a sound, stimulus intensity influenced pitch perception in a variety of experiments. Basilar membrane recordings (Rhode, 1971) suggested that basilar membrane displacement patterns at high signal levels were displaced in the basalward, or high-frequency direction, with concurrent change in an observer's rating of the pitch. Presumably, in an individual with symmetric hearing (or hearing loss), the intensity effect would be approximately equal in both ears, minimizing the likelihood of diplacusis occurring. However, in cases of asymmetric loss, or unilateral hearing loss, the influence of such basilar membrane shifts on the ensuing pitch event would be less predictable; an experienced listener (i.e., musician) could detect pitch differences that would subsequently reduce the consonance of musical passages, particularly those with substantial intensity fluctuations.

Additional investigators, such as Goldstein (1973), concluded that pitch perception was drawn from temporal information related to the periodicity of the complex waveform. The aforementioned 800 to 1000 to 1200 Hz complex had a period of 5 ms, and the waveform would complete a cycle at the same rate as a 200-Hz sinusoid. A temporal theory of pitch suggested that a central auditory processing mechanism locked to a specific phase, or moment in the waveform's cycle, could be responsible for the pitch perception in the absence of sound energy at the pitch frequency. Limitations on the rate at which neurons fire was found to limit the frequency range through which temporal mechanism would contribute to pitch identity (Palmer & Russell, 1986). Taken together, the place theory and the temporal theory offered reasonable explanations for most pitch events perceived by normal-hearing listeners.

As with the place theory, the temporal theory alone could not explain the various pitch experiences and disorders that emerged in clinical and laboratory testing. Ward (1963) specified diplacusis as evidence that the waveform periodicity alone could not explain pitch perception. If one sound was presented to both ears, then both ears must be receiving identically periodic signals. The temporal theory specified that the rates of neural discharge signal pitch; however, if the same signal was presented to both ears, then the neural discharge rates must be identical. The observation that not all patients heard the same tone in both ears affirmed that the temporal theory alone could not explain all pitch-related phenomena. Further, the likelihood that peripheral loss could influence the pitch mechanisms further limited the putative contribution of a central, temporal processing system.

Not surprisingly, subsequent findings supported the notion that pitch extraction relied upon the complimentary action of peripheral and central mechanisms. Van den Brink and colleagues (1974, 1976) performed a number of experiments in which test subjects were presented, simultaneously, different tones in each ear (e.g., 1000 Hz in the left ear, and a tone of variable frequency in the right ear). When the variable tone frequency equaled or was within 0.2 to 0.4% of the fixed tone (in this example, within 20 to 40Hz of the 1000-Hz standard; although substantial variability was found between subjects) then the participant heard a single tone. When the frequency difference was increased, the "fusion" into a single pitch heard in the two tones was no longer possible for the listener, and the percept changed to that of hearing two tones simultaneously.

The fact that two different tones would be heard as one suggested that frequency differences were not always heard as such, and that a process of fusing the two tones had occurred. This idea was supported by the observation that listeners appeared to "average" the two tones; the pitch of the emergent single "fused" tone resided somewhere between the stimulus frequencies. Because different cochlear traveling wave displacements occurred during the aforementioned two-tone stimulation, a central mechanism was involved in the fusion process. One way to conceptualize the fusion experiments would be to consider an analogous experiment in the tactile system. Two pins placed near each other on the fingertip may be indistinguishable from one pin, until the two pins are spaced further apart. At some distance, two pins can be distinguished from one pin—there is a critical distance of separation across the fingertip at which the stimulation produced by two pins cannot be fused into one.

In a sense, this central mechanism minimized the likelihood of diplacusis occurring as it reduced the relative contribution classically associated with pitch arising from the location of maximum cochlear stimulation. Recall that diplacusis manifested as the perception of different tones in the two ears despite the presentation of the same tone to each. Van den Brink et al. (1976) summarized this situation by stating that observers with "normal" hearing did not typically notice diplacusis even though all observers, regardless of hearing loss severity, had diplacusis "to some extent" (Van den Brink et al., 1976; p. 1472). This statement reiterated Licklider's (1951) assertion that "a moderate degree of binaural pitch disparity is the rule rather than the exception" (Licklider, 1951; p. 1033). Therefore, subtle changes affecting the central processor, such as those that would impair the fusion mechanism, could allow for more frequent perceptions of diplacusis in an affected individual, particularly when stimulated by environmental events that produced strong pitch perceptions, such as music. If true, then this situation would be most likely in cases of asymmetric hearing loss of cochlear origin that disrupted basilar membrane mechanics, or for individuals, such as musicians, with substantial experience involving pitch judgment.

Pitch and Musical Tones

Perception of musical intervals, or the listener's ability to evaluate the frequency difference between notes, highlights the listener's coincident use of at least the place and timing mechanisms; the reader would be safe in assuming that the listener's experience with sound and music would also influence matters. First, the pitch comparison between a note on a piano and the frequency of the note reveals a monotonic change upward as one moves toward the right side of a piano keyboard. This relation produces a sensation termed tone height (Bachem, 1950). Bachem also reports a different pitch experience related to different octaves of musical notes. For example, a C in one octave retains the pitch of a C even when played at appropriate frequencies in higher or lower registers. A note of C one octave below middle C could be matched to the same pitch as middle C even though the frequency of the former would be approximately ½ that of the latter. The consistency of pitch across octaves of a musical note, or its pitch class, is termed tone chroma. Therefore, a note with frequency of 220 Hz would have the same tone chroma as one of 440 Hz, however, the 440-Hz tone would have a greater tone height.

Other aspects of tone perception rely upon more complex processing that gives rise to a tone's quality, or its timbre. Timbre is associated with the harmonics and spectral components produced by the physical characteristics, such as length and diameter of a string (as in a harp, piano, or guitar), an open tube (as in a brass or woodwind instrument) in combination with the various constrictions or other physical modifications to the flow of air displaced by the instrument's sounding. Because of these physical differences, a musical note, say the concert A of 440 Hz, will sound different when played on a violin compared to a trumpet. Although the two instruments play the same note, it *sounds* different because of the instruments' physical differences. Timbral differences exist in the presence of pitch similarities (or differences) and may be influenced, as with other perceptual events, by disorders of pitch perception.

It is worth noting that many patients reporting diplacusis are musicians, or music enthusiasts. Schubert (1957) and others have commented that the pitch sensation associated with diplacusis might not be evident, or obvious, to an individual without musical training; they might not report the problem as it does not interfere with their livelihood or related recreational activities. This situation will be illustrated in cases reviewed at the end of the chapter. The experience of diplacusis, and the influence it exerts on the enjoyment of music, bears consideration and begs the question: if a person experiences diplacusis from an early age, is it possible that music never "sounds right" to that individual, and would that person be one who states that there is no particular form of music that they enjoy, and that, indeed, they have never been interested in listening to music?

Causes of Diplacusis

The reliance on mechanisms both peripheral (place theory, contributing primarily to tone height) and central (temporal theory, contributing primarily to tone chroma) suggests that pitch perception could be impaired via injury or disruption to several diverse and seemingly unrelated elements of the auditory pathway. Cochlear hearing loss could give rise to changes in, or losses of, audibility that would preclude pitch perception (i.e., Gaeth & Norris, 1965). Neural damage could interfere with timing cues or synchronous neural activity necessary for pitch extraction that relies upon temporal processing, or phase-locking in the analysis of a sound's spectrum. In order to make sense of patient complaints regarding pitch anomalies, such as diplacusis, it is important to consider changes to auditory function that have the potential to impair the pitch perception process. The first consideration will be cases in which a single tone is perceived as noticeably different in the two ears.

Cochlear Damage

Early mentions of diplacusis were related to patients with unilateral or asymmetric sensorineural hearing loss. Schubert (1957) summarized much of the earlier work related to investigations of pitch-related impairments as he reported that its causes included, among other insults to auditory mechanism infection, head trauma (he specified "accidents or war injuries"), atrophy of the brain, and otosclerosis surgery. Schubert also conveyed that the literature regarding diplacusis did not specify the mechanisms by which the unusual perception arose.

Schubert (1957) presented two cases upon which he built an argument for a cochlear/labyrinthine source of the inaccurate pitch event. In the first case, he described a 37-year-old male patient, a musician, with unilateral hearing loss and the presence of diplacusis in the right ear. The loss was determined to be sensorineural, and the presence of diplacusis of 3-week duration prior to Schubert's examination. Differential diagnosis included tuning fork tests, bone-conduction testing, and medical examination ruled out allergy, infection, circulatory system disorder, as well as alcohol and nicotine abuse. Because the patient was a musician, he was able to identify the specific pitch region that was affected; his complaints arose from difficulties tuning his instrument, an act that put him at odds with his colleagues in the orchestra.

Given the patient's medical history, Schubert (1957) speculated labyrinthine edema, or fluid retention in the inner ear, was at the source of the patient's reported problems. He used an intravenous glucose administration as an agent to promote dehydration in the cochlea twice daily. Diplacusis "disappeared but recurred a few days after treatment was stopped. This repeated itself several times" (p. 4) as Schubert managed the patient's case. Schubert's direct treatment of the cochlea's condition, and the ensuing diplacusis fluctuations experienced by the patient, suggested cochlear site of lesion for the diplacusis phenomenon. Schubert's intervention, in retrospect, resembled the common use of steroids for sudden hearing losses of cochlear origin believed to arise from inflammatory processes as would occur in a case of inner ear autoimmune disorder.

The association between inflammatory processes and diplacusis also was discussed by George Shambaugh Sr. (1920; cited in Albers & Wilson, 1968) and by George Shambaugh, Jr. (1940; 1959). In his 1959 text, Shambaugh, Jr. discussed the influence of labyrithitis on cochlear function. He indicated that the edema associated with an inner ear infection would affect primarily perception of high frequency sounds and could result in both distorted hearing and diplacusis, echoing Schubert's (1957) work.

Other investigators speculated regarding the importance of cochlear mechanisms to the development of diplacusis as they discussed cases similar to those reported by Schubert.

Gaeth and Norris (1965) described five patients with unilateral sensorineural hearing loss who reported diplacusis-like sound experiences. As with prior investigators, Gaeth and Norris reported that pitch variances were most prevalent in the region of hearing loss. The general findings they reported and reviewed indicated that, in fatigued (i.e., ears displaying temporary threshold shift), or damaged ears, patients experienced an upward shift in pitch, and distorted quality of hearing. They also noted, however, that an individual with normal hearing (one in their study, several historically) exhibited similar anomalous findings.

Gaeth and Norris (1965) tested patients in monaural (either the better ear or the poorer ear) and binaural listening conditions. After test subjects completed practice trials in which all stimuli were presented to normal-hearing ears, their pitch matches were assessed in other, more challenging conditions and the deviation in Hz from the initial perceived pitch in the better ear was measured. Pitch matches in the participants' poor ears were less consistent, and revealed that impaired ears perceived stimuli to be of higher pitch than nonimpaired ears. For example, the poor ear pitch matches using stimuli presented to one ear at a time (monaurally) were to frequencies consistently higher than those in normal ears when the two were compared. When test subjects with unilateral hearing loss were assessed using stimuli presented to both ears simultaneously (binaurally) the results indicated processing more similar to, but not reaching that of normal hearing ears; listeners provided intermediate pitch values that settled between the normal and abnormal matches. When stimuli levels were increased from 40 dB (as above) to 80 dB, the pitch matches in hearing-impaired ears improved, that is, pitch was matched to tone frequencies that were closer to the reference stimulus than when tested at the lower stimulus level; nevertheless, the pitch was still perceived as a higher frequency than the stimulus.

To clarify, an example of this experimental approach could be described as follows. First, a patient with unilateral hearing loss was presented a tone in the good ear, and then the patient adjusted a tone in the poorer ear until it matched the pitch of the tone in the better ear. The two frequencies that were matched in pitch by the listener were compared, and in the vast majority of cases, the listener ascribed a higher-frequency tone in the poor ear as one that matched the frequency in the better ear. In this example, it might be that a 2000-Hz tone in the better ear was equal in pitch to a 2200-Hz tone in the poorer ear. When the same person was stimulated in both ears by the same tone, and then asked to match the pitch of the tone, the participant matched the tone to an intermediate frequency. In this example, a 2000-Hz tone presented to both ears might be matched to a comparison tone of 2100 Hz.

Although cochlear damage with related hearing impairment, and diplacusis often co-occurred in clinical reports, their relation was not readily determined. Obviously not all individuals with hearing loss would experience diplacusis, and on occasion, diplacusis appeared in individuals with normal hearing (Gaeth & Norris, 1965). Knight (2004) examined a case of sudden unilateral hearing loss in which the patient complained of diplacusis, and was treated after one week's time with anti-inflammatory steroids. He compared the patient's threshold change to their otoacoustic emission (OAE) characteristics with additional consideration of the diplacusis reports. The patient displayed a slight decrease in low frequency sensitivity that did not reach clinical significance (i.e., the thresholds changed, but remained in the normal range and returned to preshift thresholds within three weeks of onset), a mild threshold shift at 8kHz that recovered as well, but over a longer time frame, and a severe threshold shift at 12 kHz that did not return to normal; in sum, thresholds over time returned to normal at frequencies through 8 kHz, but remained elevated at 12 kHz. Note that baseline data were not available, therefore thresholds that improved over time to the normal range may not have returned to preloss values.

The patient's reports of diplacusis worsened during the first week the hearing loss was present even though the hearing thresholds did not worsen during that time. Diplacusis was reportedly most pronounced in higher frequencies, associated by Knight with the possibility that infection spread from the middle ear into the basal (high-frequency) region of the cochlea. His measure of OAEs linked the cochlea's health to the reported changes in sensitivity. Emissions provoked by broadband signals (transient OAEs) displayed different recovery time courses from recovery associated with pure tone thresholds and diplacusis. Therefore, the OAE behavior was presumably related to mechanisms different from those that produced the diplacusis perception. However, Knight also used frequency-specific stimuli facilitating measures of the OAE's fine frequency structure; results of these measures were related over time and in the frequency region of interest, to patient reports of diplacusis. Although the amplitude of the OAEs was not correlated with patient reports, the spectral energy of the emission fine structure, once the emissions reappeared late in the first week following the sudden hearing loss, changed in conjunction with the patient's reports of anomalous pitch experiences. Knight indicated that the emission behavior, coupled to the patient's experience, was evidence that cochlear traveling wave mechanics had been altered, and that traveling wave peaks in the cochlea were displaced toward the base of the organ when the hearing loss was still present. A basalward displacement of the cochlear traveling wave would account for several aspects of diplacusis reported previously with a shift in pitch upward the most obvious example. As depicted in cases at the end of this chapter, diplacusis associated with sudden hearing loss resulting from cochlear damage may resolve over time as the cochlea's function improves.

Central Mechanisms

Cochlear dysfunction provided a reasonable explanation for perception of diplacusis associated with hearing loss, particularly in those cases when the loss was temporary, asymmetric, and the diplacusis experience decreased as hearing improved. However, it was also the case that individuals with normal hearing could experience pitch anomalies. Further, pitch processing that resulted in diplacusis or other undesirable auditory outcomes was often a concern for cochlear implant recipients and their audiologists. In a sense, the binaural fusion described by Van den Brink et al. (1976) might not be available, or may require training and experience, in order to be of benefit to some CI recipients.

Reiss and colleagues (2007, 2016) demonstrated that CI patients displayed changes in pitch over time with CI use, and that well-established mechanisms of pitch extraction, such as those described by van den Brink et al. (1976) could not adequately explain pitch processing and changes as demonstrated by such patients. Reiss et al. (2007) tracked changes in monaural CI users' perceived pitch and found that experience with the implant influenced pitch judgments over time. Three of five subjects who compared electrical stimuli to acoustic (in their better ear) displayed decreases in pitch matches of up to two octaves within 2 to 5 years of implant use. It should be noted that the changes in pitch were not always accompanied by similarly substantial changes in word recognition ability. The investigators indicated that mechanisms of peripheral processing that contributed to patients' pitch and frequency resolution, as well as intensity cues, could not on their own explain the observed changes in patient performance.

Perhaps a more dramatic piece of evidence supporting a dissociation between pitch perceptions with CIs was reported by Reiss et al. (2011) as a case study. A patient with profound high frequency hearing loss was implanted with a short, 10-mm electrode. Two years later, the patient's residual hearing in both ears was lost to an autoimmune disorder; the patient was implanted in the other ear with a full-length, 24-mm electrode. The differences in electrode length required distinct frequency allocations across electrode sites because the two electrodes terminated at substantially different cochlear locations. The patient was asked to compare the pitch of binaurally-presented electrical stimuli. Although the electrodes stimulating auditory nerves were of different length, their putative frequency coordinates in the cochlea allowed for predictions regarding pitch evaluations. Within three years after implantation of the second electrode, the investigators found a "large mismatch" between the cochlear locations assumed to be associated with the stimulus frequency and the resulting pitch sensation. That is, electrode pairs across the two ears that stimulated nerve fibers synapsing at substantially different cochlear regions ended up producing similar, matched, pitches in the two ears. The lack of correspondence between cochlear place and pitch suggested that CI recipients developed, from experience, adaptation strategies that relied upon central mechanisms in order to minimize or reconcile pitch/spectral differences between ears. Reiss et al. (2011) raised the interesting possibility that central mechanisms may "realign" disparate inputs, or abnormal pitch experiences, despite gross differences in cochlear areas and fiber populations stimulated. Indeed, the authors did not assert that the patient's adaptation had normalized pitch absolutely, but rather had developed the means to provide the kind of binaural fusion between the two ears discussed by van den Brink et al. (1976).

Management of Diplacusis

Management of diplacusis must consider the roles to pitch perception provided by both cochlear (i.e., place) and neural (i.e., timing) systems. Given that some degree of diplacusis is demonstrated by listeners who do not complain about the symptom, it is clear that the phenomenon is, at least in its least objectionable form, a by-product of normal auditory function. The well-established effects of listening experience, as described by Burns, Van den Brink, Reiss, and colleagues, provide hope that the diplacusis perceptions, although disturbing and perhaps career-changing, may not be permanent.

Because the majority of patients with diplacusis display hearing loss, specifically asymmetric high-frequency hearing loss, a hearing aid fit to the poorer ear should improve the situation by restoring audibility in the damaged frequency region. Unfortunately, hearing aids do not restore normal function, they merely amplify environmental sounds, and patients (such as the one examined below in case #1) report that the devices do not normalize pitch experiences. Although hearing aids may facilitate communication and localization of sound, they do not appear to reconcile the interaural differences in processing that generate two distinct pitch perceptions. This shortcoming of hearing aid fitting related to diplacusis complaints affects individuals regardless of their listening experience; musicians and non-musicians stand to receive similar benefit from hearing aid fitting, at least with regard to diplacusis complaints.

Musicians and music enthusiasts have a different set of listening experiences, and clearly a more personal relationship to music, than do non-musically inclined individuals. A person's relationship with music may be profound and cherished. Compromising or distorting that source of succor and enjoyment has the potential to ruin a life. Musicians faced with giving up their occupation often use brute force—memorization of muscle action that produces a pitch when singing, for example—in order to maintain their ability to perform or share music with peers. Such an adjustment is admirable, but frustrating to have to maintain, and many musicians curtail their activities as a result.

This situation is regrettable, particularly when we consider the importance of experience in the judgment of pitch. Age of hearing loss onset, and duration of hearing aid use, increase the likelihood that listeners will display binaural fusion across a wide range of frequencies (Reiss et al., 2017). This finding extends to Reiss and colleagues' work with patients who receive CIs in that fusion of two different tones presented to the ears occurs across a broad frequency range. Experience with devices, whether acoustic or electric, accesses or exploits plasticity in the auditory system that fuse pitch experiences for some listeners. Unfortunately, the range of frequencies through which fusion would occur in CI patients may be far greater than would be found with normal hearing listeners. Additionally, what is not clear at present is whether musicians or music lovers can exploit the fusion event to extract a pitch sensation that is accurate, or that improves the listeners' ability to practice, perform, and share music. Indeed, Reiss et al. (2016) reiterated previous reports that such fusion may actually reduce word recognition ability and lead to errors of absolute pitch judgment.

Cases

Two cases in which individuals with backgrounds in music are reviewed below. The first case involves a musician and composer, a piano player who has several recordings to his credit. Mr. C was first seen at our clinic in August 2015, at which time he was 81 years old. He served in the military, however, he reported his hearing as normal upon discharge. The patient's medical history includes type II diabetes which he indicated is controlled effectively.

The patient first noticed hearing loss in 2003, more pronounced in the left ear, and he completed a fitting with personal amplification. He used a standard hearing aid (no fitting information was available) monaurally for several years. In 2009 he was fit with a new device at a Veteran's hospital; however, throughout this time period, the patient was able to play, record, and perform music as a soloist as well as with different groups. In 2013, he was fit with a second hearing aid. It was shortly after that time that he began to notice changes in his hearing and in his ability to process pitch.

First, in the spring of 2014, on a Sunday night, he realized that he was struggling to distinguish musical notes. The notes sounded "fuzzy" and "noisy" but did not retain their pitch. However, if he played a note, one reportedly sustained for 30 to 45 seconds, the tonality would change, and the sensation of pitch would become more salient. He noticed that the severity of this problem changed day to day; there was no steady improvement, rather steps forward and backward over the course of several months.

He set about mapping the changes in pitch, and his findings were consistent with those reported by Schubert (1957) and others. Specifically, he observed that in the third octave above middle C, the note G was heard as A (that is, a full tone higher in pitch), and the sensation was obvious in the left ear. Other pitches in the same octave were similarly affected, but not to that degree. In the next octave up, the pitch sensation returned to normal for all notes. He assured us that his hearing had not changed since the time he noticed the pitch anomaly provided results from a recent audiogram.

Our time in the clinic focused on assessing specific pitch events rather than monitoring hearing. Upon completion of his intake interview, we asked whether the patient would be willing to spend some time in the audio suite "playing around." He brought with him a harmonica and was eager to experiment. First, we tried to determine whether the presence of a low-level masking noise presented to each ear in turn, and then bilaterally (both narrowband and white noise were used) would eliminate or modify the pitch perception; it did not. During this testing, the patient stated that his difficulties were most pronounced when listening to chords, or when trying to ascertain an interval separating notes. He also reported that he heard a minor third on occasion when sounding a single note, for example, when he played an E, he also heard a minor third, or a G, mixed in with the note he was playing. The patient indicated that this distortion occurred on occasion, but not at all times.

Upon interviewing the patient, it was clear that he was avoiding listening to and playing music that sounded abnormal and unpleasant to him, and he also reported that not all music produced the same response. However, he also admitted that he likely would not have noticed this event were it not for his experience with music. This final point was used as a way to help the patient shape his listening experiences and environment (see Chapter 15 for a sample listening protocol).

He was encouraged to find music that posed the minimum challenge to his enjoyment, and to try to increase his inventory of musical selections over time. Our intent was to facilitate the reintegration of music as a prime motivator and positive experience for this patient. He understood the logic of minimizing his attempts to shield himself from bothersome music (i.e., avoid avoidance), and rather to gravitate, over time, to passages that he anticipated would be difficult.

It is now two years from our initial contact. The patient reports his situation is less dire, but he is not back to where he was prior to the changes in hearing. He notes improvements not just with listening and playing music, but also with sound localization. He remains binaurally amplified, and still has a substantial asymmetric hearing loss. It is likely that this patient suffered from a sudden hearing loss sometime in the spring, 2014, that exacerbated his pre-existing loss. Perhaps the pre-existing loss, gradual in nature, had allowed for the patient to adjust unconsciously over time and to maintain reasonably accurate pitch judgments. The sudden change in 2014 likely did not recover fully, hence the patient's prior ability to adjust and manage the loss could not be repeated, producing the observed and durable changes in pitch processing. His case remains open and he will continue to be followed.

The second case centers on an individual (the chapter's author, MF) with little musical training, but a rich experience throughout his lifetime listening to and playing music. He hesitates to call himself a musician, rather, he plays bass. Until 2012, he had normal hearing bilaterally, but at about that time, he observed that he often could not hear the monitor tone from the audiometer through headphones at 6 to 8 kHz in only the right ear. Measures at that time revealed a mild, high frequency, asymmetric hearing loss. On March 15, 2016, that situation changed.

On the previous evening, the ear felt full, but not alarmingly so. During the night, however, with the left ear facing the pillow, the patient was startled when the family dog jumped on the bed. Normally, this event would be prefaced by the old dog getting a running start, scrambling across the floor, signaling the jump to come. However, on this night, the dog's nails on the floor were inaudible, hence the landing on the bed alarming.

Upon waking the next morning, it was clear that the right ear had experienced a substantial decrease in sensitivity. Running water, voices, the car, everything sounded foreign and unclear. MF was reminded of complaints he had heard in the clinic, of patients who stated that some voices sounded as though they were being spoken through cellophane; scratchy, tinny, crinkled, and distorted. While these patient impressions had, in such clinical encounters, been difficult to imagine, their veracity was now apparent.

A hearing test later that morning revealed a sensorineural hearing loss in the right ear with thresholds 10 to 30 dB worse than previously; thresholds at 4, 6, and 8 kHz were 55, 60, and 65 dB, respectively. As a patient, MF was seen later that day in a local ENT physician's office, and after an exam was prescribed prednisone. The balance of the day was spent at work, as the auditory event was not accompanied by vertigo, nor any other symptoms. Note that MF worked with the patient described above prior to the sudden hearing loss onset.

Following MF's brief experience with the patient described in case 1, he decided to experiment by listening to familiar music as a means to assess the effect of the sudden hearing loss on music appreciation. He picked an album that contained clear and simple vocal harmonies, but also distorted guitars in order to assess the effect of the hearing loss on the ability to resolve chords and accurately process complex and distorted signals. The music, as all sound at that time, sounded unusual although it remained familiar. Most striking, however, was the observation that when MF plugged his "good" ear, the pitch of the recording immediately changed, as though someone had modulated the frequency of all instruments and voices upward by approximately a full tone. This observation was repeated numerous times, including instances when MF sang along to the music with the poor ear plugged, then switched to plug the good ear, with the result that he observed the key in which he was singing was flat, or a lower pitch than the music. The process worked in reverse as well; he could plug the good ear, sing along, and when switching to plug the bad ear, his singing was now a full tone sharp as heard in the good ear. The change in pitch was immediate upon switching plugged ears, and when the maneuver was performed during an instrumental section prominently featuring guitar, the sound of the guitar changed as though the guitarist was using a so-called "whammy bar," which is a metal arm attached to the bridge of the instrument that increases or releases tension on the strings, thereby raising or lowering pitch, when it is pulled up or pressed down, respectively.

The sensation produced by sound during the next 48 hours can be described in many ways, and it was clear that a naïve patient could easily catastrophize the event. It was also clear that a person with a gratifying relationship with music would feel the change in hearing as a personal loss, perhaps a loss that compelled grieving, anger, or self-recrimination. Such were the patient narratives recalled by MF in the past; of course, at this point, such patient reports took on new meaning. Over the next few days, MF experimented with music, listening and playing. By the third day post-onset, hearing improved, and the sensation of diplacusis abated. Although the hearing did not return completely, the pitch sensation normalized.

The two cases illustrated common findings in patients with diplacusis: asymmetric hearing loss, sudden onset hearing loss, and an awareness of the disorder that was likely related to a person's listening experience. It is also likely that the patient who is able to coexist with the unusual sounds, and continue to accept exposures to such sounds, has the potential to experience improvement. Such advice, in lieu of an evidence-based cure, should be an important element of counseling and management.

References

Albers, G. D., & Wilson, W. H. (1968). Diplacusis. I. Historical review. *Arch Otolaryngol.*, *87*(6), 601–603.

Bachem, A. (1950). Tone height and tone chroma as two different pitch qualities. *Acta Psychologica*, *7*, 80–88.

Colin, D., Micheyl, C., Girod, A., Truy, E., & Gallégo, S. (2016). Binaural diplacusis and its relationship with hearing-threshold asymmetry. *PLoS ONE*, *11*(8), e0159975. doi:10.1371/journal.pone.0159975.

Gaeth, J. H., & Norris, T. W. (1965). Diplacusis in unilateral high-frequency hearing losses. *J. Speech Hear. Res.*, *8*, 63–75.

Gfeller, K., Turner, C., Mehr, M., Woodworth, G., Fearn, R., Knutson, J. F., . . . Stordahl, J. (2002). Recognition of familiar melodies by adult cochlear implant recipients and normal-hearing adults. *Cochlear Implants International*, *3*(1), 29–53. doi:10.1002/cii.50.

Goldstein, J. L. (1973). An optimum processor theory for the central formation of the pitch of complex tones. *J. Acou. Soc. Am.*, *54*, 1496–1516.

https://search.proquest.com/docview/878064162/fulltext/150F97DE184D49C0PQ/1?accountid=10771.

Jansen, E. J. M., Helleman, H. W., Dreschler, W. A., and de Laat, J. A. P. M. (2009). Noise induced hearing loss and other hearing complaints among musicians of symphony orchestras. *Int. Arch Occup. Environ. Health*, *82*, 153–164.

Jastreboff, P. J., & Jastreboff, M. M. (2015). Decreased sound tolerance: Hyperacusis, misophonia, diplacousis, and polyacousis. In G. G. Celesia & G. Hickok (Eds.). *Handbook of clinical neurology; the human auditory system*; Vol. 129 (3rd Series). Edinburgh, U.K.: Elsevier.

Knight, R. D. (2004). Diplacusis, hearing threshold and otoacoustic emissions in an episode of sudden, unilateral cochlear hearing loss. *International Journal of Audiology*, *43*, 45–53.

Licklider, J. C. R. (1951). Basic correlate of the auditory stimulus. In S. S. Stevens (Ed.). *Handbook of experimental psychology*. New York, NY: John Wiley & Sons.

Palmer, A. R., & Russell, I. J. (1986). Phase-locking in the cochlear nerve of the guinea pig and its relation to the receptor potential of inner hair cells. *Hearing Research*, *24*, 1–15.

Pantev, C., Elbert, T., Ross, B., Eulitz, C., & Terhardt, E. (1996). Binaural fusion and the representation of virtual pitch in the human auditory cortex. *Hearing Research*, *100*, 164–170.

Plomp, R. (1967). Pitch of complex tones. *J. Acou. Soc. Am.*, *41*, 1526–1533.

Reiss, L. A. J., Turner, C. W., Erenberg, S. R., & Gantz, B. J. (2007). Changes in pitch with a cochlear implant over time. *J. Assoc. Res. Otolaryngol.*, *8*(2), 241–257.

Reiss, L. A. J., Lowder, M. W., Karsten, S. A., Turner, C. W., & Gantz, B. J. (2011). Effects of extreme tonotopic mismatches between bilateral cochlear implants on electric pitch perception: a case study. *Ear Hear.*, *32*(4), 536–540. doi:10.1097/AUD.0b013e31820c81b0

Reiss, L. A. J., Eggleston, J. L., Walker, E. P., & Oh, Y. (2016). Two ears are not always better than one: Mandatory vowel fusion across spectrally mismatched ears in hearing-impaired listeners. *J. Assoc. Res. Otolaryng.*, *17*, 342–356. doi: 10.1007/s10162-016-0570-z

Reiss, L. A. J., Shayman, C. S., Walker, E. P., Bennett, K. O., Fowler, J. R., Hartling, C. L., . . . Oh, Y. (2017). Binaural pitch fusion: Comparisons of normal-hearing and hearing-impaired listeners. *J. Acoust. Soc. Am.*, *141*(3), 1909–1920.

Rhode, W. S. (1971). Observations of the vibration of the basilar membrane in squirrel monkeys using the Mossbaurer technique. *J. Acoust. Soc. Am.*, *49*, 1218–1231.

Schouten, J. F., Ritsma, R. J., & Cardozo, B. L. (1962). Pitch of the residue. *J. Acou. Soc. Am.*, *34*, 1418–1424.

Schubert, K. (1957). "On pathological pitch perception," in *Translations of the Beltone Institute for Hearing Research*, edited by C. Lightfoot. Beltone Institute for Hearing Research; Chicago, IL Vol. 5, pp. 1–12.

Shambaugh, G. E. Jr. (1940). Diplacusis: A localizing symptom of disease of the organ of Corti. *Arch. Otol.*, *31*, 160.

Shambaugh, G. E. Jr. (1959). *Surgery of the ear*. Philadelphia, PA: WB Saunders.

Terhardt, E. (1974). Pitch, consonance, and harmony. *J. Acou. Soc. Am.*, *55*, 1061–1069.

van den Brink, G. (1974). Monotic and dichotic pitch matchings with complex sounds. In E. Zwicker & E. Terhardt (Eds.). *Facts and models in hearing* (pp. 178–188). Berlin, Germany: Springer.

van den Brink, G., Sintnicolaas, K., & van Stam, W. S. (2017). Dichotic pitch fusion. *J. Acoust. Soc. Am.*, *59*, 1471–1476.

Ward, W. D. (1963). Diplacusis and auditory theory. *J. Acou. Soc. Am.*, *35*, 1746–1747.

SECTION IV

Management

13

Increased Sound Sensitivity in Children

Veronica Kennedy, Claire Benton, and Rosie Kentish

Introduction

Increased sensitivity to sounds, often termed hyperacusis, is a common experience for many children. For most children affected, this is a transient problem lasting for the duration of the sounds, for others it can be a distressing experience which limits the child's activities and those of the child's family. There is currently no consensus on the definition of hyperacusis. Nevertheless, different writers have converged on similar terminology, such as "an unusual (low) loudness discomfort level associated with annoyance from normal sounds" (Coelho, Sanchez, & Tyler 2007), "an abnormal lowered tolerance to sound" (Baguley & Andersson, 2007), an "increased sensitivity to sound in levels that would not trouble a normal individual" (Katzenell & Segal, 2001), or simply "a heightened awareness of sounds" (Phillips & Carr, 1998). Jastreboff and Jastreboff (2014) proposed two components of what they termed decreased sound tolerance (DST): the first, hyperacusis, was described as a negative reaction to the physical characteristics of a sound, and the second, misophonia, was described as an abnormally strong reaction to a sound with a specific pattern and/or meaning to an individual. Klein (1990) also used a definition describing the reaction to sound rather than the perception of sound as, "consistently exaggerated or inappropriate responses to sounds that are neither threatening nor uncomfortably loud to a typical person."

The lack of a consensus about a definition is likely a reflection of the heterogeneity of the symptoms associated with hyperacusis. Phillips and Carr (1998) proposed that disturbances in loudness perception could arise from a variety of physical and psychological sources, and that the differences in underlying pathophysiology would be reflected behaviorally.

The above definitions imply that hyperacusis arises from a disordered process, whereas in the case of young children, sensitivity to sounds may be an element of developmental or maturational experience which normalizes as the child gets older. Misophonia, loudness recruitment, which is an abnormally steep loudness growth for given increments in stimulus intensity, and is pathognomic of cochlear hearing loss (Phillips & Carr, 1998) and sound-provoked seizures (Tibussek, 2006) are explored in Chapter 8. In this chapter we will consider the effects of hyperacusis on children by defining hyperacusis as an increased sensitivity to routinely experienced sounds resulting in distress to the child or an adverse impact on the activities of the child.

Prevalence of Hyperacusis in Children

While the prevalence within a general school-aged population is reported as between 3.2 and 17.1%, the prevalence can be much higher, up to 95%, in specific populations. This variation may be explained by the ways in which children were questioned about their experiences, the definitions used by the investigators, the setting of the studies, the number of children involved, the age of the studied population, study tools, and associated conditions (Table 13–1). For example, in a study on children with Williams syndrome, Klein, Armstrong, and Greer (1990) reported a prevalence of hyperacusis of 95%. Other studies investigating children with autism spectrum disorder (ASD) reported prevalence that varied between 18% and 50% (Rosenhall et al., 1999; Hall et al., 2015).

Different age ranges have been used across the studies of children with hyperacusis. In the studies across the entire pediatric age range (0 to 19 years), the commonest age of presentation was 3 to 4 years (Settal, 2009; Myne & Kennedy, 2017). There was no consistent reported gender effect. In some studies (Coelho et al., 2007; Widen & Erlandsson, 2004), females comprised the majority of children with hyperacusis. Conversely, Hall et al. (2015), Myne and Kennedy (2017), and Settal (2009) reported a higher proportion of males with hyperacusis. Some of these differences may relate to the developmental status of the child. Developmental problems such as ASD tend to be more common in males and children thus affected may not be proportionately represented in a mainstream school study.

Associated Conditions

While hyperacusis can occur in isolation, many associated conditions have been reported in pediatric and adult populations. While adults demonstrate a high association between tinnitus and hyperacusis, less information is available in the pediatric population. Hall et al. (2015) reported that 41.9% of the children with hyperacusis also had tinnitus. Coelho et al. (2007) reported 50% of children with hyperacusis had tinnitus, while tinnitus was present in 17.8% of the children without hyperacusis. In a study on children with tinnitus, Baguley et al. (2013) reported that 39% had hyperacusis. Hearing loss has been associated with hyperacusis including conductive hearing loss due to otitis media with effusion (OME) (Coelho et al., 2007; Myne & Kennedy, 2017), and high frequency hearing loss seen in Williams syndrome (Klein et al., 1990; Miani et al., 2001; Levitin et al., 2005) or after exposure to loud music (Rodrigues et al., 2015; Landälv, Malmström, & Widén, 2013). Acoustic trauma (Remenschneider et al., 2014) and semicircular canal dehiscence (Thabet, 2014) have also been reported.

Additional medical conditions associated with hyperacusis are summarized in Chapter 7 and include migraine (Tkachuk et al., 2003), Bell's palsy (Lee et al., 2013), Lowe syndrome (Recker et al., 2015), and Laron syndrome (Attias et al., 2012). Associated neurodevelopmental conditions include ASD (Gomes, Rotta, Pedroso, Sleifer, & Danesi, 2004; Hall et al., 2015; Khalfa et al., 1999), Fragile X syndrome

Table 13–1. Overview of studies of hyperacusis in children.

	Prevalence	Age Range	No of Children (with Hyperacusis/ in Study)	Study Tools	Associated Conditions
Coelho et al. (2007)	Bothered by sound; 42% Hyperacusis 3.2% Phonophobia 9%	5–12 years;	16/499	Interview (child), questionnaire (parents) otoscopy, tympanometry, audiometry, LDLs	Tinnitus, otitis media with effusion
Khalfa et al. (2004)	63%	9–17 years	11/11	LDLs	Autistic spectrum disorder
Klein et al. (1990)	95%	1–28 years Mean age: 8 years	65/65	Questionnaire to parents	Williams syndrome
Hall et al. (2015)	3.68%	11 years	261/7093	Interview (child), audiometry, tympanometry, acoustic reflexes, otoacoustic emissions (OAE)	In the 29 children with Autistic spectrum disorder, 41.4% had hyperacusis
Myne & Kennedy (2017)	–	0–19 years	61 children with hyperacusis	Interview, audiometry, tympanometry, oto-acoustic emissions	Autistic spectrum disorder, cerebral palsy, ADHD, glue ear
Oen et al. (1997)	50%	0–6 months	25/50 Control: 19	Interview, questionnaire	Spina bifida
Rosenhall (1999)	18%	8 years	111/57	ABR, audiometry	Autistic spectrum disorder
Sattar (2009)	–	0–16 years Peak age 3–4 years	100 children with hyperacusis and no hearing loss	Interview, audiometry, tympanometry, oto-acoustic emissions	Autistic spectrum disorder, ADHD, meningitis, migraine, perinatal problems related to prematurity
Widen & Erlandsson (2004)	17.1%	13–19 years	220/1285	Questionnaire	Tinnitus

(Mott & Sun, 2014), ADHD (Mangeot et al., 2001), and spina bifida (Oen, Begeer, Staal-Schreinemachers, & Tijmstra, 1997). Hyperacusis has also been reported with problems associated with prematurity including cerebral palsy and hydrocephalus (Sattar, 2009; Myne & Kennedy, 2017).

Presenting Symptoms

Most children disturbed by sounds respond by covering their ears for the duration of the sound. Others can get quite distressed, report pain in the ears, cry, or run away from the sound, heedless of danger (Gomes et al., 2004; Sattar, 2009; Myne & Kennedy, 2017). In some cases, a phobic response occurs and the child seeks to avoid situations in which the distressing sound may be present, often with marked disruption to their family's day-to-day life (Klein et al., 1990; Stiegler & Davis, 2010; Hall et al., 2015; Myne & Kennedy, 2017). The troublesome sounds include children shouting or screaming, alarms, sirens, hand or hair dryers, vacuum cleaners, and traffic (Coelho et al., 2007; Myne & Kennedy, 2017). Hall et al. (2015) reported 42.9% of the children with hyperacusis displayed avoidance behaviors. Similarly, Stansfield (1992) investigated highly noise-sensitive and low noise-sensitive women and observed that individuals who reported greater sensitivity tended to pay more attention to sounds, were more likely to perceive sounds as threatening, and reported less control over potentially disturbing situations. There are similarities with findings seen in the pediatric population, particularly those children with ASD. While the child is generally not averse to making noise, it is the unpredictability of a sound made by others or the lack of control over a sound that can cause distress. As an example, consider the 8-year-old child who reports needing to frequently monitor the clock in class so as not to be surprised by the school bell.

The child's reactions to sounds can have a substantial impact on the child's activity and the activities of the family (Carter, Ben-Sasson, & Briggs-Gowan, 2011). Household chores such as vacuuming or shopping may be deferred until the child is absent. Outings may be avoided or limited because of the child's refusal to use a public bathroom in case someone switches on the hand dryer. The refusal to use a public bathroom can in turn lead to wetting. The avoidance behavior may influence the child's development of social skills and friendships as playgrounds and cafeterias are avoided (Stiegler & Davis, 2010; Myne & Kennedy, 2017). In a misguided attempt to help, ear defenders are sometimes provided to these children by parents or teachers (Stiegler & Davis, 2010; Hall et al., 2015; Myne & Kennedy, 2017) who are unaware of the negative impact that this can have on central auditory gain (see Chapters 6 and 8).

Categorizing Hyperacusis in Children

Based on the different presentations of hyperacusis in children, we propose the following categories of possible mechanisms:

- Immature but normally developing auditory system
- Temporary auditory deprivation
- Disorder within the auditory system
- Disorder of sensory processing

The categories are not exclusive as, in some children, there may be a combination of mechanisms across categories, for example, hyperacusis in a child with Williams syndrome and otitis media with effusion.

Immature but Normally Developing Auditory System

Although hyperacusis is commonly seen in young children, its presence and impact typically decrease over time. This suggests either habituation to the troublesome sounds or an auditory developmental process that requires maturation and experience. Moore (2002) reported that myelination of the thalamic fibers of the thalamocortical auditory system progresses from ages 1 to 4 years old with further axonal myelination through to ages 5 to 10 years. The maturation process also contributes to improvements in auditory sensitivity thresholds. Fior and Bolzonello (1982) reported maturation of intensity discrimination through at least 10 years of age. Trehub, Schneider, and Endman (1980) reported development as a gradual process throughout childhood with maturation in high frequency regions (4 and 10 kHz) before age 5 years but after 10 years of age for 1 kHz. Another developmental mechanism may be the maturation of sensory gating, the process the brain uses to inhibit "distracting," or non-relevant auditory information (Davies, Chang, & Gavin, 2009) which occurs between ages 7 and 13 years. During this age range, there is also progressive maturation of the frontal cortex resulting in a decrease in susceptibility to interference from irrelevant environmental stimuli (Marshall, Bar-Haim, & Fox, 2004).

Møller and Rollins (2001) studied the nonclassical auditory pathways involved in loudness perception in children. These pathways respond to somatosensory as well as auditory stimuli and project to different regions of the brain including the limbic system and the amygdala. Because the limbic system is involved with emotional reactions and the amygdala controls the fight or flight response, this pathway may explain the severity with which a child sometimes responds to aversive sounds. The involvement of these pathways in routine auditory processing diminishes with increasing age through childhood.

Temporary Auditory Deprivation

Reduced sound input, even from a temporary cause, can lead to an increase in central auditory gain as spontaneous and sound-evoked firing rates increase (Pienkowski et al., 2014). In children, the most common cause of temporary hearing loss is otitis media with effusion. While some children and their parents express relief if the child is less sensitive to sounds during a period of active infection, there may be an increase in hyperacusis once the condition resolves. Increased central auditory gain may result from pathology-related deprivation that appears to "turn up" the subjective loudness of sounds. Nigam and Samuel (1994) reported that 47% of children complained of hyperacusis after ventilation tubes were inserted to treat chronic otitis media with effusion. The hyperacusis was of varying degrees and lasted between 2 and 40 days. Temporary auditory deprivation may also lead to hyperacusis by other mechanisms. Based on a study of young rats, Sun et al. (2011) proposed that conductive hearing loss may impair sound tolerance by reducing GABA-related inhibition in the inferior colliculus. Therefore, changes in loudness tolerance may be viewed as a manifestation of reduced central inhibition in addition to the aforementioned central gain. Deprivation can also influence the processing of sounds in the auditory brainstem and temporarily lower acoustic reflex thresholds (Formby, Sherlock, & Gold, 2003; Munro, Turtle, & Schaette, 2014).

Disorder Within the Auditory System

In addition to transient changes in hearing sensitivity, disorders involving the peripheral and/or central auditory systems can play a role in hyperacusis. Peripheral dysfunction includes, for example, the high frequency hearing loss seen in children with Williams syndrome (Gothelf et al., 2006). In response to the peripheral auditory dysfunction, the central auditory system processing may change in ways consistent with increased auditory gain and/or decreased inhibition. As increased central gain is also thought to be one of the mechanisms for tinnitus, such processing changes may explain the co-morbidity of hyperacusis and tinnitus (Coelho et al., 2007; Baguley et al., 2013). Other studies have found the stapedial reflexes to be deficient or of reduced amplitude (Klein et al., 1990; Katzenell & Segal, 2001; Gothelf et al., 2006), or that hyperacusis may be due to impairment of the auditory efferent system (Phillips & Carr, 1998; Attias et al., 2008).

Regarding the central auditory system, Matsuzakiet et al. (2012) proposed that the primary auditory cortex was the focal site promoting sensitivity to sounds in children with ASD. Using a magnetoencephalographic assessment, they reported that children diagnosed with ASD had significantly delayed M50/M100 peak latencies suggesting neurological immaturity or functional abnormalities. Funabiki, Murai, and Toichi (2012) used changes in blood oxygenated hemoglobin (OxyHb) measured using fMRI in the prefrontal and temporal cortices to determine a hyperacusis locus. They proposed that the affected areas were not in the auditory but in the prefrontal region, a finding that could account for the selective listening (or inattention) to some sounds and sensitivity to others. Marriage and Barnes (1995) proposed that the neurotransmitter serotonin (5HT) may be implicated in hyperacusis as this neurotransmitter inhibits modulation of central responses to sensory stimuli. It must also be noted, however, that both increased and decreased serotonin levels have been noted to produce a heightened startle response in animals (Fletcher et al., 2001).

Disorder of Sensory Processing

Hyperacusis may also be related to sensory processing disorders involving modalities other than hearing. Problems in the sensory gating system, perhaps associated with delayed maturation, can lead to difficulties with selective inhibition of irrelevant or distracting information (Davies et al., 2009). This in turn can result in the processing of inappropriate sensory stimuli or difficulty with integrating sensory stimuli. Hall et al. (2017) reported that many children with hyperacusis also had other sensory sensitivities. Sensitivity to light/colors was noted in 8.4% while sensitivity to touch, smell, taste, and pain were 6.5%, 5.4%, 3.8%, and 3.5%, respectively. Sensory processing or modulation disorders have been widely reported in children particularly those with developmental disabilities. Ben-Sasson and Carter (2009) noted that sensory over-responsivity (SOR), a sensory modulation disorder manifested by intense behavioral responses, interfered with routine activities in 5 to 16% of school age children. SOR was also described in children with a range of neurodevelopmental conditions (Adamson, O'Hare, and Graham, 2006; Mangeot et al., 2001; Rogers, Hepburn, & Wehner, 2003). The children with SOR may experience a "sensory overload" effect in situations where there are a number of sensory stimuli such as the auditory, visual, tactile, olfactory stimuli of a children's party. Parents of children with SOR reported many restrictions in family life (Carter et al., 2011). Møller and Rollins (2001) suggested that failure of maturation of the non-classical auditory pathways may account for some of the sensory symptoms seen in children with developmental disorders.

Assessment

It is important to conduct a thorough interview with the child and family to elicit the main reason(s) they are seeking help. The key, however, is doing this in a manner that encourages the child to engage in the consultation (Tinnitus in Children Practice Guidance, 2015). Information gathering should include details about the troublesome noises, the situations the child finds troublesome, reactions of the child and family, and the impact on the child and family. Although there is no validated hyperacusis questionnaire for children, an estimation of the level of severity can be obtained by applying the following descriptors to the response to the troublesome sounds:

- Level 1: Dislike of sounds
- Level 2: Distress caused by sounds
- Level 3: Fear of sounds with anticipatory anxiety or avoidance of situations where the troublesome sounds may be present

It is important to determine whether the child experiences other sensory problems, as well as to identify coping strategies that have been helpful or unhelpful. If the family members have already accommodated the child's challenges, then it is important to note the degree to which their routine has been restricted or has changed. It may be relevant to explore the hyperacusis in other settings such as school or during extracurricular activities. It is also important to note the use of safety behaviors, such as avoidance of situations or the use of ear defenders, as these are often unhelpful in the long run. Background information should include audiological/otological history, medical history (medical conditions, developmental disorders), and educational history (progress, additional academic support accessed or needed).

Audiological Assessment

Each child should have a full audiological assessment to determine their hearing thresholds and middle ear status using age- and ability-appropriate techniques in a suitable pediatric setting. Children with hyperacusis may be anxious about testing, so clinicians should be prepared to allow plenty of time. Because the audiology test suite may seem foreign or unnerving, pediatric patients benefit from clear instructions and reassurance to support their confidence regarding the test protocol. Creating a friendly environment for the child and family should improve the reliability of test results.

Determining uncomfortable loudness levels (ULLs) in the assessment of hyperacusis in adults is commonplace; however, in their review, Fackrell, Fearnley, Hoare, and Sereda (2015) conclude that the evidence for their use is mixed. The test-retest reliability of ULLs is questionable in adults (Baguley & Andersson, 2007), and it is likely to be more so in children. Because the management strategies for a child with hyperacusis are based on the impact of their symptoms, such as the "distress," "dislike," and "fear" indicated above, establishing ULLs may add little to the management plan. It also seems somewhat unfair at best, and cruel at worst, to ask a child, who has come to the clinic because of sound-provoked distress, to sit and listen to loud sounds; the role of the audiologist relies at least in part on the practitioner's ability to build a relationship of trust with that child.

Management Strategies

Following assessment of auditory status and the behavioral impacts of hyperacusis, the management plan to be implemented will depend on the age and the developmental stage and/or cognitive ability of the child as well as the impact of hyperacusis on the child and family. The initial step should be to provide a clear explanation of hyperacusis. The framework of the Child Friendly Tinnitus Model (Emond & Kentish, 2013) can be adapted to hyperacusis and used as a basis for counseling and management. For some families, an explanation may be all that is needed; this can include exploring how anxiety and the child's sound sensitivity may reinforce one another and lead to negative emotions and avoidance behaviors. Part of the management process is to enable the child and/or family to develop expectations and strategies that are meaningful to them. Usually reassurances can be given that the level of sounds to which the child is sensitive will not harm the child's hearing. This can allay both child and parental anxiety.

Although the use of ear defenders or ear plugs to reduce the volume of sounds seems to be commonsense to those seeing a child distressed by loud sounds, this strategy should be actively discouraged. Evidence shows that the ensuing auditory deprivation, although well-intentioned, can actually sensitize the auditory system (Munro & Blount, 2009). It can be difficult to explain to families that a strategy that offers apparent instant relief to their child is possibly exacerbating the problem. If a child has become reliant on the wearing of ear defenders, a careful consideration of the child's activities and interests is needed to reduce their use while minimizing the child's anxiety. However, when hyperacusis is related to very loud sounds such as class music lessons (Rodrigues et al., 2015), school discos, or other noisy events, advice on noise risk reduction should be provided, and, in these situations, it may be appropriate to use ear defenders.

It is important that the strategies set for any child are achievable for that child and family and are consistently applied both at home and at school or nursery. This often involves a multidisciplinary approach to ensure that all caregivers are using similar strategies. The aim is to improve a child's confidence around the sounds that cause distress and to give the child a sense of control over the situation. In the case of a young child or a child with developmental delay, it can be particularly helpful to involve the child in the activities related to the sound, for example, leading the class in starting and stopping a singing activity, or ringing the school bell, as this can help maintain a sense of control. Another strategy is to divert the child's attention from the sound to something that might be of interest, perhaps the reason for the sound, or a characteristic of the sound ("That's the bell for lunch. I wonder what's for lunch? What do you think it will be?" "Do you think that siren is from an ambulance or police car? Let's see."). In situations where multiple sensory stimuli can be overwhelming, such as a birthday party, the child may be helped to focus attention on something manageable ("Let's find John and play with him, can you see him?"). Older children may be able to engage in rationalizing the impact of sounds, such as the necessity for some sounds (e.g., alarms) to be loud even if they are unpleasant. When possible, engage the child's cooperation in the development of coping strategies that will meaningful and effective for that child; such interactions can sometimes uncover great imaginative skills on the part of the child.

Relaxation Strategies for Children

Relaxation techniques can support coping strategies and enable a child to change their behavior around the sounds causing distress. Such techniques can be useful in situations in which these sounds are anticipated as well as to help children to become calm when startled. Relaxation can be a useful adjunct in supporting desensitization strategies. There are a variety of resources that may help develop age or ability appropriate relaxation techniques, and different families will have different preferences as to what suits them. It is important to note that children and families will need support in the monitoring of using these techniques to ensure they are successful. Breathing exercises can be carried out in a variety of situations, and, once learned, can be useful in reducing symptoms associated with anxiety. For example, for younger children, the simple exercise of blowing bubbles can be used, whereas older children can, with practice, learn diaphragm or deep breathing techniques. Again, a variety of resources are available to help with this.

Sound Therapy/Wide Band Sound Generators

A formal desensitization approach can be difficult for some children and families. Desensitization may be impaired because of difficulty engaging with strategies that address anxiety or because the child is affected by a substantial developmental or language delay. In such cases, clinicians may find it helpful to try the option of sound/wideband noise generators (WNG). Despite the lack of unequivocal supporting evidence, the use of WNG in adults with hyperacusis is common and often beneficial to the patient. The use of WNGs may improve the child's ability to tolerate the problematic sounds by modifying auditory system activity associated with hyperacusis. Formby et al. (2003) reported improved sound tolerance after 2 weeks of exposure to a moderate (50 dB SPL) level of noise. The exact mechanisms at work in that research were not clear; however, the use of such devices may help improve a child's sense of control over a situation, such as school, where the option of moving away from the sound source might not possible.

WNGs are worn either at ear level or behind-the-ear, similar to hearing aids, and are widely available. It is important to fit them with a large vent, an open ear mold, or with a slim tube, open-fit, as the child needs access to all external sounds. Binaural fitting is recommended as the hyperacusis is rarely attributed to just one ear. It is also important to ensure the child can still hear normal speech while wearing the devices. The volume of the WNG should be set at a just audible level and if the child is able to manage it, the volume control can be activated. There are no published guidelines describing how a child should use the WNG, however, support can be requested from the audiologist or the companies providing the devices.

Case Example

James was 6 years old when he first came to the clinic; he was having difficulty tolerating noise in school. He had a complex medical history and high levels of anxiety. After trying some behavioral techniques, it was decided James needed further support as his anxiety around school remained difficult to manage. He was fitted with bilateral WNGs on slim tubes, with the wide band noise set at an output of 55 dB SPL. He wore them all day at school and found his ability to cope much improved. In particular, when there was building work near his classroom, he was still able to comfortably take part in lessons. His parents felt that the WNGs gave James a sense that he could do something for himself. This helped him manage his hyperacusis and in turn improved his confidence in situations he found difficult.

Psychological Approaches to Hyperacusis Management

Management approaches for adults with hyperacusis typically include components of education, sound therapy, and counseling. In a recent randomized, controlled trial, cognitive behavior therapy (CBT) was found to be a promising intervention (Jüris, Andersson, Larsen, & Ekselius, 2014). To date, psychological approaches to hyperacusis management in children have not been evaluated, but clinically, both adults and children with hyperacusis often describe similar responses to sound: annoyance, distress, fear, sensations of pain, belief that sound exposure will harm them, and avoidance of sounds and contexts in which offending sounds occur. Given the similarities in presentation between adults and children, it is reasonable to assume that as part of a multidisciplinary approach to the management of hyperacusis, CBT will benefit children and adolescents too, particularly when there is an element of sound-related fear or anxiety. CBT has been shown to be effective in reducing a range of psychological difficulties, including chronic pain in children and adolescents (Ecclestone, Morley, Wiliams, Yorke, & Mastroyannopoulou, 2002; Velleman, Stallard, & Richardson, 2010) and as a treatment for fears and anxiety in children (Davis et al., 2011).

With children, any intervention approach must take into consideration developmental factors. Typically, younger children require an approach focused more upon behaviors and their management than older children who are better able to manage a combined cognitive behavioral approach. Parental support is essential, as is the involvement of a child's school when hyperacusis is experienced in that context. Baguley and Andersson (2007) describe a CBT approach for patients reporting hyperacusis. This includes identifying safety behaviors, relaxation methods, advice regarding sound and sound levels, graded exposure to everyday sounds, and goal setting. In CBT, the cognitive component involves identifying and challenging thoughts and responses, for example, that the feared sound is associated with danger.

From a behavioral perspective, specific fears and phobias are often maintained because of an avoidance of exposure to the feared stimuli. As a result, there is no opportunity for a child to learn that, over time, their fear can diminish if they do not avoid or try to escape the sounds, and that the outcomes they dread often do not come true or are not as terrible as imagined. Fear-provoked avoidance occurs when a patient does not enter a situation at all or enters the situation but chooses not to experience it fully. Exposure therapy is often considered an important therapeutic ingredient in CBT to address fears and anxiety. Such therapy can take many forms but most commonly involves gradually exposing individuals to a hierarchy of feared stimuli, starting with the less threatening ones and progressing to more challenging ones until the stimuli are well tolerated. This approach, employing "small manageable steps," is referred to in self-efficacy training as "mastery experience" through which a patient becomes more confident, following small victories, that the aversive situation can be managed acceptably. Imaginal exposure combines the use of fear-evoking images and thoughts with in-vivo exposure to actual feared stimuli in real life. In systematic desensitization the exposure is paired with relaxation or another physiologic state that is incompatible with fear in order to decrease the fear response. Some children, and/or their parents, report apprehension that the troublesome sound will damage hearing, and they cannot tolerate such fear or the pain caused by offending sounds. These thoughts can be challenged by gradually and carefully exposing the child to mildly troublesome or feared sounds to confront the inaccurate beliefs as the child finds the sounds can be tolerated. As the child learns to tolerate sounds, it builds confidence in the ability to tolerate other sounds the child fears or finds painful. This newfound self-confidence is empowering and an important tool in the process of change.

In systematic desensitization with children, therapy involves a number of steps:

> *Step one*: Identifying a hierarchy of feared sounds, with those most easily tolerated at the bottom and those most disliked or feared at the top. Parent, therapist, and child develop this together, and the younger the child, the greater the amount of guidance required. Children often understand and like this approach when it is presented as a ladder, with the most easily tolerated sounds placed on the lower rungs, and those most disliked and feared toward the top. When children are asked to rate sounds again during the course of treatment or at the end of treatment, this image also provides a simple and useful pre- and post-treatment measure, with progress identified as sounds move down the ladder.
>
> *Step two*: Learning relaxation and coping strategies. Children are taught simple relaxation techniques and other coping strategies, such as identifying and maintaining positive thoughts that can be used when exposed to the feared stimuli (sound). Younger children often rely upon the use of imaginary characters or "superheroes" to help them manage their anxiety or combat fears during exposure (Bouchard, Mendlowitz, Coles, & Franklin, 2004). It is essential that relaxation techniques or other coping strategies are fully mastered before the child is exposed to the troublesome sounds.
>
> *Step three*: A graded, step-by-step exposure to the sound or feared stimuli. This may be accomplished first through imaging the feared stimuli, looking at pictures, listening to the sound on the computer at gradually increasing levels and, finally, in-vivo exposure to the real sound while the child utilizes relaxation and other coping strategies to help them manage fear and anxiety. Again, it is important for the child to be involved wherever possible in drawing up the steps, starting with ones that they identify as easily manageable and can succeed at.

In practice, these techniques can be extremely effective in cases when sound hypersensitivity is combined with a high level of fear and anxiety. The exposure technique for use with children is described in detail by Bouchard et al. (2004). They stress the importance of making the treatment fun and playful, establishing a strong rapport with the child, ensuring that the child is motivated to undertake this challenging work, and rewarded for progress made. Directly observing a sound exposure gives important information not only about the child's response, but also about the parent's behavior; the latter may unintentionally convey fear themselves, or reinforce avoidance behavior. Desensitization can fail if relaxation or coping strategies are not firmly established; if the initial goal is too difficult, then the resulting failure may make the child reluctant to participate further. Progressing through the hierarchy of goals too fast and before each step has been mastered also risks the child's anxiety becoming overwhelming. Bouchard et al. (2004) stress that practice and repetition of each step are the keys to success. In each situation, the child should be able to persevere long enough that their feared beliefs can be tested out and evaluated. Finally, it is important to remember that there are some sounds such as school bells that will remain intolerably painful for a child with hyperacusis and that repeated exposure to these situations would be unethical. In such cases, alternative ways of supporting the child must be established.

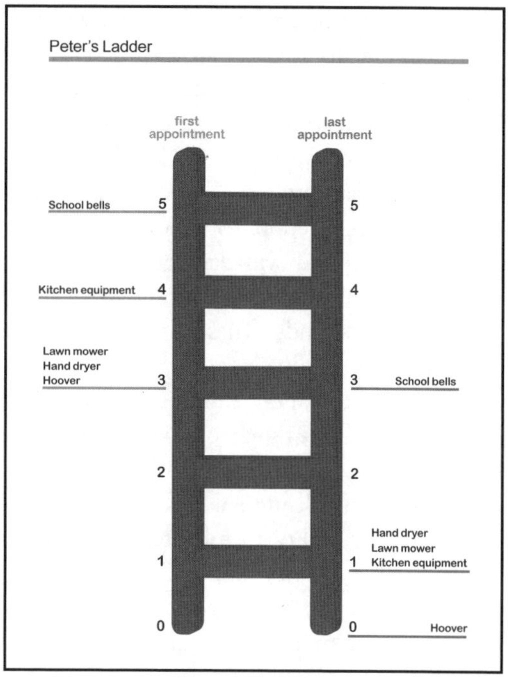

Figure 13–1. Peter's ladder. *Source*: © Medical Illustration RNTNEH 020 3456 5103 Unique Code: 33205. Reprinted with permission from University College London Hospitals NHS Foundation Trust.

Case Example

Nine-year-old Peter described pain and fear in response to a range of sounds including "hoovers," lawnmowers, kitchen food processors, and school bells. His mother made sure that he was not exposed to these sounds at home and at school he wore ear defenders for much of the day, and sometimes avoided going to school altogether. If he did hear any of these sounds he would "go into meltdown" because he believed these sounds would damage his hearing. Peter and his therapist drew up a ladder or hierarchy of sounds (Figure 13–1) from those that he would find easiest to tolerate to those he found most difficult. Hoovers were placed at the bottom of his ladder and we agreed to start with this. The first desensitization goal was then broken down into smaller steps, with Peter first looking at the hoover when not working, then standing upstairs in the house while his mother hoovered for 5 minutes and gradually moving downstairs and finally into the room where his mother was "hoovering." To acknowledge his work passing each step, Peter was given his chosen reward, picture cards of his favorite football team players. Peter was taught some simple relaxation techniques and some coping thoughts ("I can do this," "I'm brave," "Remember, the sound won't damage my ears") were written onto small cards which he kept in his pocket as a reminder. Peter and his mother practiced every day, and after two weeks, Peter had not only overcome his fear of hoovers, but was able to do the hoovering for his mother. Peter and his mother then went on to apply the same techniques to lawnmowers and kitchen appliances. At school, and with support from his teachers, Peter was able to tolerate the sound of the school bell without his headphones, provided he was given notice of when the school bell was to go off and he was not standing too close to it.

Conclusion

Hyperacusis can be distressing for children and their families. There is a need for prospective studies in children to explore underlying mechanisms and effective management techniques. However, despite the lack of validated assessment tools or outcome measures, there is a lot that can be done to help children who are distressed by sounds. An awareness of the different categories of hyperacusis can guide discussions on prognosis and management plans. Children who have an immature but normally-developing auditory system are likely to "outgrow" the problem. Those with wider sensory issues are likely to have a more persistent course and require a multimodal approach including sound therapy, behavioral and/or desensitization strategies. It is important to have a holistic approach to management, selecting aims that are acceptable and achievable with a consistent approach to be used across all the child's environments, such as home and school. It is also important to engage the child and family in the management process. While children may present with a range of hyperacusis-related problems, after appropriate explanations and guidance, it is often the children who come up with the most successful strategies. Being mindful of the concerns of the child and family and incorporating strategies meaningful to them is important in the development of an effective management plan.

References

Adamson, A., O'Hare, A., & Graham, C. (2006). Impairments in sensory modulation in children with autistic spectrum disorder. *Br. J. Occup. Ther.*, *69*(8), 57–364.

Anari, M., Axelsson, A., Eliasson, A., & Magnusson, L. (1999). Hypersensitivity to sound. Questionnaire data, audiometry, and classification. *Scand. Audiol.*, *28*, 219–230.

Attias, J., Raveh, E., Ben-Naftali, N. F., Zarchi, O., & Gothelf, D. (2008). Hyperactive auditory efferent system and lack of acoustic reflexes in Williams syndrome. *J. Basic Clin. Physiol. Pharmacol.*, *19*(3–4), 193–207.

Attias, J., Zarchi, O., Nageris, B. I., & Laron, Z. (2012). Cochlear hearing loss in patients with Laron syndrome. *European Archives of Oto-Rhino-Laryngology*, *269*(2), 461–466.

Baguley, D., & Andersson, G. (2007). *Hyperacusis: Mechanisms, diagnosis, and therapies.* San Diego, CA: Plural.

Baguley, D. M., Bartnik, G., Kleinjung, T., Savastano, M., & Hough, E. A. (2013). Troublesome tinnitus in childhood and adolescence: Data from expert centres. *Int. J. Pediatr. Otorhinolaryngol.*, *77*(2), 248–251.

Ben-Sasson, A., Carter, A. S., & Briggs-Gowan, M. J. (2009). Sensory over-responsivity in elementary school: Prevalence and social-emotional correlates. *J. Abnorm. Child Psychol.*, *37*(5), 705–716.

Bouchard, S., Mendlowitz, S. L., Coles, M.E., & Franklin, M. (2004). Considerations in the use of exposure with children. *Cognitive and Behavioural Practice*, *11*, 56–65.

British Society of Audiology. (2015). *Tinnitus in children: Practice guidance.* Retrieved from http://www.thebsa.org.uk/.

Carter, A. S., Ben-Sasson, A., & Briggs-Gowan, M. J. (2011). Sensory over-responsivity, psychopathology, and family impairment in school-aged children. *J. Am. Acad. Child Adolesc. Psychiatry.*, *50*(12), 1210–1219.

Coelho, C. B., Sanchez, T. G., & Tyler, R. S. (2007). Hyperacusis, sound annoyance, and loudness hypersensitivity in children. *Prog. Brain Res.*, *166*, 169–178.

Davies, P. L., Chang, W., & Gavin, W. J. (2009). Maturation of sensory gating performance in children with and without sensory processing disorders. *Int. J. Psychophysiol.*, *72*(2), 187–197.

Davis, E., May, A., & Whiting, S. E. (2011). Evidenced-based treatment of anxiety and phobia in children and adolescents: current status and effects on the emotional response. *Clinical Psychology Review*, 31592–31602.

Ecclestone, C., Morley, S., Wiliams, A., York, L., & Mastroyannopoulou, K. (2002). Systematic review of randomised controlled trials of psychological therapy for chronic pain in children and adolescents, with subset meta-analysis for pain relief. *Pain*, *99*, 157–165.

Emond, A., & Kentish, R. (2013). Tinnitus counselling with children. *Audacity*, (2), 26–29.

Fackrell, K., Fearnley, C., Hoare, D. J., Sereda, M. (2015). Hyperacusis questionnaire as a tool for measuring hypersensitivity to sound in a tinnitus research population. *BioMed Research International*, 290425, 1–12.

Fior, R., & Bolzonello, P. (1988). An investigation on the maturation of hearing abilities in children. *Ear and Hearing*, *8*(6), 347–349.

Fletcher, P. J., Zoë, F. S., Azampanah, A., & Sills, T. L. (2001). Reduced brain serotonin activity disrupts prepulse inhibition of the acoustic startle reflex: Effects of 5,7-dihydroxytryptamine and p-chlorophenylalanine. *Neuropsychopharmacology*, *24*, 399–409. doi:10.1016/S0893-133X(00)00215-3.

Formby, C., Sherlock, L. P., & Gold, S. L. (2003). Adaptive plasticity of loudness induced by chronic attenuation and enhancement of the acoustic background. *J. Acoust. Soc. Am.*, *114*(1), 55–58.

Funabiki, Y., Murai, T., & Toichi, M. (2012). Cortical activation during attention to sound in autism spectrum disorders. *Research in Developmental Disabilities*, *33*(2), 518–524.

Gomes, E., Rotta, N. T., Pedroso, F. S., Sleifer, P., & Danesi, M. C. (2004). Auditory hypersensitivity in children and teenagers with autistic spectrum disorder. *Arq. Neuropsychiatr.*, *62*(3–B), 797–801.

Gothelf, D., Farber, N., Raveh, E., Apter, A., & Attias, J. (2006). Hyperacusis in Williams syndrome: Characteristics and associated neuroaudiologic abnormalities. *Neurology*, *66*(3), 390–395.

Hall, A., Humphriss, R., Baguley, D. M., Parker, M., & Steer, C. D. (2016). Prevalence and risk factors for reduced sound tolerance (hyperacusis) in children. *Int. J. Audiol.*, *55*(3), 135–141.

Jastreboff, P. J., & Jastreboff, M. M. (2014). Treatments for decreased sound tolerance (hyperacusis and misophonia). *Semin. Hear.*, *35*(2), 105–120.

Jüris, L., Andersson, G., Larsen, H. C., Ekselius, L. (2014). Cognitive behaviour therapy for hyperacusis: A randomized controlled trial. *Behav. Res. Ther.*, *54*, 30–37. doi: 10.1016/j.brat.2014.01.001. Epub 2014 Jan 24.

Katzenell, U., & Segal, S. (2001). Hyperacusis: Review and clinical guidelines. *Otol. Neurotol.*, *22*, 321–327.

Khalfa, S., Bruneau, N., Rogé, B., Georgieff, N., Veuillet, E., Adrien, J. L. . . . Collet, L. (2004). Increased perception of loudness in autism. *Hearing Research*, *198*(1–2), 87–92.

Klein, A. J., Armstrong, B. L., Greer, M. K., & Brown, F. R. III. (1990). Hyperacusis and otitis media in individuals with Williams syndrome. *J. Speech Hear. Disord.*, *55*(2), 339–344.

Landälv, D., Malmström, L., & Widén, S. E. (2013). Adolescents' reported hearing symptoms and attitudes toward loud music. *Noise & Health*, *15*(66), 347–354.

Lee, H. Y., Byun, J. Y., Park, M. S., & Yeo, S. G. (2013). Effect of aging on the prognosis of Bell's palsy. *Otology & Neurotolog.*, *34*(4), 766–770.

Levitin, D. J., Cole, K., Lincoln, A., & Bellugi, U. (2005). Aversion, awareness, and attraction: Investigating claims of hyperacusis in the Williams syndrome phenotype. *J. Child Psychol. Psychiatry.*, *46*(5), 514–523.

Mangeot, S. D., Miller, L. J., McIntosh, D. N., McGrath-Clarke, J., Simon, J., Hagerman, R. J., & Goldson, E. (2001). Sensory modulation dysfunction in children with attention-deficit-hyperactivity disorder. *Dev. Med. Child Neurol.*, *43*(6):, 399–406.

Marriage, J., & Barnes, N. M. (1995). Is central hyperacusis a symptom of 5-HT dysfunction? *J. Laryngol. Otol.*, *109*, 915–921.

Marshall, P. J., Bar-Haim, Y., & Fox, N. A. (2004). The development of P50 suppression in the auditory event-related potential. *Int. J. Psychophysiol.*, *51*(2), 135–141.

Matsuzaki, J., Kagitani-Shimono, K., Goto, T., Sanefuji, W., Yamamoto, T., Sakai, S., . . . Taniike, M. (2012). Differential responses of primary auditory cortex in autistic spectrum disorder with auditory hypersensitivity. *Neuroreport*, *23*(2), 113–118.

Miani, C., Passon, P., Bracale, A. M., Barotti, A., & Panzolli, N. (2001). Treatment of hyperacusis in Williams syndrome with bilateral conductive hearing loss. *Eur. Arch Otorhinolaryngol.*, *258*(7), 341–344.

Miller, E. E., Grosberg, B. M., Crystal, S. C., & Robbins, M. S. (2015). Auditory hallucinations associated with migraine: Case series and literature review. *Cephalalgia*, *35*(10), 923–930.

Moore, D. R. (2002). Auditory development and the role of experience. *Br. Med. Bull.*, *63*(1), 171–181.

Mott, B., & Sun, W. (2014). Firing property of inferior colliculus neurons affected by FMR1 gene mutation. *Journal of Otology*, *9*(2), 86–90.

Munro, K. J., & Blount, J. (2009). Adaptive plasticity in brainstem of adult listeners following earplug-induced deprivation. *Journal of Acoustical Society of America*, *126*(2), 568–571.

Munro, K. J., Turtle, C., & Schaette, R. (2014). Plasticity and modified loudness following short-term unilateral deprivation: Evidence of multiple gain mechanisms within the auditory system. *J. Acoust. Soc. Am.*, *135*(1), 315–322.

Myne, S., & Kennedy, V. (2017). Clinical profile of children with hyperacusis. Annual Conference of British Association of Audiovestibular Physicians, Chesham, England.

Nigam, A., & Samuel. P. R. (1994). Hyperacusis and Williams syndrome. *J. Laryngol. Otol.*, *108*(6), 494–496.

Oen, J. M., Begeer, J. H., Staal-Schreinemachers, A. I., & Tijmstra, T. (1997). Hyperacusis in children with spina bifida; a pilot-study. *Eur. J. Pediatr. Surg.*, *7*(Suppl.1), 46.

Orekhova, E. V., Stroganova, T. A., Prokofyev, A. O., Nygren, G., Gillberg, C., & Elam, M. (2008). Sensory gating in young children with autism: Relation to age, IQ, and EEG gamma oscillations. *Neurosci. Lett.*, *434*(2), 218–223.

Pienkowski, M., Tyler, R. S., Roncancio, E. R., Jun, H. J., Brozoski, T., Dauman, N., . . . Moore, B. C. (2014). A review of hyperacusis and future directions: Part II. Measurement, mechanisms, and treatment. *Am. J. Audiol.*, *23*(4), 420–436.

Phillips, D. P., & Carr, M. M. (1998). Disturbances of loudness perception. *J. Am. Acad. Audiol.*, *9*, 371–379.

Recker, F., Zaniew, M., Bockenhauer, D., Miglietti, N., Bokenkamp, A., Moczulska, A., . . . Ludwig, M. (2015). Characterization of 28 novel patients expands the mutational and phenotypic spectrum of Lowe syndrome. *Pediatric Nephrology*, *30*(6), 931–943.

Remenschneider, A. K., Lookabaugh, S., Aliphas, A., Brodsky, J. R., Devaiah, A. K., Dagher, W., . . . Quesnel, A. M. (2014). Otologic outcomes after blast injury: the Boston Marathon experience. *Otology & Neurotolog.*, *35*(10),1825–1834.

Rodrigues, M. A., Amorim, M., Silva, M. V., Neves, P., Sousa, A., & Inacio, O. (2015). Sound levels and risk perceptions of music students during classes. *Journal of Toxicology & Environmental Health Part A*, *78*(13–14), 825–839.

Rogers, S. J., Hepburn, S., & Wehner, E. (2003). Parent reports of sensory symptoms in toddlers with autism and those with other developmental disorders. *J. Autism Dev. Disord.*, *33*(6), 631–642.

Rosenhall, U., Nordin, V., Sandstrom, M., Ahlsen, G., & Gillberg, C. (1999). Autism and hearing loss. *J. Autism Dev. Disord.*, *29*(5), 349–357.

Sattar, N. (2009). A study of hyperacusis in 100 normally-hearing children. *Arch Dis. Child*, *84*(Suppl 1), A98 (G251).

Stansfeld, S. A. (1992). Noise, noise sensitivity and psychiatric disorder: epidemiological and psychophysiological studies. *Psychol. Med. Monogr. Suppl.*, *22*, 1–44.

Stiegler, L., & Davis, R. (2010). Understanding sound sensitivity in individuals with autism spectrum disorders. *Focus on Autism and Other Developmental Disabilities*, *25*(2), 67–75.

Sun, W., Manohar, S., Jayaram, A., Kumaraguru, A., Fu, Q., Li, J., & Allman, B. (2011). Early age conductive hearing loss causes audiogenic seizure and hyperacusis behaviour. *Hearing Research*, *282*(1–2), 178–183.

Thabet, E. M. (2014). Ocular vestibular evoked myogenic potentials n10 response in autism spectrum disorders children with auditory hypersensitivity: an indicator of semicircular canal dehiscence. *Eur. Arch Otorhinolaryngol.*, *271*(5), 1283–1288.

Tibussek, D., Wohlrab, G., Boltshauser, E., & Schmitt, B. (2006). Proven startle-provoked epileptic seizures in childhood. *Semiologic and Electrophysiologic Variability Epilepsia*, *47*(6), 1050–1058.

Tkachuk, G. A., Cottrell, C. K., Gibson, J. S., O'Donnell, F. J., & Holroyd, K. A. (2003). Factors associated with migraine-related quality of life and disability in adolescents: A preliminary investigation. *Headache*, *43*(9), 950–955.

Trehub, S. E., Schneider, B. A., & Endman, M. (1980). Developmental changes in infants' sensitivity to octave-band noises. *J. Exp. Child Psychol.*, *29*, 282–293.

Velleman, S., Stallard, P., & Richardson, T. (2010). A review and mata-analysis of computrized cognitive behaviour therapy for the treatment of pain in children and adolescents. *Child: Care, Health and Development 36*, *4*, 465–472.

Widen, S. E., & Erlandsson, S. I. (2004). Self-reported tinnitus and noise sensitivity among adolescents in Sweden. *Noise Health*, *7*, 29–40.

14

Hearing Aids for Decreased Sound Tolerance and Minimal Hearing Loss: Gain Without Pain

Grant D. Searchfield and Caroline Selvaratnam

Introduction

Hearing loss accompanied by decreased sound tolerance (DST) can be managed by a patient-centered approach to provide hearing aid "gain without pain." Compared to the typical hearing aid fitting protocol, several additional steps are needed to fit hearing aids to the average DST patient. For patients with hearing loss, tinnitus, and DST, the first step is to manage the DST, then the hearing loss, and then tinnitus. Fitting hearing aids to this population is an iterative process that requires patience and a willingness to take small backward steps when needed to secure long-term goals.

Elsewhere in this book the types of DST and potential mechanisms have been described. Audiologists will be familiar with the issue of auditory recruitment, the abnormal loudness growth that often accompanies hearing loss, and how compression processing in hearing aids can compensate for this (Dillon, 1996; Kates, 2010). Recruitment is not the focus of the chapter; instead we concentrate on hearing aid fitting with minimal hearing loss and DST related to lowered discomfort levels or intolerance of sound. Throughout this chapter we will address our rationale with reference to existing literature where possible, but given the limited evidence in this field many of our recommendations should be viewed as opinion that is based upon an accumulation of anecdotal and clinical experience. We will present several case studies to illustrate our philosophy in managing DST.

Much of the past focus on minimal and mild hearing loss has been in the pediatric population because of concerns on its effects on language development (McKay, Gravel, & Tharpe, 2008). In adults, mild hearing loss can lead to poorer quality of life (Dalten et al., 2003). Even mild hearing loss influences the ability to filter sounds (Baker & Rosen, 2002; Moore & Glasberg, 2011), detect gaps (Leigh-Paffenroth & Elangovan, 2011; Neijenhuis, Tschur, & Snik, 2004), and localize sounds (Goverts, Houtgast, & van Beek, 2000), thereby creating issues impairing hearing in background noise (Helfer & Wilber, 1990; Pekkarinen, Salmivalli, & Suonpaa, 1990). There is concern that even mild hearing loss can contribute to deficits in cognition that occur with aging (Tun, McCoy, & Wingfield, 2009; Stewart & Wingfield, 2009). Increasing evidence also suggests that changes in hearing can occur without noticeable changes in the audiogram; such hidden hearing loss appears to arise from damage to auditory nerve synapses and fibers (Liberman & Kujawa, 2014), and leads to poorer temporal coding of sound and possibly DST (Plack, Barker, & Prendergast, 2014).

In addition to DST, tinnitus is a common co-morbidity accompanying minimal hearing loss. There is overlap in the presentation of DST and tinnitus, suggesting some common mechanisms (Schecklmann, Landgrebe, Langguth, & Group, 2014) (see Chapters 5, 6, and 8). Similar to tinnitus, DST is associated with hearing loss (Nelson & Chen, 2004) although it can also occur with normal hearing or minimal reduction in audiometric thresholds (Gu, Halpin, Nam, Levine, & Melcher, 2010). One common approach to managing tinnitus is the fitting of hearing aids (Shekhawat, Searchfield, & Stinear, 2013), and in the last decade we have reported a great deal regarding the ways in which hearing aids can be best used for tinnitus management (Searchfield, 2015). DST presents an even greater challenge to hearing aid fitting. Another layer of complexity is created by the audiological goal of amplifying sound as it conflicts with patients' beliefs that less sound is needed. We have the technology to address these conflicting goals, but the patient must buy-in to a process that they may fear. Counseling is very important to enable the person with DST to tackle their sensitivities and fears.

A Protocol for Fitting Minimal-Mild Hearing Loss Accompanied by DST

Our philosophy to manage hearing loss and tinnitus with DST has not changed a great deal over the last decade (Searchfield 2006, 2016). The overarching principle is to reduce an individual's sense of sound isolation created either by avoidance behaviors or the presence of hearing loss. We address this principle through counseling and the fitting of hearing aids. In order to accommodate reduced loudness tolerance, extra caution must be applied in selecting appropriate hearing aids and their settings. Optimal amplification of speech sounds may have to be sacrificed initially with preference given instead to comfort and amplification of soft sounds. If necessary, gain is reduced across inputs and is gradually increased as sound tolerance permits. When a patient cannot tolerate any amplification, combination instruments can be used; in such cases, low level broadband sound may be used for desensitization (Sandlin & Olsson, 1999), gradually withdrawn, and eventually replaced by amplified sounds. The fitting has to be a progressive, but measured, process that takes the individual's needs into account. It is recommended that the aids are first used in quiet environments, with exposure increasing over time (Herraiz & Diges, 2010).

A Step-Wise Approach

We employ an adaptation-based protocol in which the individual's needs are assessed and a management plan created that varies according to the person's progress. It usually consists of the following elements:

- Clinical history taking
- DST assessment
- Needs assessment, goal setting, and counseling
- Weaning from earplugs
- Hearing aid selection
- Fitting
- Transition to tolerance

1. Clinical History Taking

Along with standard audiological history taking, it is important to understand the DST problem and how it affects the person in as much fine-grain detail as possible. Here are some examples of questions to ask and how they might inform the hearing aid fitting process accompanying DST.

A. Reaction effect

i. What effect does the sound have on you?
ii. Is it painful or irritating?
iii. Does the effect persist even after the sound stops?

With these questions we provide an opportunity for the patient to express details regarding their DST. We hope to gain an understanding of effects and how quickly any management plan might proceed. A longer intervention time course might be planned when DST effects are dramatic. The nature of the impact should assist in decisions on referrals to other professions (e.g., psychology).

B. The sounds causing discomfort

i. Do all sounds cause discomfort?
ii. What are the specific sounds?
iii. Is it always the same sound?
iv. Do you have an idea why these sounds cause discomfort?
v. Is it only when that sound is very loud or does it make you feel uncomfortable even if it is not loud?

These questions enable us to evaluate sound related effects for tuning of hearing aids. In particular we want to know if the effects are primarily related to the loudness of sounds, or if the DST is more related to intolerance or annoyance to sounds (whether loud or not) (Tyler et al., 2014).

C. Situations and environments—psychosocial context

i. Where are you when the discomfort occurs?
ii. Does the same sound always cause discomfort?
iii. Does the problem occur at a particular time of day?
iv. How do your partner/family/friends react to the same sound?
v. Are they supportive?
vi. Does it change if you are busy or having fun?
vii. Does it change if you are experiencing stress?

In a family-centered context these questions are also important for the patients' significant others to answer. Clinicians need to know the effects that the DST has on family and friends as they try to determine the degree to which the complaint is sensory versus behavioral. When there is evidence of a strong psychological component to the DST, counseling takes on a greater importance than it would in less complicated cases. As with tinnitus, audiologists need to establish when psychological referral is required to either augment or substitute for audiology-based counseling.

D. Coping strategy

i. What do you do when the sounds occur?
ii. Do you wear earplugs or earmuffs? How often?
iii. Do you limit yourself or your activities socially, and has this changed?

It is important to identify existing coping strategies, and then provide expert advice regarding whether they are helpful for long-term reductions in DST and hearing aid acceptance. We should recognize and work with the strategies the person has developed; if they are maladaptive and unhelpful for recovery of sound tolerance then the clinician must find a gentle and preferably evidence-based way of turning behaviors in a positive direction. For example, lecturing a patient who is reliant on earmuffs that they must immediately stop using them will likely create a barrier to further progress. Instead the effects of sensory deprivation need to be explained and support provided to "wean" patients from their perceived, but often inaccurate need to use hearing protection.

E. Pleasant sounds

i. What are your favorite sounds?
ii. Do you listen to music?
iii. Is your work/home environment quiet?
iv. How easy would it be to introduce enjoyable sounds to your lifestyle?

The goal here is to identify sounds that may be used in the rehabilitation process. The patient is encouraged to increase exposure to "enjoyable" sounds. The spectral differences between tolerable and intolerable sounds can be estimated to indicate the contribution of frequency-specific sensitivity to the DST. With multiple channel hearing aids, it is possible to alter level-dependent gain at DST frequencies.

2. DST Assessment

While some researchers have reported positive correlations between loudness discomfort measures and hyperacusis complaint (Goldstein & Shulman, 1996) others have not (Meeus, Spaepen, de Ridder, & van de Heyning, 2009). Methods of obtaining loudness measures and their description vary (Mueller & Bentler, 2005). Terms used for the intensity of sound that patients report as being too loud or creating discomfort include: Threshold of Discomfort, Loudness Discomfort Level (LDL), and Uncomfortable Loudness Level (UCL; Mueller & Bentler, 2005). In this chapter we will use UCL to encapsulate all these measures. The overall RMS of the signal appears to determine the UCL rather than its spectrum, but that being said UCL at 750, 1500, and 3000 Hz may be the most appropriate frequencies to set hearing aid maximum output to a pure-tone sweep (Bentler & Nelson, 2001) or 1500 Hz for NBN (Keidser, Bentler, & Kiessling, 2010).

Keidser et al. (2010) importantly noted that patients react differently to laboratory stimuli compared to real-world sounds. In a similar manner to the context of tinnitus (Searchfield, 2014), sound, personality, and mood are all likely contributors to discomfort (Keidser et al., 2010). Some clinicians are very reluctant to measure UCL due to the fear that it may distress the patient and alienate them from the clinician. We believe that the benefits of obtaining the measure outweigh the risks (see hearing aid fitting), however, we approach these measurements with great caution and forewarning of the process. We always begin near threshold of the test signal, very gradually increase the sound, and stop immediately when indicated by patient feedback. Testing is not continued if the patient is distressed. UCLs are not measured if the patient finds standard audiometry uncomfortable.

A different measure of the effects of noise is the Acceptable Noise Level (ANL) (Nabelek, Freyaldenhoven, Tampas, Burchfiel, & Muenchen, 2006). The ANL is the difference (in dB) between the most comfortable level (MCL) of a speech stimulus and the highest background noise level (BNL) acceptable to the patient listening to the speech. One version of the ANL is available commercially through Frye Electronics (http://www.frye.com/wp/anl/). The ANL is not a typical DST measure as it relates less to loudness discomfort than to the annoyance of sounds (Bees, 2016). Patients who are more accepting of background noise have smaller ANLs (their MCL and BNLs are closer) than those less accepting of noise. In a small group, Levy et al. (2011) found ANLs were larger (less acceptance) in a group with various forms of DST than in a normal hearing group (Levy, Peck, & Balachandran, 2011). Importantly, in the context of this chapter, the ANL can predict success with hearing aids, as those more accepting of noise are more likely to be successful hearing aid users (Nabelek et al., 2006).

There is some preliminary evidence, in children, that the ANL is related to some measures used in the assessment of auditory processing disorder (APD) (Sheehan, Houghton, & Searchfield, 2016). We have also found that many persons referred to our clinic for DST also have symptoms of APD and fail some APD tests. We now routinely undertake APD testing when patients present with DST. Their complaints of intolerance to sound seem related to an inability to cope in social environments when surrounded by competing sound. A common description is that their brain "crashes" and they need to escape from the sound. The division between DST and APD can be blurred so a differential diagnosis to understand the full nature of the patient's complaint is worthwhile. Improvement in signal:noise is important for management of both APD and DST as we describe below.

There are several questionnaire-based indices of hyperacusis's effects on quality of life (Fackrell, Fearnley, Hoare, & Sereda, 2015; Khalfa et al., 2002). These questionnaires tend not to have been psychometrically validated to the same extent as their tinnitus equivalents. The problem with all questionnaires is their ability to be relevant to the individual undergoing assessment. For identifying the needs of patients and measuring the outcomes of DST therapy in our clinic (see also Chapter 4) we tend to prefer a version of the Client Orientated Scale of Improvement (COSI) adapted for delineation of the patient's objectives associated with tinnitus and/or DST (Dillon, James, & Ginis, 1987).

3. Needs Assessment, Goal Setting, and Counseling

Due to the heterogeneous presentation of DST, identifying individual's needs and then turning those needs into goals for therapy is very important. The modified COSI can address both patient needs and help the clinician set realistic goals for therapy. Based on the history we ask the patient their main problems, we list those, and then seek to place them in order of priority. This is a two-way process (and will be more comprehensive if family can be encouraged to participate). The patient's goal priorities can be used to create an "effect-timeline" whereby the clinician can go through each goal and explain which is achievable first and why. New goals can emanate from this conversation and should be noted.

Counseling should be undertaken whenever hearing aids are fitted, but the need is heightened with DST. Psychoeducation, or the use of psychological therapies, is very important in this process. Materials developed for tinnitus have been modified for DST, for example,

Hyperacusis Activities Treatment (Pienkowski et al., 2014) emerged from Tinnitus Activities Treatment (Tyler, Gogel, & Gehringer, 2007).

Detailed counseling suggestions are made elsewhere in this book. To be successful the patient must trust the clinician, who is essentially recommending an intervention that patients fear and that they may see as the opposite from their needs (i.e., increasing sound not decreasing it). Encourage patients to become familiar with dangerous versus safe sound levels (http://dangerousdecibels.org/). Consistency in patient-clinician contact is extremely important; ideally the patient will see the same clinician over many visits, and failing this a consistent message and protocol should be used within a clinic to avoid confusion and doubt. Patients need to be able to understand how hearing aids work, identify the sounds and situations that are most troublesome, develop strategies to manage the challenging situations as they take responsibility for their own rehabilitation. It is important for the clinician to understand the psychological state of the patient and learn their existing coping strategies in order to create a safe environment for the reintroduction of sound (Westcott, 2002).

4. *Wean from Earplugs*

Some DST patients develop an unhealthy dependence on hearing protection. A not too uncommon sight in our waiting room is a person reading a magazine while wearing earmuffs. Reducing this reliance on ear protection must be managed with empathy, it should not be rushed; overcoming this barrier to adaptation is a key to future success.

A. Instruct appropriate use of protection

Hearing protection use is appropriate when sound is damaging. Patients need to be given the tools to understand this. For some patients, Vernon (2002) instructed use of a sound-level-meter (SLM) to determine when sound was damaging, and only use of earplugs when it was (Vernon, 2002). SLM apps are now available for smartphones (many examples are available from iTunes and google play). If used appropriately, patients can challenge themselves to experience higher levels of sound, but care needs to be taken so that obsessive use of SLMs does not replace one maladaptive coping strategy with another.

B. Nonlinear or active earplugs

The use of nonlinear or active plugs to provide level-dependent attenuation can assist weaning off earplugs. These earplugs provide greater attenuation as sound levels increase (Dancer & Hamery, 1998), they are often marketed for shooters or motorbike riders and consist of a small acoustic filter in a silicon plug either available off-the-shelf or in custom versions. More expensive electronic active earplugs are also available (e.g., http://www.etymotic.com/consumer/hearing-protection.html). Patients feel safer being provided with a substitute for their usual earplugs, given these provide primarily high intensity attenuation they are an interim step toward recovery of sound sensitivity.

C. Reduce hours of use

Each increase in hours experienced without protection should be seen as an achievement and celebrated with the patient.

5. *Hearing Aid Selection*

Special hearing aids for DST featuring low compression thresholds, low maximum outputs, and no venting were available in the 1990s (Preves, Sammeth, Cutting, & Woodruff, 1995). These aids were primarily active electronic earplugs. They only provided sufficient amplification to reduce insertion-loss created by plugging the ear. These aids would be of minimal benefit in correcting for hearing loss, and no longer appear to be available; however, the ideal hearing aid for DST would have a similar range of compression thresholds and flexibility in selection of maximum output. Such settings would enable the user to begin using the aid at levels of amplification that, while suboptimal for speech recognition, could provide "safe" amplification as patients transition to normal prescribed targets. Here we list some of the features we prefer in hearing aids for DST, and provide brief rationales.

A. Flexible output and compression settings

The maximum output (maximum power output [MPO] or output sound pressure level [OSPL]) is the highest level that the hearing aid can produce. Output-controlled compression is designed so that a compression threshold below the patient's UCL should prevent discomfort. Appropriate output limiting is an important determinate of hearing aid success in general (Mueller & Bentler, 2005), and even more so when an individual's UCLs are lower than normal. But it should not be assumed that lowering the maximum output is the best or only solution. It is important to remember that manipulations to maximum output will only affect high-level sounds. DST may occur to sounds lower than this setting can control. Wide dynamic range compression (WDRC) is an input compression scheme with low compression threshold (40 to 50 dB SPL) and low compression ratios (1.5 to 3:1). WDRC reduces gain as sound level increases. It is important to note that WDRC is designed to provide gain to soft sounds and increases (worsens) the ANL by 1.5 dB (Wu & Stangl, 2013). If soft sounds are a problem for the listener, then the compression threshold should be raised and expansion should be activated. Expansion reduces the gain below the compression knee point; greater expansion results in less soft sound. The dynamic characteristics of compression desirable for DST would include a fast attack-time (so that the aids react quickly to increases in sound) that must be balanced against Dillon's (2012) suggestion that moderate release times provide more comfort.

B. Noise Reduction

Automatic noise reduction is unlikely to improve speech intelligibility but it can improve comfort and reduce listening effort (Dillon, 2012). Initially, high levels of noise reduction may be needed for DST. Noise reduction has been shown to improve the ANL by 1.1 dB (Wu & Stangl, 2013). As sound tolerance improves, noise reduction can be reduced. Less noise reduction should result in better sound quality and environmental awareness.

C. Directional and remote microphones

Improving the signal-to-noise ratio through directional microphone settings, and especially wireless microphones close to the sound of interest, will improve effective communication. When combined with listening strategies, for example, the patient orienting their attention away from noise sources, use of wireless microphones will reduce the influence of background noise relative to that of the signal. Wireless microphones become even more important when DST accompanies APD. Directional microphone settings improve the ANL by 2.8 dB (Wu & Stangl, 2013).

D. Transient impulse control

Transient impulse control is available in some hearing aids; this feature detects sounds that increase more rapidly in intensity than speech, and does not amplify them (Hayes, 2006).

E. Datalogging

Datalogging does not directly change the sound perceived by persons with DST. Instead, datalogging provides an insight to the use patterns of the aids. The information obtained through datalogging can guide adjustments in fitting and supplement the patient's self-report of hearing aid use.

F. Domes versus earmolds

Persons with minimal-mild hearing loss should be able to use open-fit aids. This style of aid will minimize occlusion; however, they allow essentially unimpeded passage of environmental sounds. Persons accustomed to earplugs may be best served by use of custom earmolds, and then progress to domes with time. Select-A-Vent variable diameter venting can be used to block and then progressively open the vents to allow more environment sound to pass into the ear. From open ear molds the user can transition to open-fit domes.

G. Combi devices and Bluetooth

If hearing aids with low amplification settings are not tolerated, then it is best that the focus on restoring audibility be delayed until acceptable sound tolerance is achieved. Use of constant low-level broadband noise can be beneficial for those patients who fear unexpected amplified sounds. Combination devices are ideal for providing such desensitizing sound as the sound generator can be phased out with amplification introduced in time. This strategy avoids the expense of purchasing a dedicated sound therapy device and then changing to hearing aids. Bluetooth-featured hearing aids allow the users to stream music or other sounds from their portable music players or smartphones direct to the aids. Many hearing aid manufacturers have mobile applications (apps) for tinnitus sound therapy that can be used for this purpose, and there are websites with material suitable for desensitization (e.g., www.tinnitustunes.com).

H. Volume Control

The volume control is a simple feature that has become somewhat sidelined in today's world of automatic adjustment; however, a volume control on the aids or remote can empower the user. If the audiologist is concerned that the user will just turn the volume to minimum and leave it there, avoiding sound, compliance can be checked with datalogging. A volume control minimizes the likelihood of patients having to persevere with uncomfortable sounds.

I. Programs

Most manufacturers offer multiple memories in their aids that are designed for different purposes (e.g., listening in quiet, comfort, music). Different prescriptions of amplification can be trialed in different programs. A winning prescription can be determined on the basis of self-report and datalogging. We also suggest that a program be created that has several degrees less amplification than the standard program. This so-called "safe program" is intended for loud environments where conventionally amplified ambient sounds would be intolerable. The safe program would include most of the features described above such as: strong noise reduction, expansion, a high compression ratio, directionality, and low maximum output. This setting would serve as the emergency program to enable the user to feel safe while providing some environmental awareness and sound stimulation. The safe program provides more gain than the next recommendation.

J. Off button

The reason and use of this should be self-explanatory.

6. Fitting

We use hearing aid prescriptions and real-ear measures to inform our fittings for patients with DST. However unlike normal hearing aid fittings, meeting targets created by the prescription is not the initial goal, it is the long-term goal. It is important to start with a clear strategy to select and verify initial settings for target gain and output. Hearing aids use level-dependent amplification strategies based on prescription of gain to make speech audible and maximum output to avoid discomfort (Dillon, 1996; Kates, 2010). Compression is used to compensate for recruitment (Dillon, 1996; Kates, 2010). Hearing prescriptive procedures (e.g., NAL-NL1; Byrne, Dillon, Ching, Katsch, & Keidser, 2001; NL2; Keidser, Dillon, Flax, Ching, & Brewer, 2011; DSL V5; Polonenko et al., 2010) and their implementation in hearing aids are well established and intended to manage the loss of sensitivity to low intensity sounds in patients with normal UCLs. Compression and its benefit in cases of recruitment is covered in many standard hearing aid textbooks (Dillon, 2012).

Prescription procedures and default settings in hearing aids have not been specifically developed for the less-frequent situation of abnormal discomfort levels or annoyance of sounds. To achieve the goals of hearing aid fitting with DST, the clinician must understand the technology and how to find "workarounds" to achieve the fitting goals. Prescriptive procedures utilize target gain and UCL values derived from average predictions of ideal settings based on the audiogram (Storey, Dillon, Yeend, & Wigney, 1998). Verification occurs through real-ear measures using different intensities of sound (Dillon, 2012). As DST invariably results in lower preferred levels of amplification than would be typical, the prescribed targets become end goals rather than initial targets. The different prescriptions suggest different targets for soft-loud sounds for different hearing losses (Figure 14–1). The estimated UCLs based on the audiogram may be grossly inappropriate in cases of DST. The prescriptions allow for the substitution of measured UCLs instead of average values. We believe that the measurement of UCLs is invaluable for this purpose, although as stated previously their measurement must be undertaken with caution to avoid discomfort.

Hearing aid fitting based on loudness growth measures have also been used in the past (e.g., LGOB; Allen, Hall, & Jeng, 1990) but time pressures in clinic and the putative adequacy of threshold based estimations of UCLs means threshold-based prescriptions dominate audiology. In the DST population, loudness growth measures can assist in identifying dynamic range, modify the prescription of the maximum output levels, and assist the clinician in selecting reasonable estimates of suitable gain for soft, medium, and loud inputs. Aided loudness validation (such as RESR) may be more valuable than unaided UCL measures (Mackersie, 2007), however any measurements undertaken for a person with DST must either consider *a priori* the patient's UCL or start the measurements at a low level with gradual increases. The clinician must be able to stop measurements rapidly to avoid discomfort and risk alienation of the patient. If the client has adverse reaction to even low-level sounds, it is possible to use coupler measures incorporating RECD measures as a substitute for UCLs (Dillon, 2012).

Audiologists need to be careful when using the manufacturer's software to adjust anti-feedback features. Feedback tests can create SPLs in the ear canal of 110 to 115 dB (Sankowsky-Rothe, Blau, Schepker, & Doclo, 2015), far in excess of what many people with DST will accept. If feedback occurs with the aids (the feedback can be uncomfortable in its own right), audiologists should try manual adjustment of the manufacturer's feedback

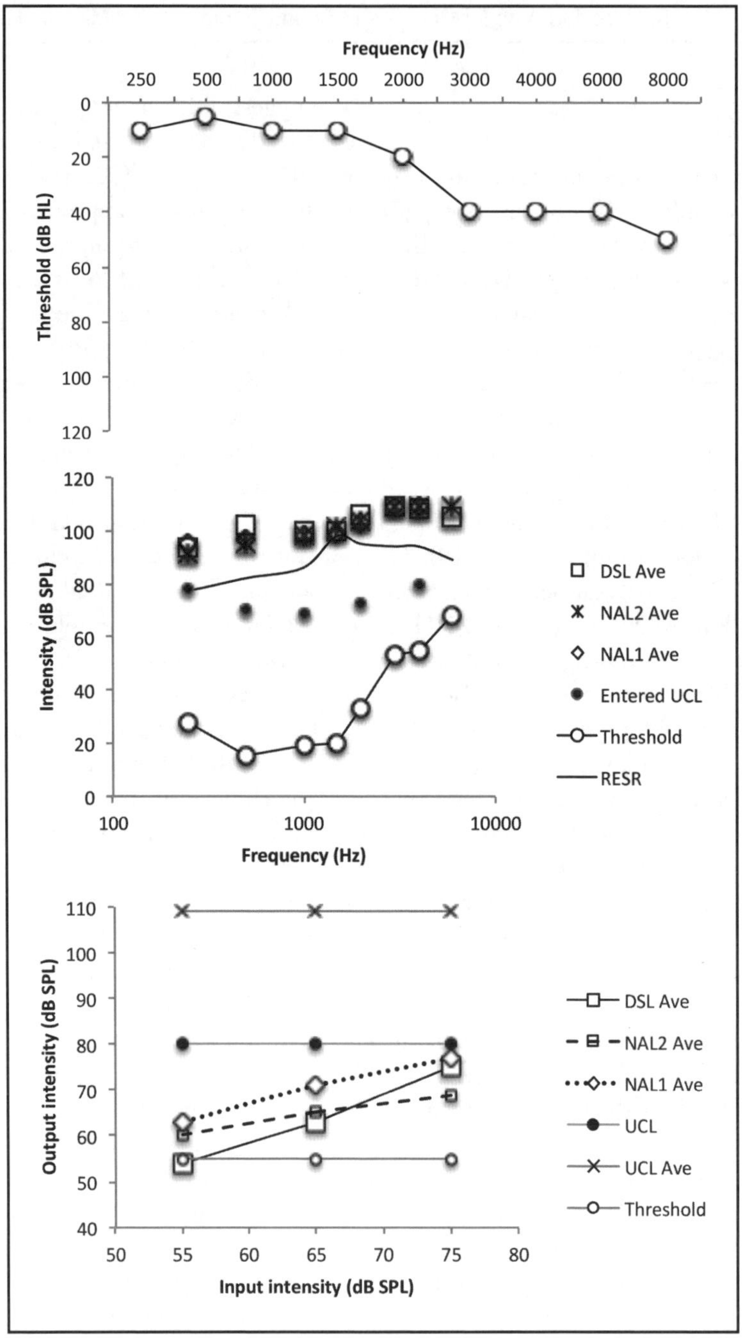

Figure 14–1. A. Audiogram from right ear of a patient. **B.** SPL-O-gram, audiogram thresholds converted to SPL, UCLs estimated for the audiogram using NAL-NI1, NAL-NL2, and DSL v 5 Adult, and measured UCL. **C.** Input-output function for the audiogram (4 kHz) based on the three prescription procedures, the UCL for the prescriptions based on the audiogram (same for all three), and the actual UCL. The prescriptions provide varying targets depending on input. The average UCL estimate by the different prescriptions is very similar, but much higher than the actual UCL in this case. The RESR is the real ear saturation response for the example hearing aid.

Table 14–1. Recommended changes to address patient complaints related to comfort.

	Problem Description							
	Background noise too loud	Voices too loud	Booming	Too loud	Sound painful	Dishes too loud	Loud sounds too loud	Sounds uncomfortable
	Potential Solultion							
1	Decrease LF gain	Decrease overall gain	Decrease LF gain	Decrease overall gain	Decrease MPO	Increase HF CR	Decrease MPO	Decrease MPO
2	Increase LF CR	Decrease LF gain	Decrease overall gain	Decrease LF gain	Increase HF CR	Decrease MPO	Increase HF CR	Decrease overall gain
3	Raise LF CT	Increase LF CR	Decrease MPO	Decrease MPO	Decrease overall gain	Decrease HF gain	Increase LD CR	
4	Decrease overall gain							

Source: Based on Jenstad, Van Tasell, & Ewert (2003).

settings, or traditional methods of reducing feedback such as less venting, or softer and tighter earmolds. We would strongly recommend not performing these feedback tests until the users tolerance to sound has normalized, and even then performing the tests should be a last resort; be ready to hit the pause button. Multichannel hearing aids have many parameters that can be adjusted to improve comfort (Table 14–1).

7. *Transition to Tolerance*

Counseling is critical for enabling the person with DST to develop improved tolerance to sound. Clinicians can center their approach around supporting goals established with the COSI. In addition to increasing passive sound exposure through generated and amplified sound there is also emerging evidence that auditory training used with tinnitus (Searchfield, Morrison-Low, & Wise, 2007) may improve acceptance of noise as measured by the ANL. Following a 3-week sound identification and localization task ("AOIL" available commercially from www.tinnitustunes.com) Morrison-Low (2006) found a 2.4 dB decrease (improvement) in the ANL. A crossover study comparing LDLs and ANLs measured in 40 participants with normal hearing, prior to and after 15 days of training and 15 days of no training (control) also found a significant training-specific decrease (improvement) in ANLs, but no change in LDLs was observed (Bees, Guan, Alsarrage, & Searchfield, 2017).

Risk of Conservative Hearing Aid Fitting

Under-amplification carries risks of rejection due to the absence of benefit to hearing. With very low maximum output, high amounts of compression, and low gain, the hearing aid will provide a narrowed dynamic range that may create distortion and minimal benefits in hearing (Formby et al., 2015). This very conservative setting of hearing aids must be considered temporary and will need to be modified as rapidly as the individual's tolerance will allow. The limitation of an initial conservative fitting strategy on the audibility of speech needs to be clearly articulated to patients. They need to understand the initial setting is just a stepping-stone to more amplification. If the patient does not have a clear understanding of the process and/or the benefit of audibility at far less than optimum levels, then the patient may reject the hearing aids.

Case Examples

Case One (M)

This 10-year-old child presented with severe reaction and distress to sound (curling into a ball on the ground and bursting into tears). The problem started one year prior to testing as a result of girls in his class screaming in his ear, and initially his strong reaction was only observed when he heard sounds that would be considered potentially damaging to his hearing. Over the space of a year, M started to become defensive to sound both within and outside the classroom and was reacting aversively to sounds that others did not consider loud. There were no concerns with regards to hearing with M's mother reporting that he had always exhibited "super" hearing for soft sounds. In the classroom M had struggled learning to read and write.

The assessment process encompassed both loudness tolerance measures and APD tests. Thresholds were within normal limits bilaterally although there was a notch in otoacoustic emissions at 4000 Hz, bilaterally. M became very distressed when asked to do loudness tolerance testing and as such his UCLs were quite limited (20 dB above threshold). Most comfortable levels (MCL) to sentences were substantially higher (70 dB above threshold), the UCL/MCL difference indicative of a significant emotional response to sound. In APD testing M exhibited delays in his ability to process temporal and tonal aspects of sound.

Dangerous decibel (http://dangerous decibels.org/) counseling was carried out with M and contact was made with the school to recommend that they participate in a dangerous decibel program. The recommendation was based on the school's suggestion that M ignore the behavior of his classmates rather than treating the incidents as an assault. Sound files were provided for use in quiet settings to reduce his awareness of external sounds, and by doing so facilitate control over his anticipatory behavior. An APD program was also designed to help develop M's temporal and tonal processing.

M was reassessed after 6 months. He was still more reactive to loud sounds than his peers but no longer anticipated discomfort and simply covered his ears when unexpected loud sounds occurred. Significant changes had been seen with his reading and writing, with APD tests showing that M was approaching normative levels.

Case Two (G)

This 61-year-old man experienced a traumatic brain injury 9 years ago that resulted in significant light and sound sensitivity, balance issues, lack of peripheral vision and changes in memory and concentration. G reported that sudden sound was more uncomfortable than steady-state noise but that all sound negatively affected his ability to concentrate on a task. Speech needed to be whispered and the radio/TV were set to a level that was below audibility for everyone else. G did work part time in the local fire station doing data logging but could only cope with this if the station was empty and there were no sirens. He was wearing off-the-shelf earplugs when he was exposed to car noise but not in quiet settings.

Testing revealed a mild high frequency sensorineural loss in both ears with UCL's 30 dBHL above threshold for low frequency sounds and 20 dBHL above threshold for high frequency sounds. APD testing was not completed because the neuropsychological assessment had already confirmed a significant cognitive impairment.

Nonlinear plugs replaced the off-the-shelf ear defenders for use in noisy settings and G was counseled regarding the impact of consistent exposure to environments with limited sound. Bilateral open fit mini BTE aids were fitted for use in quiet environments with the long-term goal being consistent hearing aid use in all settings. Noise suppression was set to maximum and given his visual issues, microphones were set to provide a low level of directionality. NAL 2 was chosen because of the level of compression and initially the aid was set to 70% of the prescriptive target. Closed domes were attached to the aid to try to reduce the amount of incidental non-processed sound reaching the ear. An FM system was provided for use in group or noise environments to support speech audibility. Counseling was required at every appointment to keep G positive and on task.

Over the space of 6 months G gradually increased his aid use to 6 hours per day. Over this time his tolerance of both expected and unexpected sounds (in quiet) improved to the point that he was able to listen to the radio/TV at a level that was audible for others. G rejected the FM because the level of sound appeared louder than the level of the aid (despite verification in the test box showing that the gain was similar) and as such he found that no improvement had occurred with his ability to tolerate sound in more dynamic environments. G continued to use ear protection appropriately.

Case Three (S)

S is a 54-year-old man who experienced a sudden hearing loss in his right ear 3 years ago. Since the sudden loss he has suffered from debilitating tinnitus, hyperacusis, and panic attacks that left him feeling very isolated. Prior to the incident he was an avid musician and played the guitar in a band. S was still able to work but at all times wore an earplug in his good ear. When at home he locked himself in his office and used ear buds with white noise to reduce his awareness of external sounds. S was taking the maximum dose of anti-anxiety medication allowed and was self-medicating with alcohol to help him cope. S came to the clinic for assessment just prior to having a cochlear implant inserted into his worse ear. At this point S was not in the care of a mental health specialist.

Hearing testing revealed that S had no residual hearing in the right ear and a mild high frequency sensorineural loss in the left. The tinnitus assessment identified that his tinnitus was localized to the right while all sensitivity issues were localized to the left. UCL's were reduced and revealed a dynamic range of approximately 50 dB for frequencies up to 6000 Hz. At 6000 Hz and above sounds were uncomfortable 5 dB above threshold. Initial recommendations were that the cochlear implant be delayed so that earplug use could be reduced first, but given that S had already tried numerous treatments in the past he felt the need to proceed with the implant as soon as possible.

The cochlear implant was successfully inserted into the right ear with settings being determined by intraoperative measures. Current levels were initially reduced so that sound was just audible and over the space of nine months settings were increased until the map was at an appropriate level. At the same time counseling was provided for appropriate ear plug use and S was encouraged to stop using the plugs when he was in a quiet setting with long-term goals being to restrict ear plug use except when S was exposed to loud noise. In the home setting S was asked to use a speaker rather than ear buds when listening to sound files so that he was less isolated, and that he move out of the office for his relaxation time when it was quiet enough for him to feel safe. Referral to a counselor was arranged to help with his anxiety and addiction problems.

Nine months after the CI was switched on, S reported that tinnitus was no longer an issue other than when he slept. He was working with a psychologist, reduced his consumption of alcohol, but still required a maximum dose of anxiety medication to function. Overall sensitivity to sound improved but was still an issue. S is now more confident interacting with people in a quiet setting and does not isolate himself in his office at the end of the day. He has gone back to playing the guitar independently and is hopeful that he will be able to play with friends in the future.

Summary

In a book chapter on the management of tinnitus with hearing aids published a little over a decade ago (Searchfield, 2006), the challenge in writing about tinnitus was similar to that we faced here writing about DST. There was little empirical evidence to support recommendations. While we do have evidence to support the benefits of hearing aids for the use of tinnitus relief (Searchfield, 2015), we now need similar evidence for DST. Clinical experience supports the recommendations made in this chapter; we firmly believe that with care, patience, and patient motivation, hearing aid gain can over time be achieved with little or no pain in cases of minimal hearing loss and DST.

References

Allen, J. B., Hall, J. L., & Jeng, P. S. (1990). Loudness growth in 1/2-octave bands (LGOB)–a procedure for the assessment of loudness. *J. Acoust. Soc. Am.*, *88*(2), 745–753. Retrieved from http://www.ncbi.nlm.nih.gov/pubmed/2212299.

Baker, R. J., & Rosen, S. (2002). Auditory filter nonlinearity in mild/moderate hearing impairment. *J. Acoust. Soc. Am.*, *111*(3), 1330–1339. Retrieved from http://www.ncbi.nlm.nih.gov/pubmed/11931310.

Bees, K., Guan, D., Alsarrage, N., & Searchfield, G. (2017). The effects of auditory object identification and localization (AOIL) training on noise acceptance and loudness discomfort in persons with normal hearing. *Speech, Lang & Hear*, 1–8.

Bentler, R. A., & Nelson, J. A. (2001). Effect of spectral shaping and content on loudness discomfort. *J. Am. Acad. Audiol.*, *12*(9), 462–470. Retrieved from http://www.ncbi.nlm.nih.gov/pubmed/11699817.

Byrne, D., Dillon, H., Ching, T., Katsch, R., & Keidser, G. (2001). NAL-NL1 procedure for fitting nonlinear hearing aids: Characteristics and comparisons with other procedures. *J. Am. Acad. Audiol.*, *12*(1), 37–51. Retrieved from http://www.ncbi.nlm.nih.gov/pubmed/11214977.

Dancer, A. L., & Hamery, P. J. F. (1998) A new nonlinear earplug for use in high-level impulse noise environment. *J. Acoust. Soc. Am.*, *103*(2878).

Dillon, H. (1996). Compression? Yes, but for low or high frequencies, for low or high intensities, and with what response times? *Ear Hear*, *17*(4), 287–307. Retrieved from http://www.ncbi.nlm.nih.gov/pubmed/8862967.

Dillon, H. (2012). *Hearing aids* (2nd ed.). Sydney: Boomerang Press.

Dillon, H., James, A., & Ginis, J. (1987). Client oriented scale of improvement (COSI) and its relationship to several other measures of benefit and satisfaction provided by hearing aids. *J. Am. Acad. Audiol.*, *8*, 27–43.

Fackrell, K., Fearnley, C., Hoare, D. J., & Sereda, M. (2015). Hyperacusis questionnaire as a tool for measuring hypersensitivity to sound in a tinnitus research population. *Biomed. Res. Int.*, 290425. doi:10.1155/2015/290425.

Formby, C., Hawley, M. L., Sherlock, L. P., Gold, S., Payne, J., Brooks, R., . . . Siegle, G. R. (2015). A sound therapy-based intervention to expand the auditory dynamic range for loudness among persons with sensorineural hearing losses: A randomized placebo-controlled clinical trial. *Semin. Hear*, *36*(2), 77–110. doi:10.1055/s-0035-1546958.

Goldstein, B., & Shulman, A. (1996). Tinnitus—Hyperacusis and the loudness discomfort level test—A preliminary report. *Int. Tinnitus J.*, *2*, 83–89. Retrieved from file:///C|/Documents%20and%20Settings/msan020/Local%20Settings/Application%20Data/Quosa/Data/My%20Citations/e3rsbvhnkoekv3n3iejgeqa744.qpw.

http://www.ncbi.nlm.nih.gov/entrez/query.fcgi?cmd=Retrieve&db=pubmed&dopt=Citation&list_uids=10753346.

Goverts, S. T., Houtgast, T., & van Beek, H. H. (2000). The precedence effect for lateralization at low sensation levels. *Hear. Res.*, *148*(1–2), 88–94. Retrieved from http://www.ncbi.nlm.nih.gov/pubmed/10978827.

Gu, J. W., Halpin, C. F., Nam, E. C., Levine, R. A., & Melcher, J. R. (2010). Tinnitus, diminished sound-level tolerance, and elevated auditory activity in humans with clinically normal hearing sensitivity. *J. Neurophysiol.*, *104*(6), 3361–3370. doi:10.1152/jn.00226.2010.

Hayes, D. (2006). Transient impulse control for hearing aids. *The Hearing Review.*

Helfer, K. S., & Wilber, L. A. (1990). Hearing loss, aging, and speech perception in reverberation and noise. *J. Speech Hear. Res.*, *33*(1), 149–155. Retrieved from http://www.ncbi.nlm.nih.gov/pubmed/2314073.

Herraiz, C., & Diges, I. (2010). Tinnitus and hyperacusis/phonophobia. In A. R. Moller, B. Langguth, D. De Ridder, & T. Kleinjung (Eds.), *Textbook of tinnius*. New York, NY: Springer.

Jenstad, L. M., Van Tasell, D. J., & Ewert, C. (2003). Hearing aid troubleshooting based on patients' descriptions. *J. Am. Acad. Audiol.*, *14*(7), 347–360. Retrieved from http://www.ncbi.nlm.nih.gov/pubmed/14620609.

Kates, J. M. (2010). Understanding compression: Modeling the effects of dynamic-range compression in hearing aids. *Int. J. Audiol.*, *49*(6), 395–409. doi:10.3109/14992020903426256.

Keidser, G., Bentler, R., & Kiessling, J. (2010). A multi-site evaluation of a proposed test for verifying hearing aid maximum output. *Int. J. Audiol.*, *49*(1), 14–23. doi:10.3109/14992020903160876.

Keidser, G., Dillon, H., Flax, M., Ching, T., & Brewer, S. (2011). The NAL-NL2 prescription procedure. *Audiol. Res.*, *1*(1), e24. doi:10.4081/audiores.2011.e24.

Khalfa, S., Dubal, S., Veuillet, E., Perez-Diaz, F., Jouvent, R., & Collet, L. (2002). Psychometric normalization of a hyperacusis questionnaire. *ORL J. Otorhinolaryngol. Relat. Spec.*, *64*(6), 436–442. doi:67570.

Leigh-Paffenroth, E. D., & Elangovan, S. (2011). Temporal processing in low-frequency channels: effects of age and hearing loss in middle-aged listeners. *J. Am. Acad. Audiol.*, *22*(7), 393–404. doi:10.3766/jaaa.22.7.2.

Levy, M., Peck, T., & Balachandran, R. (2011). Acceptable noise levels in hyperacusic individuals. Powerpoint presentation.

Liberman, M. C., & Kujawa, S. G. (2014). Hot topics—Hidden hearing loss: Permanent cochlear-nerve degeneration after temporary noise-induced threshold shift. *J. Acoust. Soc. Am.*, *135*(4), 2311–2311. doi:doi:http://dx.doi.org/10.1121/1.4877618.

Mackersie, C. L. (2007). Hearing aid maximum output and loudness discomfort: Are unaided loudness measures needed? *J. Am. Acad. Audiol.*, *18*(6), 504–514. Retrieved from http://www.ncbi.nlm.nih.gov/pubmed/17849638.

McKay, S., Gravel, J. S., & Tharpe, A. M. (2008). Amplification considerations for children with minimal or mild bilateral hearing loss and unilateral hearing loss. *Trends Amplif.*, *12*(1), 43–54. doi:10.1177/1084713807313570.

Meeus, O., Spaepen, M., de Ridder, D., & van de Heyning, P. (2009). Correlation between hyperacusis measurements in tinnitus patients [poster abstract]. From clinical practice to basic neuroscience and back: An international conference on tinnitus: *Third Tinnitus Research Initiative Meeting*, Stresa, Italy. June 24–26, 2009. (pp. 59). Stresa, Italy: TRI.

Moore, B. C., & Glasberg, B. R. (2011). The effect of hearing loss on the resolution of partials and fundamental frequency discrimination. *J. Acoust. Soc. Am.*, *130*(5), 2891–2901. doi:10.1121/1.3640852.

Mueller, H. G., & Bentler, R. A. (2005). Fitting hearing aids using clinical measures of loudness discomfort levels: An evidence-based review of effectiveness. *Journal of the American Academy of Audiology*, *16*(7), 461–472.

Nabelek, A. K., Freyaldenhoven, M. C., Tampas, J. W., Burchfiel, S. B., & Muenchen, R. A. (2006). Acceptable noise level as a predictor of hearing aid use. *Journal of the American Academy of Audiology*, *17*(9), 626–639. Retrieved from http://www.ncbi.nlm.nih.gov/pubmed/17039765.

Neijenhuis, K., Tschur, H., & Snik, A. (2004). The effect of mild hearing impairment on auditory processing tests. *J. Am. Acad. Audiol.*, *15*(1), 6–16. Retrieved from http://www.ncbi.nlm.nih.gov/pubmed/15030098.

Nelson, J. J., & Chen, K. (2004). The relationship of tinnitus, hyperacusis, and hearing loss. *Ear Nose Throat J.*, *83*(7), 472–476. Retrieved from file:///C|/Documents%20and%20Settings/msan020/Local%20Settings/Application%20Data/Quosa/Data/My%20Citations/os2s4l7bmojkp6qbdv5t3lbmig.qpw.

http://www.ncbi.nlm.nih.gov/entrez/query.fcgi?cmd=Retrieve&db=pubmed&dopt=Citation&list_uids=15372918.

Pekkarinen, E., Salmivalli, A., & Suonpaa, J. (1990). Effect of noise on word discrimination by subjects with impaired hearing, compared with those with normal hearing. *Scand. Audiol.*, *19*(1), 31–36. Retrieved from http://www.ncbi.nlm.nih.gov/pubmed/2336538.

Pienkowski, M., Tyler, R. S., Roncancio, E. R., Jun, H. J., Brozoski, T., Dauman, N., . . . Moore, B. C.

(2014). A review of hyperacusis and future directions: Part II. Measurement, mechanisms, and treatment. *Am. J. Audiol.*, *23*(4), 420–436. doi:10.1044/2014_AJA-13-0037.

Plack, C. J., Barker, D., & Prendergast, G. (2014). Perceptual consequences of "hidden" hearing loss. *Trends Hear.*, *18*. doi:10.1177/2331216514550621.

Polonenko, M. J., Scollie, S. D., Moodie, S., Seewald, R. C., Laurnagaray, D., Shantz, J., & Richards, A. (2010). Fit to targets, preferred listening levels, and self-reported outcomes for the DSL v5.0 a hearing aid prescription for adults. *Int. J. Audiol.*, *49*(8), 550–560. doi:10.3109/14992021003713122.

Preves, D., Sammeth, C., Cutting, M., & Woodruff, B. (1995). Experimental hearing device for hyperacusis. *Hearing Instruments*, December, *34*, 37–40.

Sandlin, R. E., & Olsson, R. J. (1999). Evaluation and selection of maskers and other devices used in the treatment of tinnitus and hyperacusis. *Trends in Amplification*, *4*, 6–26.

Sankowsky-Rothe, T., Blau, M., Schepker, H., & Doclo, S. (2015). Reciprocal measurement of acoustic feedback paths in hearing aids. *J. Acoust. Soc. Am.*, *188*(4), EL399–EL404.

Schecklmann, M., Landgrebe, M., Langguth, B., & Group, T. R. I. D. S. (2014). Phenotypic characteristics of hyperacusis in tinnitus. *PLoS ONE*, *9*(1), e86944. doi:10.1371/journal.pone.0086944.

Searchfield, G. D. (2006). Hearing aids and tinnitus. In T. R (Ed.), *Tinnitus protocols*. New York: Thieme.

Searchfield, G. D. (2014). Tinnitus what and where: An ecological framework. *Front. Neurol.*, *5*, 271. doi:10.3389/fneur.2014.00271.

Searchfield, G. D. (2016). Hearing aids for tinnitus. In D. M. Baguley & M. Fagelson (Eds.), *Tinnitus: Clinical and research perspectives*. San Diego, CA: Plural.

Searchfield, G. D., Morrison-Low, J., & Wise, K. (2007). Object identification and attention training for treating tinnitus. *Prog. Brain Res.*, *166*, 441–460. doi:10.1016/S0079-6123(07)66043-9.

Sheehan, G., Houghton, J., & Searchfield, G. D. (2016). Acceptability of background noise amongst children diagnosed with an auditory processing disorder. *Speech, Language and Hearing*, *19*(3), 180–188. doi:10.1080/2050571X.2016.1182310.

Shekhawat, G. S., Searchfield, G. D., & Stinear, C. M. (2013). Role of hearing AIDS in tinnitus intervention: A scoping review. *J. Am. Acad. Audiol.*, *24*(8), 747–762. doi:10.3766/jaaa.24.8.11.

Stewart, R., & Wingfield, A. (2009). Hearing loss and cognitive effort in older adults' report accuracy for verbal materials. *J. Am. Acad. Audiol.*, *20*(2), 147–154. Retrieved from http://www.ncbi.nlm.nih.gov/pubmed/19927677.

Storey, L., Dillon, H., Yeend, I., & Wigney, D. (1998). The National Acoustic Laboratories' procedure for selecting the saturation sound pressure level of hearing aids: Experimental validation. *Ear Hear.*, *19*(4), 267–279. Retrieved from http://www.ncbi.nlm.nih.gov/pubmed/9728722.

Tun, P. A., McCoy, S., & Wingfield, A. (2009). Aging, hearing acuity, and the attentional costs of effortful listening. *Psychol. Aging*, *24*(3), 761–766. doi:10.1037/a0014802.

Tyler, R. S., Gogel, S. A., & Gehringer, A. K. (2007). Tinnitus activities treatment. *Prog. Brain Res.*, *166*, 425–434. doi:10.1016/S0079-6123(07)66041-5.

Tyler, R. S., Pienkowski, M., Roncancio, E. R., Jun, H. J., Brozoski, T., Dauman, N., . . . Moore, B. C. (2014). A review of hyperacusis and future directions: Part I. Definitions and manifestations. *Am. J. Audiol.*, *23*(4), 402–419. doi:10.1044/2014_AJA-14-0010.

Vernon, J. A. (2002). Hyperacusis: Testing, treatments and a possible mechanism. *Australian and New Zealand Journal of Audiology*, *24*(2), 68–73.

Westcott, M. (2002). Case study. Management of hyperacusis associated with post-traumatic stress disorder. In P. R. (Ed.), *Proceedings of the Seventh International Tinnitus Seminar* (pp. 280–285). Perth: University of Western Australia.

Wu, Y. H., & Stangl, E. (2013). The effect of hearing aid signal-processing schemes on acceptable noise levels: perception and prediction. *Ear Hear.*, *34*(3), 333–341. doi:10.1097/AUD.0b013e31827417d4.

15

Hyperacusis Management: A Patient's Perspective

Rob Littwin

Onset

I am a musician. In 2004, I developed hyperacusis and severe ear pain. A year later, I developed tinnitus. I created my own approach to address these challenges which enabled me to re-establish my tolerance of sound, ameliorate my ear pain, and manage tinnitus.

In April 2004, I visited a friend who owned and ran a small restaurant/grocery with his wife in a suburb of Atlanta. My friend had moved a number of wooden tables and chairs outside, behind the restaurant, and was using a pressure washer to clean them. I stood outside with him for 30 to 40 minutes watching the color and grain of the wood reveal itself. While it was very loud—both of us were standing several feet from the pressure washer without hearing protection—I didn't realize anything was wrong until I was driving home that afternoon and put on a CD. The music sounded sharper, distorted, tinny, high-pitched, and uncomfortably loud. It was also somewhat painful to hear. I shut off the CD. I tried listening to it again a few minutes later with the same results.

I took it easy for a couple days at home and rested my ears. Then I went to the gym to work out when very few people were there. The background music, which I had never paid attention to before, seemed uncharacteristically loud and high-pitched. For the first time, I felt continual pain, numbness, and pressure in my left ear.

When the ear pain and other symptoms didn't go away over the next day or two, I made an appointment with a highly regarded neurotologist. My otologic examination, which took place one week after I had been exposed to the pressure washer, was normal. My audiogram demonstrated normal hearing. One of the tests administered to me showed I had acoustic reflex decay in my left ear. In light of this result, the doctor believed there was a 40 to 50% chance I could have an acoustic neuroma and he ordered an MRI scan. He prescribed prednisone and Trental (pentoxifylline) and said he would not treat me further until the MRI results came back. I had the MRI a day or two later. My doctor failed to tell me how critically important it is to wear hearing protection during an MRI. This is particularly true for individuals with decreased sound tolerance. As a result, I wore no hearing protection and none was offered to me.

The experience was painful, but I withstood more than 45 minutes of intensely loud sound because I was concerned my symptoms might be explained by an acoustic neuroma. I also badly needed my doctor's continued help. But from that moment forward, following the MRI, my symptoms were exacerbated and my life changed. At home that evening, I turned on the television. A big-voiced contestant on a popular show at the time was singing, but rather than take pleasure in the performance, or even regard it with critical distance, the experience was like being physically assaulted by sound and I quickly turned off the TV. I was stunned.

I called my doctor a few days later. When I told him how much worse I was after the MRI and questioned him about it, he was nonchalant. He didn't believe exposure to an MRI could worsen my symptoms. Perhaps I misread it, but he seemed more invested in defending his professional acumen than in supporting his very worried patient. I fired him.

Much later, after I took the reins of my own recovery by educating myself about my challenges and doing something about them, I read the following in a book about tinnitus and hyperacusis (Jastreboff & Hazell, 2004, p. 79) that proved invaluable: "All patients being referred for magnetic resonance imaging must be advised about the need for hearing protection, as this examination involves quite high levels of sound. In those with severe decreased sound tolerance, it should be considered that the scan is delayed until significant improvement is noted." Other researchers have described the importance of wearing properly inserted earplugs during an MRI to preserve cochlear function (Radomskij et al., 2002).

In hindsight, I regard my decreased sound tolerance and accompanying ear pain following exposure to the pressure washer as moderate at best. However, after being exposed one week later to the extremely loud sound of an MRI—the auditory version of double-dipping—my sensitivity to sound became very severe and the ear pain was frequently excruciating. Normal, everyday sounds were considerably louder to me and were often painful to hear.

I had two very different kinds of ear pain. One type of pain was immediate and occurred uniformly upon the presentation of sounds that exceeded my tolerance—the aural equivalent of placing one's hand on a hot stove. Many normal sounds that I would not have characterized as remotely loud prior to exposure to the pressure washer and MRI felt physically painful or uncomfortable to hear in both ears for as long as the sound lasted. These sounds included high-frequency or resonant adult voices, a crying baby, the voices or laughter of young children, a party, the percussive sound of a glass being placed on a counter, a dog barking, a bird whistling, silverware dropped in the sink, the clatter of dishes being placed in the dishwasher, a garbage disposal or vacuum cleaner, a piano, sax, trumpet, flute, violin, or drums, my own singing, some flushing toilets, a leaf blower, a dentist's drill, shopping malls, grocery stores, movie theaters, most restaurants, announcements over a loudspeaker, a car horn, squealing brakes, and the sounds of road noise when driving.

The other type of ear pain consisted of unremitting, continuous waves of sharp, stabbing pain in my left ear that felt as if a nail or an ice pick was repeatedly driven deep into my ear. These bouts of severe pain lasted for days, weeks, or months. Unlike the other type of ear pain, which was immediate and would last for as long as the given sound was present, I would continue to feel the second type of ear pain even when I was no longer exposed to the sound or the setting in which I had heard it.

Since the MRI, I had been feeling hopeless about my prospects and I was in a kind of mourning. I felt powerless, lethargic, and prodigiously sorry for myself. I was practically looking at my life in retrospective terms, watching it recede.

Prior to developing hyperacusis, I had been working on a long and satisfying project in a recording studio where I sang, played keyboards, co-wrote horn and string arrangements, produced the sessions, and worked with some seriously fine jazz musicians. I couldn't imagine ever being able to tolerate working in a recording studio again, much less sing, or listen to or write music at home. I was very upset with the doctor who had treated me, but I realized soon enough that I had to try to let those feelings go. Feeling anger and regret was to face in the wrong direction, looking back at something that had already happened and expecting a different result. I needed to look ahead.

Fear can paralyze us or it can be a catalyst for making changes. Four months after I developed hyperacusis, I woke up one morning and realized as much as I missed experiencing sound the way I used to, I missed myself even more. I could no longer locate myself. I hadn't listened to music for months. On this morning, I resolved no matter how scared and overwhelmed I felt, I would book some time at the recording studio.

The session consisted of my engineer and me doing a lot of close listening to tracks we had previously recorded and creating "comp" (short for composite) tracks from them. I didn't think I would last more than two minutes. I discovered I had far more control in a recording studio than in other settings. We tend to think of recording studios as loud environments, and they can be, but I learned to work smart, carefully, and very quietly when I returned to the studio. Instead of using the large speakers I was accustomed to, we used much smaller speakers, a comparatively comical-looking delivery system considering all the great-sounding equipment at hand that I was unable to tolerate at the time. We also adjusted the mix by taking off some high frequencies so the music wasn't physically painful to hear. We kept the volume extremely low. The sound level was still uncomfortable to hear at times, but being back in the studio doing what I loved gave me access to something in myself that I missed and needed. On my first day back, we worked for two or three hours.

Returning to my recording project provided a huge psychological boost at a time when I needed to be reminded how important it is to look forward to things. I didn't begin desensitization therapy for eight more months, but in a sense my recovery began that day. Over the coming months I was able to continue working on the project, albeit very quietly.

For the first few months, hyperacusis had defined me. But I found it was possible, indeed essential, to take hold of a few things in my life that were meaningful to me and get busy pursuing them. None of this came easily or quickly.

If a recording studio was one of the few places I could control sound in my environment, I had little or no control in other settings. I remember trying to watch the movie *Million Dollar Baby* when it was released early in the following year. Even the narration by the soft-spoken Morgan Freeman was so loud and painful to me that I had to leave the theater.

I also worked as an independent contractor, as a business analyst, and I was often required to be onsite. The sounds of some co-worker's voices were like knives, and the particular sound quality of some male and female voices was physically very painful to hear. A printer near my office made a loud, piercing beep each time it printed a page. It too was painful to hear. Some of my symptoms were surprising. For months I felt aural fullness, as if a tiny balloon had been inflated inside my ear, and left there. I had difficulty with processed sound and in settings with a lot of echo. A conversation on the telephone lasting for more than a couple minutes would result in my feeling the presence of something in my ear that didn't belong there and lowered my tolerance of sound for several days. As a workaround, I placed a small piece of duct tape over the receiver to help modulate the volume and frequency of the sound, making it less painful to hear.

The highly processed sound of voices coming through a speakerphone during conference calls was both immediately painful to hear and resulted in my feeling continual waves of pain in my left ear. During an emergency at work, I sat in a conference room for eight hours with several co-workers, as well as others who called into a conference bridge for a call that lasted into the middle of the night. Within an hour, I began to feel sharp pain in my left ear. Over the next two months, the pain did not let up for a minute.

Diagnosis

During this time I was diagnosed with hyperacusis at the Department of Otolaryngology at the Emory School of Medicine. The doctor who examined me was the fifth doctor to do so, a frustrating experience many hyperacusic patients share in our search to obtain an accurate diagnosis. It gave me some hope to attach a name to what I was experiencing and the doctor was extremely solicitous and kind. He encouraged me to look into a program at Emory University called Tinnitus Retraining Therapy (TRT), an intervention used to manage tinnitus and hyperacusis. He advised me to wear hearing protection for several weeks at work to let my constant ear pain gradually diminish. When it did, I weaned myself off hearing protection, as my doctor had suggested, and no longer used earplugs as a routine practice.

Despite hyperacusis developing and persisting, I decided to continue working. I spent every day around sound, rather than purposely avoiding it. I didn't seek out sound that was painful, but it is axiomatic that painful sound will seek out a hyperacusic. I got out in the world to the best extent I could, despite many setbacks and daily exposure to innumerable sounds that were too loud for me and caused pain or were uncomfortable to hear. Several years later, an experienced clinician told me my decision to continue to go to work was an important step to take. To be honest, it was a decision I made out of necessity. I needed to earn a living. When I had several setbacks during which my sensitivity to sound was exacerbated, I explained my situation to my manager and to a few co-workers; my colleagues could not have been more gracious or understanding. I was encouraged to know that I had help and support at work.

Just as I encountered many sounds at work that were either physically painful or uncomfortably loud to hear, the same held true in many settings outside work. With hyperacusis, I noticed that many background sounds became foreground sounds. The beeping produced by the price scanners at the checkout in the grocery store where I shopped was painfully loud and exacerbated my sensitivity to sound for several days. For a while, driving was overwhelmingly loud. Many places I frequented were too loud and painful for me to even consider. Living with hyperacusis was a tug of war between engagement and avoidance. I put myself in settings I could handle and avoided environments that were too much for me, even as I gently tried to push the aural envelope. I didn't look for a perfect situation; I looked for environments that were tolerable. For example, I found and could enjoy a comparatively quiet restaurant where the acoustics were acceptable and echo was minimal.

When I was diagnosed with hyperacusis, I invested time in learning as much as I could about the condition and my options so that I could make an informed decision about how to proceed. I learned that hyperacusis is not well known and is often misunderstood. Many hearing healthcare clinicians are tentative or apprehensive with respect to its diagnosis and treatment. There is an abundance of confusion regarding even basic information, such as terminology and definitions, ranging from the short-lived *hyperacusis dolorosa* (Mathisen, 1969)—which speaks to the emotional impact and attendant distress and sorrow of hyperacusis sufferers—to the dismissive view that hyperacusis is an "exaggerated or inappropriate" response to sounds that "a typical person" would regard as neither a threat nor uncomfortably loud (Klein et al., 1990). Studies on the prevalence of hyperacusis in the general population have drawn widely different conclusions (Andersson et al., 2002; Rubinstein et al., 1996). The mechanisms that may explain the emergence of hyperacusis are hypothetical. When hyperacusis is described in the media, the reports are typically short on fact and long on hyperbole, and often employ the language of catastrophe.

During this period, I improved my understanding by reading Dr. Jastreboff and Mr. Hazell's book on Tinnitus Retraining Therapy (TRT), the approach recommended by the doctor who had diagnosed me. For many TRT patients, therapy included the use of wearable noise generators (WNGs). These devices emitted broadband noise and were initially intended to foster habituation in patients suffering from tinnitus. The devices were also used by individuals with hyperacusis as part of a strategy to help them become less sensitive to sound. I also learned that a highly respected clinician, Dr. Jack Vernon, was using broadband pink noise to treat his hyperacusis patients.

A company that produced well-regarded WNGs for use in TRT made available a readout of its broadband noise presentation on its website, and I worked with two colleagues in the recording studio to replicate the presentation. However, even when I played it very softly, I was unable to tolerate the broadband noise presentation used in TRT without experiencing immediate discomfort. It hurt to hear the sound, and for this reason I chose not to pursue TRT.

Dan Malcore, who founded and moderates The Hyperacusis Network (http://www.hyperacusis.net)—an Internet health support board and information website dedicated to individuals with hyperacusis and other forms of decreased sound tolerance—graciously sent me a copy of the pink noise Dr. Vernon used with moderate success to treat hyperacusic patients. Pink noise is generally perceived as less shrill than white noise. The idea of using pink noise to help re-establish sound tolerance was suggested to Dr. Vernon by a patient whose experience with pink noise affirmed that this form of broadband noise would be easier to tolerate than white noise.

Unfortunately, after auditioning the pink noise through headphones for just 10 seconds, I felt so profoundly dizzy I could barely stand up. When a mastering engineer and I examined the pink noise presentation at the studio we found it was very poorly made. Using high-end equipment to provide a visual representation of the pink noise in real time, we discovered it contained an uncountable number of artifacts throughout the entire track. These artifacts resembled a series of fence posts, each causing a momentary increase in volume. As a result, the presentation repeatedly jumped from a steady volume to a much higher volume and back again. The spikes occurred over so short a period, a listener wouldn't be able to hear it as a volume increase, but the overall effect to the listener was that the sound was harsh. We also discovered the pink noise was unfiltered and had a bandwidth of 1 Hz to 22,050 Hz, a considerably higher high end than the more moderate, filtered presentation Dr. Vernon described in his excellent book (Vernon & Sanders, 2001). Although we subsequently created a filtered pink noise presentation that matched the characteristics described in Dr. Vernon's book—200 Hz to 6 kHz—I found this presentation painful to hear as well.

I was at a crossroads. I knew I needed help, but it appeared I couldn't tolerate the commercially available options. A year had passed. I had put myself out in the world from the start and did the best I could despite daily exposure to many sounds that were too loud for me and caused pain or discomfort. Most environmental sound was uniformly louder, as if someone had reached into my auditory system and turned the gain way up. Many sounds produced discomfort, and those that exceeded my tolerance in a given frequency range and volume were immediately painful to hear. In the preceding year, my sound tolerance had barely improved.

Treatment

I decided to create a pink noise presentation I *could* tolerate, one that caused me no pain, discomfort, or annoyance. Working in the studio, we produced several trial versions of broadband noise before I found one that was well-suited for me. I was able to tolerate broadband pink noise with a low-end frequency of 30 Hz and a high-end frequency of just 3 kHz. My experience with broadband noise is atypical in this regard. It is unusual for a patient to have a difficult time tolerating unfiltered pink noise or the broadband noise presentations of in-ear wearable noise generators. For this reason, my approach to manage hyperacusis may or may not be effective or suitable for others.

We made a pink noise CD for my use and although its frequency content differed from that recommended by Dr. Vernon, and was considerably less ambitious than the broadband noise used in TRT, I was thrilled to find an acceptable and therapeutic sound. By creating broadband noise in the studio, I also had an advantage; the commercial WNGs were limited with respect to the low-end frequencies they could emit, whereas broadband noise could be produced in a recording studio that contained substantially more of the low-frequency energy I could tolerate. This gave the broadband noise a more rounded, pleasant sound, making it easy for me to use.

In terms of volume and time spent using broadband noise, I chose to not adopt Dr. Vernon's protocol to work with broadband noise at the *loudest* volume that was comfortable. I was mindful that Jastreboff and Hazell had written some particularly severe cases of hyperacusis could be permanently worsened by using broadband pink noise at a high volume. Instead, I gradually increased the volume to a level that did not cause annoyance or discomfort. More recently, Jastreboff has recommended (2014) hyperacusic patients in TRT use broadband noise at about 9 dB SL (i.e., 9 decibels above one's threshold for hearing the noise). Although I ultimately worked with the volume set higher than the TRT level, I could clearly hear external sound and was rarely aware of the broadband noise. I worked up to using the pink noise CD for eight hours a day, and achieved better results when using it for eight consecutive hours rather than dividing the time spent listening into smaller portions. I used the CD for three months, at a very low volume in the first month, slightly increasing the volume the next month, and increasing it a little more in the third month. I found it helpful to set and forget the volume at the beginning of the month and not change it until the following month.

I used good, very comfortable headphones, capable of accurately producing high-end, midrange, and low-end frequency sound. To ensure I could clearly hear sound in my immediate environment, I used open air headphones for which the headphone pads lay flat against the ears rather than fully enclosing them.

I developed a program to manage my hyperacusis using a series of graduated broadband pink noise presentations created in a recording studio. Each presentation was slightly more ambitious than the previous one. Every three months, I increased the high-frequency energy of the presentation and started again at the lower volume. In addition to using broadband noise during waking hours, I used a tabletop sound machine at bedtime so that I did not sleep in silence.

Four or five months after I began therapy, now working with broadband noise with a low end of 30 Hz and a high end of 4 kHz, I noticed a small improvement in my sound tolerance. Over time, I would extend the high end to 5 kHz, 6 kHz, 6.5 kHz, 7.5 kHz, 8.5 kHz, and above. By working in this way, the broadband noise that I was unable to tolerate at first became comfortable to use over time. I hired an experienced, smart, supportive audiologist to periodically administer an audiological test called a Loudness Discomfort Level (LDL) test to me. The test can help a hearing healthcare clinician determine the nature and extent of a person's decreased sound tolerance. When I was initially diagnosed with hyperacusis, my LDLs were in the mid-30 to mid-40s decibel range, consistent with my experiencing discomfort at low conversational levels.

In an LDL test, sound is presented through headphones using a clinical audiometer to a patient seated in an audiometric test suite. The test is used to identify the sound level that distinguishes a presented tone as loud from one that is *uncomfortably* loud. When a tone reaches a volume that is uncomfortable to hear, the patient signals the clinician to move on to the next frequency. Tones at each new frequency are initially presented at a considerably lower volume. I was always tested twice in each ear and my audiologist used the second set of readings. We used the LDL test to measure my progress and fine-tune my treatment.

I had started a new contract as a business analyst and immediately encountered a problem. Most companies keep their large servers in a closet or in an enclosed area, but this company had placed a large server in an open area where my manager and a co-worker sat. The server emitted a relatively high-pitched sound I measured at 65 dB—the only time I ever used a sound meter to measure anything. At the time, my LDLs showed my sound tolerance at 6 kHz and above was still low. Exposure to the high-frequency sound of the server hurt to hear and made me more sensitive to sound; everything sounded louder to me. I decided to leave the contract. Later, I was compelled to leave another contract when exposure to sound on site exacerbated my sound tolerance for days. My progress was slow and fitful.

A similar problem occurred on another contract at a time when the U.S. economy was terrible and contract positions, like all jobs, were hard to come by. Ever since I developed hyperacusis, I continued to have difficulty tolerating the heavily-processed sound of speakerphones on conference calls. Even at moderate sound levels, someone's voice over a speakerphone physically hurt to hear in the moment and each call caused me to feel continual stabbing ear pain. Since I participated in multiple calls per day, I was in non-stop pain for the entire contract—seven-and-a-half months. I felt waves of sharp pain in my left ear, whether I was sitting in a quiet room, driving, working, waking up, or trying to fall asleep. After the contract ended and my ear pain had time to resolve, I found that if I used broadband noise as a buffer while on a conference call, I could tolerate speakerphones without ear pain. While I was glad to find a workaround, I thought of it as an auditory Band-Aid® but not a solution.

Until that time, a major part of my therapy consisted of using sound whose spectrum was progressively widened to improve my tolerance of sound. In an LDL test administered after I had been working for three months with broadband noise with a high-end frequency of 8.5 kHz, my tolerance of sound at 8 kHz and above had improved, but less than I would have liked. It was taking longer for me to reestablish my sensitivity to sound in high-end frequencies.

There are two ways to customize broadband noise for use in the desensitization therapy I employed. One is to extend the high-end frequency, and I had been using this approach since I started therapy. The other approach is to increase the amplitude of the broadband noise presentation at specific frequencies or frequency ranges. This approach was used by companies that made wearable noise generators, and it was used in TRT to treat tinnitus and hyperacusis. I adopted the latter approach as I proceeded with desensitization therapy to manage hyperacusis.

An important difference between the broadband noise emitted by a well-regarded wearable noise generator and the filtered pink noise I had been using to this point was that the WNG contained a 10 dB increase in amplitude at 6 kHz and a smaller increase in amplitude at 2.8 kHz. These boosts in amplitude, which can be very helpful to treat hyperacusis, were absent in the broadband noise I had used to this point. We replicated the characteristics of the commercially available presentation in the studio by applying filters and a narrow band-pass. We purposely used a high end of 9.5 kHz, slightly more ambitious than the high-end frequency used by the aforementioned WNGs (Figure 15–1).

It had taken me a long time, but by working with progressively more challenging broadband noise, I was eventually able to tolerate and use a presentation with spectral characteristics that were comparable to those used in TRT. A new LDL test administered to me around this time indicated my sound tolerance at 8 kHz and 12 kHz had increased dramatically.

Later, we would create a broadband white noise presentation modeled on the characteristics of a WNG (Figure 15–2). Experienced clinicians report filtered broadband white noise is a bit more effective for hyperacusis treatment than broadband pink noise, provided the patient can tolerate it.

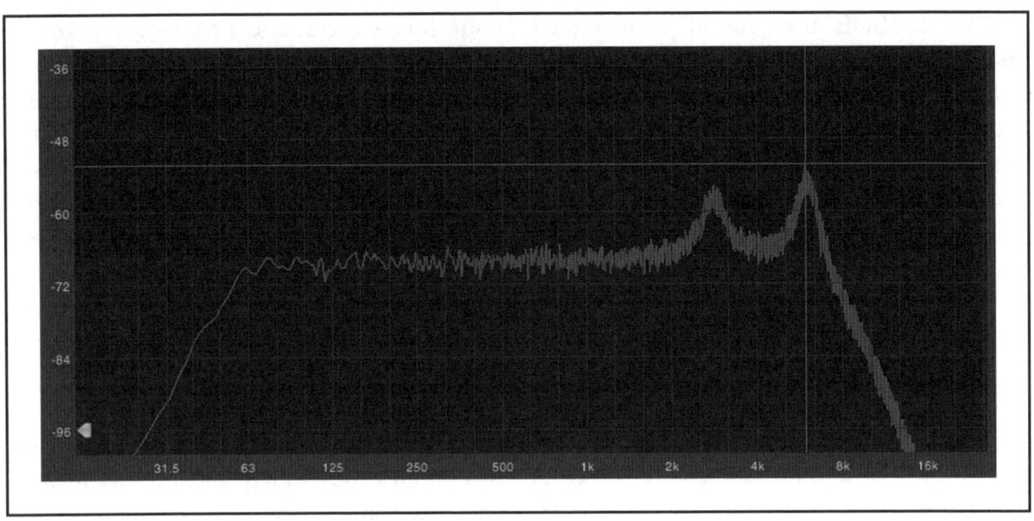

Figure 15–1. Broadband noise modeled on a wearable noise generator presentation with emphasis at 2.8 kHz and 6 kHz.

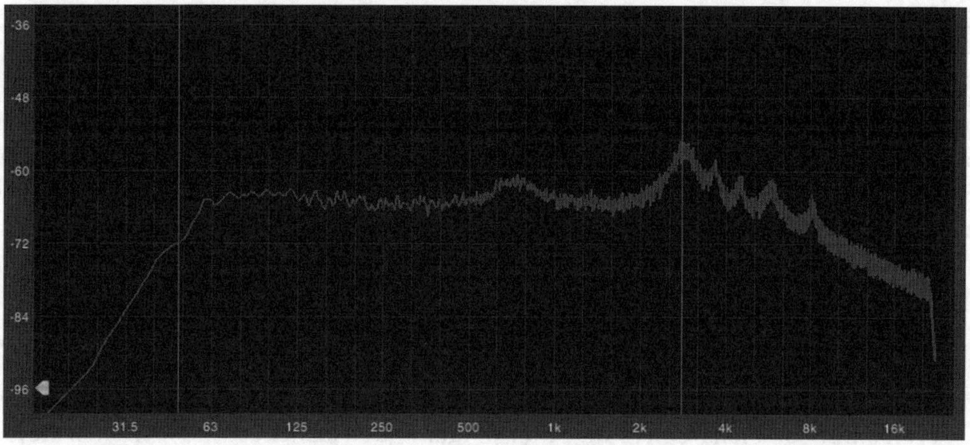

Figure 15–2. White noise from 30 Hz to 22,050 Hz modeled on a wearable noise generator presentation with six small increases in amplitude. We purposely increased the low end to round out the sound.

Emotions

The central auditory system is a master detective. When we consider a sound to be important, particularly if we regard the sound as a threat, our auditory system works hard to monitor it. The auditory system is also an effective discriminator. When a sound is no longer perceived to be of importance, our hearing system disregards it. In this way, the hearing system is selective about the sound to which it attends, which is why we can hear our name being called across a noisy, crowded room or wake up to the sound of a crying baby, but sleep through a thunderstorm.

A hyperacusic regards many sounds as a threat, hence of value and requiring attention. While it is reasonable to respond with prudence to sound that is physically painful to hear, inevitably, for the hyperacusic this results in developing strong and adverse feelings about sound. These feelings, and the resultant hypervigilance to or avoidance of sounds, are enormously powerful. Recognizing the feelings in oneself and finding a way to address them is difficult but essential.

One of the greatest barriers to success in treating individuals with severe hyperacusis is the failure to acknowledge and address the role of the emotions in their response to sound. Different terms—phonophobia (Phillips & Carr, 1998), misophonia (Jastreboff & Jastreboff, 2002), fear hyperacusis, and annoyance hyperacusis (Tyler et al., 2014)—have been used to distinguish this aspect of decreased sound tolerance. Although audiologists and hearing scientists are not in agreement on the utility of these terms, each is an attempt to describe the emotional response that accompanies hyperacusis like an uninvited dinner guest who has an inordinately large appetite.

Since starting therapy, I regarded hyperacusis as a physiological problem that had to do with the way the brain processes sound. While I was aware of the emotional impact hyperacusis exerted on me every day, I assumed all my challenges with decreased sound tolerance would be resolved by working with broadband noise, avoiding the overuse of hearing protection around normal sound, and consistently exposing myself to different external settings. However, I was wrong. The strategies I deployed, similar to those used in clinics around the world to improve LDLs, had *not* helped me resolve my continual ear pain. Like other hyperacusics, I was concerned that the pain was a symptom of irreparable damage to my auditory system. For this reason, I maintained an abiding, if unfamiliar sense of caution around sounds and in settings that could provoke these symptoms. For a long time, I didn't understand the line connecting my ear pain and aural fullness on one hand, to the fear, anxiety, and distress I experienced around some specific sounds and settings on the other.

Ear Pain

The tensor tympani and stapedius muscles reduce the power at which sound reaches the inner ear. The contraction of the tensor tympani muscle is regarded as a startle reflex. For some individuals, tensor tympani muscle activity may increase, and the muscle may eventually be fixed in a state of tonic contraction. Klochoff (1979) speculated that the overactivity of the tensor tympani is associated with several symptoms often reported by patients. These symptoms include episodic ear fullness; otalgia (i.e., ear pain); tinnitus; dysacusis consisting of murmurs, clicks, and distortion; tension headaches; and vertigo. Klochoff and Westerberg (1971) reported that increased mental stress appeared to be the common thread running through nearly every case of spontaneous tonic tensor tympani muscle activity in the ear, which they called the tonic tensor phenomenon. Due to the prevalence of these symptoms, Klochoff (1979) wrote, "it seems justified to talk of a Tensor Tympani Syndrome." For several years, some authors (e.g., Westcott, 2016) have preferred the term Tonic Tensor Tympani Syndrome (TTTS).

Hyperacusic patients who report aural fullness or pressure, ear pain, and other symptoms consistent with the involvement of the tensor tympani muscle are described by Westcott and Jastreboff. For Westcott (2016, p. 145) these symptoms were reported by patients "with an anxiety-based need to protect the health of their ears or their hearing." For Jastreboff (2014, p. 111), the "over-activation of the autonomic nervous system may, in turn, activate the tensor tympani muscle resulting in tensor tympani syndrome (e.g., fullness, pulsation, pain in the ear)."

The symptoms of Tensor Tympani Syndrome have also been reported by individuals exposed to an unexpected loud sound, typically with a short rise time that produces a so-called acoustic shock, as well as by patients with temporomandibular disorders (TMD). Patuzzi, Milhinch, and Doyle (2000) proposed that symptoms of acoustic shock injury may be attributed to an excessive startle reflex of the tensor tympani muscle. Ramirez et al. (2007, p. 97) wrote that emotional stress may play an important role in patients with TMD, noting that ear pain "can be felt by tympanic membrane tension due to constant tensor tympani muscle contracture."

Regarding therapy for Tensor Tympani Syndrome, Klochoff (1979) indicated the most important step is for clinicians to reassure patients that the symptoms relate to "psychosomatic dysfunction due to stress" and are not a sign of disease. For patients in intractable pain, Klochoff recommended physical relaxation therapy and medication such as diazepam. Westcott has reported that broadband noise desensitization therapy combined with Cognitive Behavioral Therapy, or referral to a physiotherapist or pain specialist are helpful to some hyperacusic patients with ear pain and other symptoms of TTTS. As a last resort, some patients have considered surgery to section the stapedius and/or tensor tympani muscle tendons. In a systematic review of 21 articles of mostly case reports or case series, based on the poor quality of the studies Bhimrao et al. (2012) reported there is weak evidence to support surgical tenotomy of the middle ear muscles in the treatment of middle ear myoclonus—of which Tensor Tympani Syndrome is a subtype.

Music Protocol

I had reached a point in therapy at which I needed to push the aural envelope a little further. Broadband noise has no dynamics; it is static, with no loud and soft sections, whereas everyday life is filled with such dynamics. Listening to music in a deliberate, controlled, and purposeful way would expose me to sound that varies considerably over time. I hoped it would be an effective approach to supplement the use of broadband noise and enable me to further improve my tolerance of high-frequency sound and address my challenges with severe ear pain. With these goals in mind, I created a protocol for listening to music. The last thing I wanted was to create something that felt like more "work" so I made it fun. I walk on a treadmill every day for at least 45 minutes and I thought if I used that time to listen to music, I could exercise and concentrate on enjoying music at the same time.

By pairing sound with an enjoyable activity, the music protocol helped me reevaluate the emotional response to sound that accompanied my hyperacusis and to address my anxiety and stress about sound in certain settings. I thought it was important to move *toward* my anxiety rather than away from it. That is why one of the conditions I set for myself was to listen to music through headphones. I needed to prove to myself that even with sound right up against my ears, there was nothing to be concerned about.

Until that time, I had been able to work with music in the controlled environment of a recording studio. The music protocol enabled me to give myself control over sound in a different setting, feel less tentative around sound, and slowly prove to myself, consciously and unconsciously, that I could let go of the feelings and beliefs I had developed about the dangers of sound. Exposure to normal sound could not hurt me.

The music protocol helped me completely resolve the continual bouts of severe ear pain I felt and helped me to further improve my LDLs. I have used the protocol twice: once to manage hyperacusis and severe ear pain and again when I was exposed to a loud, sudden sound at work that clinicians characterized as an acoustic shock. Following the acoustic incident, I felt earache, aural fullness, pressure, tingling, and slight pain—comparatively mild symptoms. Over time, these symptoms decreased and then fully resolved as I continued to use the music protocol week after week.

The protocol consists of three phases. In phase 1, the baseline setting is the *lowest* possible volume the listener can hear. In phase 2, the baseline setting is the *most comfortable* volume the listener chooses. In phase 3, the baseline setting is the *loudest* volume the listener can tolerate without being uncomfortable. See Tables 15–1, 15–2, and 15–3.

Phase 1 should be used for nine weeks, phase 2 for 18 weeks, and phase 3 for 12 weeks; however, individual needs and differences may dictate that modifications are indicated.

- Every day, listen to an entire CD (i.e., between 40 and 75 minutes per session depending on the recording used in that day's session).
- Choose any type of music, regardless of style and dynamic range, from Beethoven to Hendrix, Miles Davis to Judy Collins, rap to country music. The key is to play music one enjoys and wants to hear.
- Actively listen to the music.

- It is very important to introduce the music as directly and consistently as possible to one's auditory system. Therefore, listen to the music via headphones rather than through external speakers.
- The only requirement about the headphones is for the music to sound pleasing when played through them. Noise cancellation headphones can be used, if preferred.
- Use CDs, LPs, or files that have been downloaded in the WAV or AIFF format.
- Do not use MP3 files, as their sound quality may be degraded and less pleasant.
- Do not use the typical ear buds that come with iPods. There are commercially available ear buds with much better fidelity, although they are far more expensive.
- If listening to a certain style of music feels too ambitious during the first couple of months, it is fine to listen to any style of music that is relaxing.
- If the music hurts or is uncomfortable at any time, lower the volume. If the music continues to hurt, stop and play something else. The music should never be physically painful or uncomfortable.
- For the first few weeks, the volume will be extremely low. It may seem that no progress is being made, but during this time one is learning to treat sound as nonthreatening.
- Do not use broadband noise during a listening session.
- Use the music protocol for nine months.

Table 15–1. Phase 1.

Week	Instructions
1	Each day of the week, set the volume of the CD so it is at the lowest possible volume that can be heard (i.e., at one's threshold for hearing sound). Listen to the entire CD. By design, the listener will strain to hear the music. Relax and pay attention.
2	Each day of the week, set the volume of the CD so it is at the lowest possible volume that can be heard. Then, increase the volume to a level that is slightly louder. Listen to the entire CD. If the music feels painful at any time, even at this low volume, slightly lower the volume so that it is at the threshold for hearing sound.
3	Each day of the week, set the volume of the CD so it is at the lowest possible volume that can be heard. Then, increase the volume to a level that is slightly louder. Then, increase the volume slightly more. Listen to the entire CD. If the music feels painful at any time, slightly lower the volume. If the listener feels worried or uncomfortable, try to hang in there. If these feelings persist, slightly lower the volume so that it is at the threshold for hearing sound.
4–9	Listen to an entire CD each day of the week. Set the volume to a level that is slightly louder than the previous week. For example, during week 4 the volume should be slightly louder than it was for week 3, in week 5 the volume should be slightly louder than it was for week 4, and so on. Listen to the entire CD. If the music feels painful at any time, slightly lower the volume. If the listener feels worried or uncomfortable, try to hang in there. If these feelings persist, slightly lower the volume a little more.

Table 15–2. Phase 2.

Week	Instructions
10	Each day of the week, set the volume of the CD so it is at the most comfortable volume. Listen to the entire CD. If the volume is set to a level that is lower than the volume used in the previous week, it is fine. Relax, pay attention, and enjoy the music. If the music feels painful at any time, or if the listener feels worried or uncomfortable, slightly lower the volume.
11	Each day of the week, set the volume of the CD so it is at the most comfortable volume. Then, increase the volume to a level that is slightly louder. Listen to the entire CD. If the music feels painful at any time, or if the listener feels worried or uncomfortable, slightly lower the volume.
12	Each day of the week, set the volume of the CD so it is at the most comfortable volume. Then, increase the volume to a level that is slightly louder. Then, slightly increase the volume a bit more. Listen to the entire CD. If the music feels painful at any time, or if the listener feels worried or uncomfortable, slightly lower the volume.
13	Repeat the steps described in week 10.
14	Repeat the steps described in week 11.
15	Repeat the steps described in week 12.
16	Repeat the steps described in week 10.
17	Repeat the steps described in week 11.
18	Repeat the steps described in week 12.
19	Repeat the steps described in week 10.
20	Repeat the steps described in week 11.
21	Repeat the steps described in week 12.
22	Repeat the steps described in week 10.
23	Repeat the steps described in week 11.
24	Repeat the steps described in week 12.
25	Repeat the steps described in week 10.
26	Repeat the steps described in week 11.
27	Repeat the steps described in week 12. By now, individuals may find the volume at which one is most comfortable listening to music is a little louder than it was during the first several weeks of using the music protocol. This is to be expected and indeed is a positive sign.

Table 15–3. Phase 3.

Week	Instructions
28	Each day of the week, set the volume of the CD so it is at the most comfortable volume. Listen to the entire CD. If the volume is set to a level that is lower than the volume used in the previous week, it is fine. Relax, pay attention, and enjoy the music. If the music feels painful at any time, or if the listener feels worried or uncomfortable, slightly lower the volume. At the end of the session, choose any song on the CD. Set the volume so it is uncomfortably loud and then lower the volume until it is no longer uncomfortable to hear. Each day during the week, listen to one song at the *end* of the session at this volume. If the chosen volume is louder than normal, it is fine provided it is neither painful nor uncomfortable. As always, the listener should lower the volume anytime he or she feels uncomfortable or afraid.
29	Each day of the week, set the volume of the CD so it is at the most comfortable volume. Then, increase the volume to a level that is slightly louder. Listen to the entire CD. At the end of the session, choose two songs on the CD. Set the volume so it is uncomfortably loud and then lower the volume until it is no longer uncomfortable to hear. For each day during the week, listen to two songs at the *end* of the session at this volume. If the chosen volume is louder than normal, it is fine provided it is neither painful nor uncomfortable. As always, the listener should lower the volume anytime he or she feels uncomfortable or afraid.
30	Each day of the week, set the volume of the CD so it is at the most comfortable volume. Then, increase the volume to a level that is slightly louder. Then, slightly increase the volume a bit more. Listen to the entire CD. At the end of the session, choose three songs on the CD. Set the volume so it is uncomfortably loud and then lower the volume until it is no longer uncomfortable to hear. For each day during the week, listen to three songs at the *end* of the session at this volume. If the chosen volume is louder than normal, it is fine provided it is neither painful nor uncomfortable. As always, the listener should lower the volume anytime he or she feels uncomfortable or afraid.
31	Repeat the steps described in week 28.
32	Repeat the steps described in week 29.
33	Repeat the steps described in week 30.
34	Repeat the steps described in week 28.
35	Repeat the steps described in week 29.
36	Repeat the steps described in week 30.
37	Repeat the steps described in week 28.
38	Repeat the steps described in week 29.
39	Repeat the steps described in week 30.

After using the music protocol, working with broader spectrum noise presentations that contained increases in amplitude at certain frequencies (similar to the broadband noise used in TRT), and continuing to put myself out in the world, the last time my LDLs were administered, they were in the 90 dB HL to 100 dB HL range, which hearing healthcare clinicians regard as within the range of normal LDLs for non-hyperacusic patients (Knobel & Sanchez, 2006).

There is a lot we do not know about hyperacusis. Rather than focus on the unknowns, I chose to focus on what *could* be done, on what I could do to help myself. No matter how frustrated I was by repeated setbacks, or the number of adjustments I made to my treatment or in my thinking, I focused on getting better. At times, improvements were hard to come by because hyperacusis could be unpredictable. One afternoon, after working quietly in the recording studio, my sound tolerance collapsed for days. Therapy did not progress in a straight line, and exposure to normal sound could repeatedly cause sound in general to be louder for days or longer. Still, I did not allow "I can't recover from this" to be part of my vocabulary.

I have come a long way in re-establishing my sound tolerance. There are many activities in which I can engage that I never imagined I would be able to do again. I can go to movies, many restaurants, and even some clubs without fear or concern. While I have not recovered 100% of my sound tolerance, my LDLs are once again in the normal range and I function normally, comfortably, and with pleasure in many aural settings. My sound tolerance continues to improve as I expose my auditory system to a broader range of sound. The continual ear pain I felt and the sense of aural fullness have completely resolved.

Intuition

A bat and a ball cost $1.10. The bat costs $1.00 more than the ball. How much does the ball cost? ____ cents

When this puzzle was presented to students at Harvard, MIT, and Princeton, as part of a Cognitive Reflection Test, more than half gave the intuitive answer, 10 cents (Frederick, 2005). When students at less selective colleges and universities tried to solve the puzzle, more than 80% reached the same conclusion. This answer, which comes easily and immediately to mind, is wrong. (The correct answer is 5 cents.) Notably, when students answered correctly, in many cases they considered the intuitive answer first before crossing it out and solving the puzzle.

The bat-and-ball puzzle demonstrates two cognitive processes at work—one process is performed quickly, automatically, and effortlessly, with little conscious thought; the other process is performed more slowly, reflectively, and deliberately. The processes, named System 1 and System 2 (Stanovich & West, 2000), are the focus of many studies in cognitive and social psychology, and have enormous relevance for sufferers of tinnitus, hyperacusis, and ear pain.

An intuitive answer can be regarded as the first thought that comes to mind. Just as the bat-and-ball puzzle evokes an intuitive response, the same can be said of a patient's response to tinnitus and hyperacusis. I had developed tinnitus a year after I developed hyperacusis and, at first, I was miserable. Like many other tinnitus sufferers, I focused on how loud and inexorable tinnitus was. Tinnitus was inimitable, unlike any other sound, and I was constantly aware of it.

If my tinnitus could be likened to an opera composed by a thousand hyperactive mosquitos trapped in a blender set to the highest speed, then my thinking about tinnitus could be reasonably compared to the accompanying libretto. When I acquired tinnitus, my mind kept up a running commentary about it and I drew unremitting, dire conclusions about my prospects. For example, I thought life as I knew it was over, I would never be happy again, and I would never feel differently. These beliefs and judgments, the first thoughts that had entered my mind on a subject I knew nothing about—I had never discussed tinnitus with a doctor or read anything about it—were arrived at with assurance and I subscribed to each one.

Over time, I realized my thoughts about tinnitus were contributing to and energizing how bad I felt. I was used to trusting my own thinking, but on the subject of tinnitus, I decided to take a counterintuitive approach: I accepted that whatever I thought about tinnitus was probably wrong and rather than endorse the thought, I would dismiss it. This realization was liberating. The key to managing tinnitus had less to do with the sound of tinnitus and a great deal to do with my thinking about tinnitus.

People often make decisions and base their actions about intrusive tinnitus on little more than intuitive thinking. When the first thing that comes to mind seems plausible, the thought is endorsed, even if it isn't in one's best interest and when following the first thing that comes to mind serves to make one miserable. We can't shut off that part of ourselves, but we don't have to take these thoughts seriously or pursue them.

I have a vivid memory of working in the recording studio the day after I had this realization. I had a lot of close listening to do and was concerned I wouldn't be able to concentrate. For a while during the session, when my overly assured "inner expert" began to pontificate about tinnitus, I short-circuited his commentary by silently reminding myself I didn't know what I was talking about. I ended up having a very productive session in the studio.

An individual's intuitive thinking about tinnitus can have a profound negative influence on one's attempts to manage the condition; less attention has been paid to how a person *thinks* about hyperacusis (McKenna, Baguley, & McFerran, 2010). Human beings are predisposed to making intuitive, quick judgments about sensory experiences, and sound is no exception. An ambulance runs its siren, and anyone driving nearby *automatically* reacts, essentially without thinking. Indeed, the siren sound is composed in a manner that ensures an automatic reaction in anyone within hearing distance. When individuals develop hyperacusis, they continue to make reflexive judgments about sound. Unfortunately, routine sounds of moderate level can cause them to feel endangered, and the patients may respond automatically to these sounds in a manner resembling a prior, and normal, response to a considerably louder sound such as a siren. Thus, the impact of everyday and undamaging sound levels on people with hyperacusis changes dramatically and the meaning they assign to their sound experiences changes as well.

Those who experience a sensation of physical pain or discomfort when exposed to moderate sound levels develop a strong accompanying emotional response to such sounds that may, in turn, influence their beliefs about sound and the decisions they make. These emotions are consistent with the reactions of individuals who struggle with intrusive tinnitus who also may believe that many routine and innocuous environmental sounds are dangerous and can further worsen their condition.

When individuals with hyperacusis are exposed to sound that is perceived as painfully loud, a series of interconnected ideas, emotions, and behaviors are evoked. Exposure to a painful sound triggers surprise, fear, and anxiety, perhaps evoking memories of similar exposures, which, in turn, trigger a tendency to avoid the painful sound, thereby intensifying the emotions to which this behavior is linked, and further reinforcing the affected individual's inaccurate analysis regarding the dangers of sound. This self-reinforcing, interconnected series of events, called associative activation, is a feature of System 1 that occurs automatically, and is notable for its coherence and internal consistency, despite potential inaccuracies. Thoughts, emotions, beliefs, and actions that are "activated by the associative context" are given considerably more weight than they deserve, whereas other highly relevant information, such as others in the environment displaying no discomfort at the sound's presence, is underweighted or ignored (Morewedge & Kahneman, 2010; Kahneman, 2011).

For these reasons, hyperacusics are not well-served by making intuitive, automatic judgments about sound, and the choices they make as a result of these judgments (e.g., the overuse of hearing protection, disinclination to seek treatment, a preference for silence and seclusion, etc.) may not be in their best interest. Modifying automatic thinking about sound is difficult because it is natural and essential for people to trust their judgments about what they hear. Moreover, mood influences the ability to think intuitively (Bolte et al., 2003); when a hyperacusic feels uncomfortable, anxious, or fearful around sound, it can have a strong impact on intuitive performance.

A patient's belief that sound is damaging is persuasive; the belief may compel a patient to modify lifestyle and routine activities. That said, there is no evidence to support the belief that a hyperacusic's auditory system is more susceptible to damage than someone who does not have hyperacusis. A sound may be very uncomfortable or physically painful to hear, but it is important for patients with hyperacusis to distinguish between sound that is loud enough to cause physical damage and sound that they perceive *feels* that way.

Getting Help

Hyperacusis is manageable; even individuals with severely decreased sound tolerance can make progress, if they work at it. As a first step, it is very important to be evaluated and diagnosed by a neurotologist, otoneurologist, or audiologist who is experienced in successfully diagnosing and treating hyperacusis. It is also important to explore whether a medical condition explains the presence of hyperacusis. If there is a medical explanation, a medical intervention may be possible.

Every day, individuals with hyperacusis are well-advised to engage in an activity that gets them out of their homes and to do so without hearing protection so that they begin to associate safety with environments other than their own home. The auditory system thrives on sound, and this is as true for individuals with hyperacusis as it is for people who do not have hyperacusis.

Loudness Discomfort Levels

While there is general agreement among hearing healthcare professionals that LDLs are decreased in patients with hyperacusis, there is no international consensus on how to administer or evaluate LDLs. At a minimum, individuals should be tested at .5 kHz, 1 kHz, 2 kHz, 3 kHz, 4 kHz, 6 kHz, and 8 kHz. A frequency-specific LDL test that begins at .5 kHz and tests up to 12 kHz is ideal.

The LDL test (also referred to as a test to measure uncomfortable loudness levels, or ULLs) is regarded as risky by some patients and clinicians. However, if the test is properly administered and the directions are clearly stated and followed, then no one who takes an LDL test is subjected to a painful sound; it is a loudness *discomfort* level test and not a loudness *pain* test. There is also a significant difference between a sound that is uncomfortable to hear and one that is dangerous to hear. Sounds of dangerous levels are not presented to patients during an LDL test when the clinician and patient communicate effectively. The LDL test can also offer hope to patients as therapy proceeds because it gives measurable proof of progress and provides valuable information about frequency regions in which progress occurs more slowly.

Desensitization Therapy

The use of broadband noise for the purposes of desensitization has enabled many hyperacusics to significantly improve their tolerance of sound. As indicated above, white noise may be more effective than pink noise; however, some hyperacusic patients find white noise too harsh. In those cases, a pink noise presentation will be more easily accepted, and hence considerably more effective; few patients will use broadband noise that is painful or uncomfortable, but most patients will accept a neutral signal they can easily ignore. For best results, desensitization therapy should be done with the guidance of a knowledgeable hearing healthcare professional who has successfully diagnosed and treated other patients who have hyperacusis. The clinician should be conversant with the options available to manage hyperacusis and help the patient determine the best course for his or her needs. If it isn't possible to locate a knowledgeable clinician near one's home, it is important to be willing to travel to a clinician who can help.

I was approached several years ago by Dan Malcore to create an original recording of unfiltered pink noise for The Hyperacusis Network. I made the Network's pink noise CD with two colleagues, Larry Anthony and Marty Kearns, and donated it to The Hyperacusis Network. The pink noise CD is about 74 minutes in length and the recorded sound covers a range from 30 Hz to 22.05 kHz. By placing one's listening device in "repeat" mode, individuals can offer themselves virtually uninterrupted, unfiltered broadband noise. The file can be downloaded to an iPod, but should be converted to the WAV or AIFF audio formats. The iPod supports both formats.

Background Sound

Playing gentle, neutral, relaxing background sound at bedtime and at other times (e.g., reading at home, working in the office) is an important part of desensitization therapy for hyperacusis. The background sound should be set to a low volume so that it isn't intrusive and doesn't keep one awake at bedtime. A table-top sound machine or a recording with nature sounds (e.g., forest, rain, ocean, etc.) are effective options.

Hearing Protection

When sound becomes shocking, loud, or painful, it is logical for people with hyperacusis to want to protect themselves from it. Common sense tells us that if a car horn blows unexpectedly in a parking lot, and produces a sensation of immediate pain in a passerby, then the sound can be avoided the next time by wearing earplugs in parking lots. If street noise is uncomfortable or painful to hear, logic dictates discomfort can be avoided by wearing hearing protection when walking down the street. When these beliefs are extended, hyperacusics may wear hearing protection *in anticipation of loud sound regardless of the probability that such sounds may not occur* to limit what these individuals regard as the risk of further auditory system damage.

The use of hearing protection is seductive because it allows a hyperacusic to feel less pain and discomfort around sound and provides a measure of control. Although it is counterintuitive, hyperacusis is improved not by playing defense against sound but through purposeful and consistent exposure to sound. Overuse of hearing protection is detrimental to individuals with hyperacusis and typically makes one more, not less, sensitive to sound. When Formby et al. (2003) investigated the impact of hearing protection versus the use of wearable noise generators on loudness perception for individuals with no hyperacusis, they concluded that subjects who used hearing protection became more likely to display reduced LDLs over time, while subjects who used in-ear noise generators displayed increases in LDLs during the same period.

Hyperacusics and non-hyperacusics alike *should* wear hearing protection in settings when ambient sound levels require individuals to speak loudly in order to communicate with someone standing next to them. Earplugs purchased in a pharmacy or grocery store provide hearing protection that attenuates some frequencies more than others, which is why sound is muffled or appears unnatural when using store-bought earplugs. Foam earplugs with a Noise Reduction Rating (NRR) of 32 or 33 provide excellent protection; the NRR is listed on the package. Musician's earplugs may provide less protection; however, they attenuate sound more evenly across a wide range of frequencies. As a result, environmental sounds, and in particular music, will sound natural. Because they are custom-fitted for one's individual ears, musician's earplugs are also much more expensive than store-bought earplugs.

Travel

Noise cancellation headphones are excellent at blocking out the low-frequency rumble of airplane engines and are ideal for a hyperacusic when flying. Care should be taken to select a well-reviewed and reputable product. Individuals with hyperacusis may find it helpful to request a seat that is closer to the front of the plane and away from the engines.

Support Groups

Some kind, thoughtful, and generous people contribute to Internet patient support groups in which hyperacusis and other forms of decreased sound tolerance are discussed. There is also a lot of misinformation about hyperacusis in the patient community; in particular, that hyperacusis is caused by ear damage and exposure to normal sound is dangerous for hyperacusics. Substantial negative counseling and counterproductive thinking occur on these sites.

A newcomer to a support site will soon discover that accurate information competes for space alongside inaccurate information. Thus, one will read about viable treatments for hyperacusis, such as broadband pink noise therapy and Tinnitus Retraining Therapy (TRT), but one will also read about the overuse of earplugs. The best way for a newcomer to distinguish practical, worthwhile information about hyperacusis from happy talk and misinformation is to discuss all suggestions one learns about on the Internet with one's audiologist or doctor.

Ineffective, insufficient, or dangerous treatments for hyperacusis are often endorsed by support groups. These include the application of low level laser therapy (LLLT) to treat hyperacusis when numerous placebo-controlled studies have failed to show efficacy (Klienjung, 2011); a surgical procedure for round and oval window reinforcement that results in minor improvement in LDLs (Silverstein et al., 2015); and the use of dangerous anti-epileptic drugs to treat hyperacusis based on an anecdotal report on the Internet. The reception these approaches have received on support sites may be indicative of the mere exposure effect (Zajonc, 1968), in which repeatedly exposing an individual to a stimulus creates a positive attitude for it.

Support groups can be frequented by individuals who have chosen to *not* get the help they need to manage hyperacusis. Some never get out of the starting blocks, while others become frustrated when setbacks occur and decide to avoid sound rather than to engage it. This is understandable, as people can be powerfully motivated to protect themselves when they feel threatened. It also explains why experienced hearing healthcare clinicians generally advise patients with hyperacusis to limit the time spent on support sites or avoid them altogether during treatment.

Three heuristics are frequently encountered on Internet support settings. A heuristic is a mental short-cut individuals use when making intuitive judgments about uncertain events. Heuristics help people to find "adequate, though often imperfect, answers to difficult questions" by substituting a question that is easier to answer (Kahneman, 2011).

When participants on a hyperacusis support board evaluate the frequency or probability of an event, such as the number of cases in which hyperacusis has not improved with proper intervention, or the chances that exposure to moderate sound levels has caused damage to the auditory system, frequency and probability are assessed "by the ease with which instances or occurrences can be brought to mind." Because these topics are often discussed on hyperacusis support boards, instances may be recalled more easily, and hence seem more numerous to participants than they really are. This is known as the availability heuristic (Tversky & Kahneman, 1973, 1974).

The representativeness heuristic (Kahneman & Tversky, 1972, 1974) is used to make an intuitive judgment about the probability of an event "by the degree to which it is similar in essential properties to its parent population." In support settings, ear pain is often incorrectly assessed as physical damage to the auditory system because the symptoms are similar to (i.e., representative of) an individual's mental model of physical damage.

The affect heuristic (Slovic et al., 2002) is frequently observed on hyperacusis support boards, on which people's judgments and choices are strongly influenced by their emotions. One's evaluation of sound and the decisions a person makes to approach or avoid it are guided by a reliance on feelings rather than on more deliberate, analytical thinking. Slovic et al. (2002) suggest that "affect may serve as a cue for many important judgments."

Clinicians

When desensitization therapy is not helpful to patients, or not helpful enough, in some cases it is because the emotions associated with decreased sound tolerance were not identified or not considered an important element of intervention. When patients are asked to consider that there may be an emotional component to hyperacusis or ear pain, they sometimes dismiss it or view it as an insult. They may wonder why it isn't clear to others that they are describing a purely physical challenge and their responses to it are self-evident and natural. It is important for clinicians to be sympathetic to patients in this regard, while at the same time help patients acknowledge the strong feelings that unavoidably develop about the experience.

The physiological responses associated with hyperacusis are so powerful that it may be difficult for patients to understand and attribute the impact of hyperacusis on one's beliefs and decisions. A hyperacusic's beliefs about sound can be deep-rooted and often difficult to change. Hence, it is important for clinicians to uncover a hyperacusic patient's beliefs and behaviors regarding exposure to normal sound. These beliefs, which patients may be resistant or reluctant to share or challenge, can influence the decisions patients make with regard to exposing themselves to sound.

Patients should discuss with their providers any concerns they may have that exposure to normal sound can cause permanent damage to their auditory system. These questions are not trivial and a full discussion will likely uncover fears and concerns about offending sounds that are worth exploring. Patients may interpret the pain or discomfort they feel around normal sound to be evidence of damage to the auditory system, and they may strongly believe continued exposure to sound will further damage their hearing. Cognitive Behavioral Therapy (CBT) may be helpful in challenging catastrophic thinking about decreased sound tolerance; however, in my view, CBT should be undertaken in concert with a desensitization program that involves the use of broadband noise to help re-establish one's tolerance of sound. In a randomized controlled trial on the use of CBT to treat hyperacusis (Jüris et al., 2014), LDL tests were only administered up to 4 kHz and improvement in LDLs was less than 10 dB in both ears.

If prospective hearing healthcare clinicians take a "by-the-numbers" or "cookbook" approach to treating hyperacusis, most likely it won't fulfill them and it certainly won't help their patients. On the other hand, if clinicians place a value on listening to patients, empathizing with and being responsive to them, and respectful of them, and are invested in making a hard-earned difference in people's lives, a significant number of patients with these challenges will benefit from their guidance.

References

Andersson, G., Lindvall, N., Hursti, T., & Carlbring, P. (2002). Hypersensitivity to sound (hyperacusis). A prevalence study conducted via the Internet and post. *International Journal of Audiology, 41*, 545–554.

Bhimrao, S., Masterson, L., & Baguley, D. (2012). Systematic review of management strategies for middle ear myoclonus. *Otolaryngology—Head and Neck Surgery, 146*, 698–706.

Bolte, A., Goschke, T., & Kuhl, J. (2003). Emotion and intuition: Effects of positive and negative mood on implicit judgment of semantic coherence. *Psychological Science, 14*, 416–421.

Formby, C., Sherlock, L. P., & Gold, S. C. (2003). Adaptive plasticity of loudness induced by chronic attenuation and enhancement of the acoustic background. *Journal of the Acoustical Society of America, 114*, 55–58.

Frederick, S. (2005). Cognitive reflection and decision making. *Journal of Economic Perspectives, 1*(4), 25–42.

Jastreboff, M. M. & Jastreboff, P. J. (2002). Decreased sound tolerance and Tinnitus Retraining Therapy (TRT). *The Australian and New Zealand Journal of Audiology, 24*(2), 74–84.

Jastreboff, P. J. & Hazell, J. (2004). *Tinnitus retraining therapy*. Cambridge, UK: Cambridge University Press.

Jastreboff, P. J. & Jastreboff, M. M. (2014). Treatments for decreased sound tolerance (hyperacusis and misophonia). *Seminars in Hearing, 35*(2), 205–120.

Jüris, L., Andersson, G., Larsen, H., & Ekselius, L. (2014). Cognitive behaviour therapy for hyperacusis: A randomized controlled trial. *Behaviour Research and Therapy, 54*, 30–37.

Kahneman, D. (2011). *Thinking fast and slow.* New York, NY: Farrar, Straus and Giroux.

Kahneman, D. & Tversky, A. (1972). Subjective probability: A judgment of representativeness. *Cognitive Psychology, 3*, 430–454.

Klein, A. J., Armstrong, B. L., Greer, M. K., & Brown III, F. R. (1990). Hyperacusis and otitis media in individuals with Williams syndrome. *Journal of Speech and Hearing Disorders, 55*, 339–344.

Klienjung, T. (2011). Low-level laser therapy. In Moller, A., Langguth, B., De Ridder, D., & Kleinjung, T. (Eds.), *Textbook of tinnitus* (pp. 749–752). New York, NY: Springer.

Klochoff, I., Lindholm, L., & Westerberg, C. E. (1971). Spontaneous impedance fluctuation—a "tensor tympani syndrome" with special reference to tension headache. *Nordisk Medicine, 85*, 577.

Klochoff, I. (1979). Impedance fluctuation and a "tensor tympani syndrome." In R. Penha & P. Pizarro (Eds.), *Proceedings of the Fourth International Symposium on Acoustic Impedance Measurements* (pp. 69–76). Lisbon, Portugal: Universidad Nova de Lisboa.

Knobel, K. & Sanchez, T. (2006). Loudness discomfort level in normal hearing individuals. *Pró-Fono Revista de Atualizacão Cientifica, 18*(1), *31–40.*

Mathisen, H. (1969). Phonophobia after stapedectomy. *Acta Oto-Laryngologica (Stockholm), 68*, 73–77.

McKenna, L., Baguley, D., & McFerran, D. (2010). *Living with tinnitus and hyperacusis.* London, U.K.: Sheldon Press.

Morewedge, C. & Kahneman, D. (2010). Associative processes in intuitive judgment. *Trends in Cognitive Sciences, 14*(10), 435–440.

Patuzzi, R., Milhinch, J., & Doyle, J. (2000). Acute aural trauma in telephone headset and handset users. *Neuro-otological Society of Australia Annual Conference*, Melbourne.

Phillips, D. P. & Carr, M. M. (1998). Disturbances of loudness perception. *Journal of the American Academy of Audiology, 9*, 371–379.

Radomskij, P., Schmidt, M. A., Heron, C. W., & Prasher, D. (2002). Effect of MRI noise on cochlear function. *The Lancet, 359*(9316), 1485–1486.

Ramirez, L. M., Ballesteros, L. E., & Sandoval, G. P. (2007). Tensor tympani muscle: Strange chewing muscle. *Medicina Oral Patologia Oral y Cirugia Bucal, 12*, E96–E100.

Rubinstein, B., Ahlqwist, M., & Bengtsson, C. (1996). Hyperacusis, headache, temporomandibular disorders and amalgam fillings—an epidemiological study. In Reich, G. E. & Vernon, J. A. (Eds.), *Proceedings of the Fifth International Tinnitus Seminar* (pp. 657–658). Portland, OR: American Tinnitus Association.

Silverstein, H., Wu, Y., & Hagan, S. (2015). Round and oval window reinforcement for the treatment of hyperacusis. *American Journal of Otolaryngology—Head and Neck Medicine and Surgery, 36*, 158–162.

Slovic, P., Finucane, M., Peters, E., & MacGregor, D. (2002). The affect heuristic. In Gilovich, T., Griffin, D., & Kahneman, D. (Eds.), *Heuristics and biases: The psychology of intuitive judgment* (pp. 397–420). New York: Cambridge University Press.

Stanovich, K. & West, R. (2000). Individual differences in reasoning: Implications for the rationality debate? *Behavioral and Brain Sciences, 23*, 645–726.

Tversky, A. & Kahneman, D. (1973). Availability: A heuristic for judging frequency and probability. *Cognitive Psychology, 5*, 207–232.

Tversky, A. & Kahneman, D. (1974). Judgment under uncertainty: Heuristics and biases. *Science, 185*(4157), 1124–1131.

Tyler, R., Pienkowski, M., Roncancio, E., Jun, H., Brozoski, T., Dauman, N., Coelho, C., Andersson, G., Keiner, A., Cacace, A., Martin, N., & Moore, B. (2014). A review of hyperacusis and future directions: Part 1. Definitions and manifestations. *American Journal of Audiology, 23*, 402–419.

Vernon, J. A. & Sanders, B. (2001). *Tinnitus questions and answers* (pp. 132–139). Allyn and Bacon.

Westcott, M. (2016). Middle ear myoclonus and tonic tensor tympani syndrome. In Baguley, D. M. & Fagelson, M. (Eds.), *Tinnitus: Clinical and research perspectives* (pp. 145–162). San Diego, CA: Plural.

Zajonc, R. (1968). Attitudinal effects of mere exposure. *Journal of Personality and Social Psychology*, *9*, 1–27.

16

Hyperacusis: Past, Present, and Future

Marc Fagelson and David M. Baguley

Introduction

Despite patient experiences with hyperacusis and other disorders of sound tolerance reported for hundreds of years, the conditions have taken a long time to attract any significant scientific, clinical, or public interest. As indicated in Chapter 3, there have been sporadic mentions in various categories of literature, but it was only in the early 2000s that patient narratives and therapeutic options received any substantial attention. One reason for the unfortunate lack of interest was that many current auditory scientists, and audiology or otology clinicians, completed their training with nary a mention of decreased sound tolerance. That this situation is improving is due to a concerted effort, and the pioneering interest of several individuals, whose names populate the reference lists of each chapter, and who contributed chapters to this book.

It is difficult to know why a symptom that can be severe, and is apparently prevalent in the modern world, has attracted so little attention. Issues may include the fact that audiologists and otologists have been extremely busy diagnosing and managing hearing loss (and tinnitus and imbalance) and so have had insufficient time to dedicate to reduced sound tolerance. Also, it may be the case that in previous generations the rigours of everyday life were such that decreased sound tolerance was neither a rehabilitative imperative nor a priority. Although it may be a modern conceit that we consider ourselves to have an easier life than previous generations, a patient's sensory experiences, both positive and negative, remain by-products of the ubiquitous media, entertainment, and occupational advances we expect and routinely employ. While emerging technology, modern medical care, and food availability are all great blessings in the present day, access to these is by no means predictable, hence the stress imposed by the environment upon individuals can be difficult to ascertain. Further, a professional working week can presently be longer than at other times in history, challenging both patients with sensory disruptions, and the clinicians charged with addressing their needs. It may be that hyperacusis is a modern disorder, relatively rare in previous times, but derived now from twenty-first century lifestyles whose quality is challenged by the proliferation of stress-related disorders: without a time machine, or the adventitious discovery of some legacy data this cannot be ascertained.

The unique and evolving listening requirements and environmental-sound challenges faced by many individuals likely contributes to the problem. Most of us are confronted numerous times in any day by sounds that are loud, incessant, or annoying; ironically, it is also the case that sounds appearing as negative to one person will be equally pleasing to the next. The experience of sitting in traffic listening to another driver's music is common; if the music is enjoyed, then the two drivers may share a smile and nod of the head, if the music is not enjoyed, then windows are raised along with associated anger. Alarms and sirens are intended to remind us of tasks or warn us of approaching danger, and these sounds are intended to be the center of attention, they are designed for maximum detectability (Patterson, 1990). It is no surprise that some individuals find the sounds irritating; indeed, this irritating nature is intentional and contributes to the difficulty one has ignoring them. If individuals with normal tolerance limits find such sounds intrusive, then we, as clinicians, must consider the powerful effect the sounds would have on an individual with hypersensitivity or a low tolerance. While not all environmental sounds serve the purpose of a warning signal, the tendency over time appears to favor the public use of attention-grabbing sound, not just for caution, but for advertising and recreation. The ubiquity and obnoxiousness of such noise compels many people to avoid situations and places.

It is only recently that people with hyperacusis are finding, or being allowed, their voice in public. The success and popularity of communities based around hyperacusis.net, and hyperacusisreasearch.com, and various decreased sound tolerance Facebook communities, indicates that a public conversation is underway, and this is unlikely to decrease over time—as with the noises with which we share the world, the proliferation of patients with concerns and the networks that can serve them are rather more likely to increase.

Where We Are Going

Several improvements must be made with respect to the clinical assessment of disordered sound tolerance. Greater consensus than currently exists regarding measures of loudness in particular must be developed and implemented if we are to distinguish auditory pathologies, particularly those to which other clinical tests are insensitive, from one another. The replicability of such measures must be addressed, and improvements would facilitate audiologists maximizing the benefit of hearing aids for patients with sound tolerance issues, and to detect changes over time, perhaps as linked to intervention, for the patients served.

The proliferation of smartphone applications to measure hearing, along with the increased availability of over the counter hearing aids and personal sound amplification products suggests that patients who would in the past have accessed audiologic rehabilitation through an audiologist may in the near future try to manage their hearing health care needs on their own. The probability is high, however, that these individuals will seek services to maximize the benefit provided by their generic devices at some point. This statement is not intended as an indictment of self-fitting amplification, and audiologists will likely be compelled to walk a fine line between dismissing the self-fitting process and patients who practice it altogether with offering support and assistance to those patients (who may have rejected the audiologists' help initially). Clearly, as with any clinical endeavor, many things can go wrong with a patient testing their own hearing and self-fitting a hearing aid. The situation is exacerbated by the lack of orientation and counselling that comprise an essential element of audiologic rehabilitation, but that would not be available to such patients, unless an audiologist with an interest in rehabilitation steps up to help. Of particular concern for such patients would be the possibility that their assistive device's effectiveness would be minimized because of an obscure and difficult-to-detect sound tolerance problem.

As indicated in Chapter 2, reliable measures of loudness tolerance remain a challenge for routine clinical practice; for a self-fit hearing aid, a patient may be unaware of loudness tolerance issues, have no accurate or replicable test to obtain such information, and therefore endure a fitting with a device whose benefit will be limited from the start. A patient experiencing such problems will have options, of course. They can return the device, or, because its price was modest to begin with, they can use the device sparingly without experiencing undue remorse that might accompany the purchase of something expensive, but little used. Limiting use of amplification, especially for a person with loudness tolerance issues, may exert a negative influence on desensitization to various sound levels, as described in Chapters 7 and 9. Some degree of desensitization would be expected to occur following routine exposures to amplified sound; ideally, such exposures would, over time, ameliorate some of the loudness tolerance problems. Unfortunately, the patient can wear the device, but at output levels too low to provide adequate amplification or consistent benefit; in such cases, patients would be likely to minimize device use as well.

Another option would focus on seeking help from a professional. In this instance, patients may find themselves asking an audiologist or hearing instrument specialist about fitting parameters that could be adjusted to improve the device's effectiveness. Here it will be essential for the audiologist to advise and support the patient even in the possible circumstance that the patient declined hearing aids from the audiologist in the past.

Hearing health care for patients with disorders of sound tolerance must incorporate effective counseling and strategies to ease a patient's adjustment to amplification. All patients receiving amplification benefit from such counseling, although some patients adjust to personal amplification relatively easily. Our concern is for the patient who, with the best of intentions, acquires a product that does not initially suit their needs. Audiologists will adhere to their professional responsibilities and provide care and information in these cases, or they will be brushed aside as the patient either gives up on the device or seeks help elsewhere. Clearly, the interests of patient and provider are most reasonably met when the audiologist helps the patient obtain their money's worth, even if the device's purchase is not from the audiologist. While this situation may be most common in the United States, it serves as a reminder that it may be our counseling and communication skills, our ability to troubleshoot fitting problems, and our understanding of technology and its interface with our patients that confirms our value as an essential element of the patient's hearing health care. This book's intent is to improve the clinician's understanding of the varieties and manifestations of disordered sound tolerance as one way to improve the audiologist's ability to provide information, counseling, and adaptation strategies for patients experiencing difficulty with amplification.

Hearing protection devices present similar challenges in that their use requires careful consideration of the patient's motivation, strategies, and rationale for protecting hearing.

Patients are clearly in need of accurate information regarding options, benefits, and limitations related to hearing protectors. As noise levels and warning signals in the environment increase, we can be certain that a proportion of the population will experience aversive responses during routine occupational and recreational activities. If patients are willing to test their own hearing to purchase amplification devices, then it is certain that they will continue to make their own decisions regarding hearing protection. As discussed in Chapters 3, 6, 7, and 8, hearing protection can be overused and exacerbate the negative sound experience that triggers their use in the first place. This situation should be avoidable in most cases; however, providers must have an understanding of the neural mechanisms at work in order to counsel effectively when patients experience loudness tolerance issues that restrict dynamic range and, by extension, activities the patient might routinely carry out.

Another issue relates to the various patient groups that experience frequent exposures to some of the most toxic environmental sounds. Emergency medical technicians, firefighters, officers of the law, and military populations have unique exposures that require hearing protection; however, the rigors of the jobs and frequent need to communicate may contraindicate routine use of protective devices or earplugs. Little is known regarding the prevalence of workers whose sound intolerance compels them to retire or find new employment rather than continuing work in these important areas. An additional consideration relates to the risk members of these populations face regarding concussion or traumatic brain injury (TBI). Patients recovering from TBI often experience hypersensitivities to a variety of sensory inputs, particularly visual, auditory, and olfactory inputs, whose effects are exacerbated when unexpected, or when serving as reminders of traumatic exposures (Alwis et al., 2012).

Cochlear implantation influences a patient in many ways, and it may be that training derived from various psychophysical test strategies can improve outcomes with the devices. The pitch changes over time reported by Reiss and colleagues (2011, 2016) and in Chapter 12 are reminders that, even in drastically modified peripheral systems, the same rules of central adaptation and compensation that apply to normal-hearing individuals may be accessed by cochlear implant users, hence the potential value in honing assessments that are sensitive to such change.

Hyperacusis will likely receive more attention in the lab and literature in the future. Therefore, its use as a term may require more specificity and care than is exercised at present, a concept advanced by several investigators, Tyler et al. (2014) for example, and as discussed in Chapter 3. In particular, the use of hyperacusis to connote extreme sensitivity regarding absolute threshold should be reconsidered. One disorder in particular, superior semicircular canal dehiscence (SSCD), has as the typical clinical sign of unusually low bone-conduction thresholds, particularly in the low frequencies. The thresholds often appear as clinically relevant air-bone gaps despite normal hearing via air conduction testing. This situation, described in Chapter 6, has been termed "conductive hyperacusis" (e.g., Minor, 2005), in which the hyperacusis label indicates better than average sensitivity rather than what we would suggest as the preferred use, connoting loudness intolerance. Perhaps hypersensitivity or hypersensitive bone-conduction thresholds could be applied to patients' results during SSCD testing; the possibility that a patient with SSCD could experience both conductive hyperacusis, meaning extremely sensitive bone-conduction thresholds, and loudness hyperacusis simultaneously should be motivation enough to clarify terminology and usage.

One example of an opportunity to improve matters would relate to the development of a clinic practice guideline for the management of patients with disordered sound tolerance. The American Academy of Otolaryngology offers dozens of well-crafted and thorough practice guidelines covering specialty areas from pediatric middle ear management to benign paroxysmal positional vertigo, to tinnitus. At present, no guideline is offered for disorders of sound tolerance, although hyperacusis is mentioned in the guidelines for tinnitus (Tunkel et al., 2014) and Bell's palsy (Baugh et al., 2013).

It is possible that the physicians and practitioners who contribute to practice guideline development are confounded by patient complaints of disordered sound tolerance. The literature regarding sound-evoked pain, for example, as summarized in Chapter 9, is in its infancy and may be years from translation into clinical practice. In this regard, the current state of disordered sound tolerance management resembles that associated with tinnitus management some 10 to 15 years ago; a variety of clinical approaches with minimal supporting evidence applied to a distressed population of patients who struggle to get answers or assistance from their traditional medical sources. Professionals in our field must commit to improving the situation, and the development of a practice guideline would compel communication between physicians, audiologists, and psychologists with the ultimate goal of standardizing terminology, diagnoses, and components of patient care.

Research Priorities

From the issues raised above it will be clear that there are many opportunities for research into hyperacusis. A summary of those research questions deemed to be priorities was proposed by Baguley and Hoare (in press), and can be found in modified form in the bulleted list below. It will be seen that these span basic, behavioral, and clinical science. While the fact that the research questions are so plentiful, and so broad is an indication that our knowledge regarding hyperacusis really is sparse, it is also an indication that this is an area in which research opportunities abound.

Unanswered research questions in disordered sound tolerance (modified from Baguley and Hoare, in press):

- What is the prevalence of hyperacusis in adults and children?
- What are the risk factors associated with hyperacusis?
- What is the natural history of hyperacusis?
- How is "pain hyperacusis" perceived?
- What mechanisms are involved in hyperacusis?
- What is the relation between hyperacusis and tinnitus?
- Can a questionnaire be developed that accurately measures the impact of hyperacusis, and can be used as a treatment outcome measure?
- What treatments, alone or in combination, are effective for hyperacusis?

A multidisciplinary approach to hyperacusis research would be valuable, as the tinnitus field has benefited from an additional linkage (Hall et al., 2013), drawing patients into the discussion about tinnitus research through a formal process led by the James Lind Alliance in the United Kingdom (http://www.jla.nihr.ac.uk/priority-setting-partnerships/tinnitus/). The result of the process was a list of research priorities in tinnitus, with the aim of increasing the traction of funding applications for tinnitus research, with independent verification that the topic chosen was of both scientific and public interest. A similar program is underway for hyperacusis, again involving the James Lind Alliance, and led by Dr. Kathryn Fackrell in the

United Kingdom. Additionally, the growing dialogue between patient communities such as those based around the Hyperacusis Network and Hyperacusis Research and the scientific and clinical communities is welcome.

Two things are missing, however. The first is the absence of any formal patient organization, such as exist for tinnitus (the American and British Tinnitus Associations, for example): these perform an invaluable role in patient advice, support, and advocacy, and in fundraising for research. While these tinnitus associations acknowledge that there is some overlap between tinnitus and hyperacusis, neither has sought a significant role with hyperacusis patients, and there is no indication that this is likely to develop.

The second missing element is that of a substantial funding stream, such as is available for hearing loss, and becoming more available for tinnitus. The absence of research resources will hamper progress in hyperacusis until this is remedied.

Closing Words

While opportunities are evident for progress in understanding the mechanisms of hyperacusis, the natural history, and in developing optimal treatments, some significant constraints are also apparent. It is our hope that in editing this book we will have contributed toward the embedding of hyperacusis into the mainstream of audiology, and of auditory neuroscience, which is essential if the field is to develop. Patients with disorders of sound tolerance are numerous, and the burden on them as individuals, their families, and upon the societies in which they live, is substantial. If the reader is motivated to contribute to the development of this fascinating and important field, then we will have succeeded in our aims.

References

Alwis, D. S., Yan, E. B., Morganti-Kossmann, M.-C., & Rajan, R. Sensory cortex underpinnings of traumatic brain injury deficits. *PLoS ONE 7*(12), e52169. https://doi.org/10.1371/journal.pone.0052169.

Baguley, D. M., & Hoare, D. J. *Hyperacusis: major research questions*. HNO, in press

Baugh, R. F., Basura, G. J., Ishii, L. E., Schwartz, S. R., . . . Vaughan, W. (2013). Clinical practice guideline: Bell's palsy. *Otolaryngology—Head and Neck Surgery*, 149, 3 suppl, S1–S27.

Hall, D., Mohamad, N., Firkins, L., Fenton, M., & Stockdale, D. (2013). Identifying and prioritizing unmet research questions for people with tinnitus: The James Lind Alliance Tinnitus Priority Setting Partnership. *Clinical Investigation, 3, 1*, 21–28, doi: 10.4155/cli.12.129.

Minor, L. B. (2005). Clinical manifestations of superior semicircular canal dehiscence. *The Laryngoscope, 115*, 1717–1727. doi:10.1097/01.mlg.0000178324.55729.b7.

Patterson, R. (1990). Auditory warning sounds in the work environment. *Philos. Trans. R. Soc. Lond. B Biol. Sci., 327*(1241), 485–492.

Reiss, L. A. J., Lowder, M. W., Karsten, S. A., Turner, C. W., & Gantz, B. J. (2011). Effects of extreme tonotopic mismatches between bilateral cochlear implants on electric pitch perception: a case study. *Ear Hear., 32*(4), 536–540. doi:10.1097/AUD.0b013e31820c81b0.

Reiss, L. A. J., Eggleston, J. L., Walker, E. P., & Oh, Y. (2016). Two ears are not always better than one: mandatory vowel fusion across spectrally mismatched ears in hearing-impaired listeners. *J. Assoc. Res. Otolaryng., 17*, 342–356. doi: 10.1007/s10162-016-0570-z.

Tunkel, D. E., Bauer, C. A., Sun, G. H., et al. (2014). Clinical practice guideline: Tinnitus. *Otolaryngology—Head and Neck Surgery, 151*, S1–S40. doi: 10.1177/0194599814545325.

Tyler, R. S., Pienkowski, M., Roncancio, E. R., . . . , Moore, B. C. J. (2014). A review of hyperacusis and future directions: Part I. Definitions and manifestations. *Am. J. Aud.*, (23), 402–419.

Index

Note: Page numbers in **bold** reference non-text material.

D

E

F

G

H

N

O

P

Q

R

S

U

V

W

Y